BEFORE
YOU CALL
THE DOCTOR

BEFORE YOU CALL THE DOCTOR

A family guide to diagnosing common symptoms

DR HILARY JONES

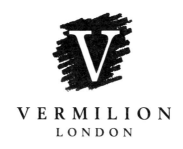

VERMILION
LONDON

To Sarah

*Without the love, support and impressive typing skills of my
wife Sarah, this book would never have been completed.*

I am also indebted to Caroline Johnson for her painstaking
and meticulous work in editing the manuscript.

❖

5 7 9 8 6 4

First published in the United Kingdom in 1994 by
VERMILION
an imprint of Ebury Press, Random House
20 Vauxhall Bridge Road, London SW1V 2SA

A CIP record for this title is available from the British Library

Designed by Terry Jeavons/Bridgewater Book Company
Typeset by Chris Lanaway

ISBN 0 09 1784239

Printed and bound in Great Britain by
Butler & Tanner Ltd, Frome and London

CONTENTS

INTRODUCTION

Symptoms can be a pain. Quite literally. But they can range from a pins-and-needles kind of sensation to blindness to one eye, from a tremor to a sudden weakness. They can come in the shape of lumps and bumps, they may appear in different colours, as in the yellow tinge of jaundice and the ashen whiteness of anaemia, and you can see, feel, taste and or smell them. They may be localized, affecting only a tiny part of the body, or generalized, causing exhaustion, loss of appetite and weight loss.

Everybody experiences symptoms at one time or another, from the trivial right through to the serious and disturbing. The problem is, how to read them? For example, how long should a headache last before it becomes abnormal? When is a lump in the breast dangerous? What is the difference between a twinge of chest pain and a heart attack? When is a child's temperature a sign of impending meningitis? Symptoms such as these are the characteristic sensations of a medical disorder, the means by which our bodies tell us something is wrong, and as such they are very valuable.

So really we should welcome symptoms. Without them we would remain blissfully unaware of any health problems developing within us. As small children, the symptom of pain teaches us to withdraw our hand from something hot, thereby protecting us from a severe burn. On the other hand, people who have lost sensation as a result of a nervous disease or poor blood supply constantly injure themselves because they unwittingly continue to walk on damaged joints or fail to realize that the infection they have picked up is spreading. We need these early-warning signals to keep us well. Look what happens when diseases are present that do not cause symptoms. Although high blood pressure, for example, is extremely common, people rarely know about it until they have their blood pressure measured. Yet hypertension commonly leads to heart attacks and strokes, and these can be disabling or even fatal. One of the commonest treatable causes of blindness in this country is glaucoma, which may have no symptoms at all. Diabetes and brittle-bone disease can be equally 'silent', yet claim thousands of lives every year.

Fortunately, however, most problems affecting our health soon let us know they are there and symptoms are the most important clues of all in establishing medical diagnosis and treatment. Through symptoms alone, 90 per cent of all medical problems can be diagnosed, without the need for medical examinations, intricate scientific tests or laboratory investigations, and yet their meanings remain largely unknown or misunderstood by most people. This book aims to make sense of them, helping people to decide for themselves whether or not something is genuinely serious and if it should be referred urgently to the doctor. As a practising GP, I know that any abnormality is worrying, especially when it remains unexplained. Where understanding exists, fear and anxiety are lessened.

One of the reasons I wanted to write this book was because I receive so many letters from people who are terrified by what is happening to them and want to deny that there is any problem, or who want to obtain more information about their health problems but are frustrated in their search for it. Most medical books deal with diseases under disease headings. They talk about myocardial infarction, gallstones and multiple sclerosis. But people don't go to their doctors with these conditions. They do go to their doctors with chest pain, dark-coloured urine, or numbness. And they want to know what their symptoms mean. They want to know what makes one kind of headache a migraine and another a brain tumour. They want to know the difference between blood in the urine due to cystitis and blood in the urine due to a kidney stone, when to report those swollen glands to the doctor, and how soon.

That is why I have written this book. So you can look up your symptoms without first having to see the doctor to learn what your diagnosis is likely to be. Unfortunately, most medical books can only be used when you already have that diagnosis and I think that is illogical as well as rather dangerous. Illogical because anyone learning that skin cancer begins with a pigmented mole will panic about mere freckles. And dangerous because in the case of certain diseases, especially cancer, detection at the earliest possible stage is vital for a cure to be achieved. So, if you have ever worried about dizziness, wheezing, intense tiredness or your child's incessant crying, this book will not only reassure and interest you, it will also make you feel a great deal better.

Before You Call the Doctor is not intended to be a comprehensive guide to all human afflictions, nor a substitute for professional medical consultation. Symptoms alone are the most important factors in evaluating disease, but their significance should always be confirmed by a full physical examination and medical investigation. However, with the help of this book, which includes all the commonest symptoms you or your family are ever likely to experience in any one lifetime, you will at least be able to make an educated guess about the probable nature of the ailment and wisely decide not only whether you should call for expert assistance, but also how soon.

1
GENERAL SYMPTOMS

By general symptoms, I mean unexplained changes in weight, loss of appetite, fever and tiredness. These symptoms are often highly significant but very nonspecific. They are good indicators of a vast number of different medical problems, but in themselves provide little specific help to aid diagnosis.

Almost any medical condition can lead to these constitutional upsets. Thus the lay-person can easily and perhaps wrongly assume that weight changes and/or loss of appetite are due to problems within the digestive system when thyroid irregularities, depression, infection or the side effects of medication could just as well be responsible. In the same way, fatigue is often simply put down to lack of sleep or to overwork when it could in fact represent anaemia, diabetes, glandular fever or heart disease. Although sometimes difficult to make sense of, these general symptoms nevertheless desperately need to be investigated and treated. Accompanying symptoms are therefore particularly important in providing essential clues as to the nature of the underlying problem.

FEVER

One of the human body's most remarkable abilities is its automatic control of body temperature within very narrowly defined limits. A normal temperature ranges from 97.5 to 99°F (36.4 to 37.2°C), which is the optimum level at which the vast majority of bodily functions work most efficiently. Having said that, however, there are a number of factors that affect normal temperature regulation which do not signify disease at all.

For example, normal body temperature is lowest first thing in the morning, reaching a peak between 6 and 10 pm. In a hot climate the resting temperature is likely to be a little higher. After a hot bath or exercise the temperature will be temporarily raised, and for women a 1°F (0.4°C) rise after ovulation is common. These are all normal physiological variations. When the temperature is constantly above 99°F (37°C) for 24 hours, however, that person can safely be said to have a fever. From the moment that conclusion is reached, both patient and doctor should start to think about a possible cause. To summarize, these are what certain temperature levels mean:

97.5–99°F (36.4–37.2°C): normal
99°F (37.2°C) and above: fever
107°F (41.6°C) and above: hyperpyrexia (abnormally high)
98°F (36.6°C) and below: subnormal
95°F (35°C) and below: hypothermia (abnormally low)

HOW TO TAKE A TEMPERATURE

In the old days, physicians used to place the back of their hand on a patient's forehead to see how warm the skin was. Unfortunately the results were often inaccurate and highly misleading. It is quite possible for someone with a normal internal temperature to feel quite cold and clammy to the touch; someone with true hypothermia can have quite warm skin.

There are three main ways of taking someone's temperature, and all vary slightly in their results. The commonest is with an oral thermometer, which is simply a glass cylinder containing a column of mercury. It is important to leave the thermometer under the tongue long enough for the true reading to be represented, and modern thermometers should indicate how long they should be left in place. A low-reading thermometer where the mercury can be shaken down to below 95°F (35°C) is worth buying because low temperature can sometimes be seen, especially in an elderly person who has collapsed or become comatose as a result of a stroke or heart attack. Whilst the temperature is being monitored, it is important that the patient firmly closes his or her lips around the thermometer and desists from talking, as air passing through the mouth during the reading will give a falsely low result. Having said that, an oral temperature will give a slightly higher reading than a temperature taken from the armpit or groin, and a slightly lower reading than one taken rectally.

With children it can often be difficult to take an oral temperature, so a reading taken from the armpit or groin can be taken instead. The thermometer should be placed at the top of the armpit with the arm then firmly brought down on the thermometer against the side of the chest. If a groin reading is taken, the thermometer should be placed in the crease of the groin with the front of the thigh brought up against the abdomen. When left long enough, the thermometer will pick up a true fever, although the reading in these areas is generally 1°F (0.4°C) lower than it would be orally.

Finally, for the most accurate and reliable reading of all, a special rectal thermometer may be used which reflects the body's true inner temperature. The reading here will generally be 1°F (0.4°C) higher than the oral temperature. There are newer electronic digital thermometers and special plastic fever strips available, but although these are easy to use and are fine for everyday needs, they are not really suitable for monitoring serious disease.

NORMAL HEAT REGULATION
The body regulates its temperature by balancing heat production against heat loss. Even at rest the various functions of the body such as circulation of the blood, the action of the liver and the work of the muscles will all produce steady heat. When the temperature rises above normal, blood is diverted to the skin through the widening of blood vessels. The radiation of heat and the cooling effect of sweat evaporating from the surface of the skin allow the body to cool down. In people who have become hypothermic, however, where the body temperature has fallen below 95°F (35°C) the body will be furiously trying to conserve heat. The skin will usually be pale and blanched because the blood vessels will automatically have been closed off to prevent further heat loss, and it will also be dry as there will be no sweating. Unless heat production comes from within from digestive processes, from muscle movement or from external warming, the temperature will continue to fall and life itself will be at risk.

HEAT REGULATION IN FEVERS
When a fever is present, the mechanism controlling heat regulation is set at a higher level than normal as a result of the disease process acting on the brain itself. Paradoxically, despite having a raised internal temperature, the sufferer can experience violent shivers or 'rigors' and feel very cold. The explanation for this is simple. Because the body's thermostat is temporarily at a higher level, the body will try

to conserve heat by constricting the blood vessels in the skin. The skin consequently feels cold and goose pimply, and its fine little hairs will stand on end. Later, when the higher temperature is reached, the heat-loss mechanisms come into play again and the skin becomes hot and sweaty: the familiar, recognizable signs of fever.

OTHER SYMPTOMS OF FEVER

As well as having a temperature, the patient's skin may look and feel flushed, and there may be aching in the muscles and joints. Headache and sweating usually accompany a temperature, and loss of appetite is common. Small children may not be able to describe exactly how they feel, but they may demonstrate the problem by becoming irritable, crying incessantly, exhibiting feeding problems or rubbing their ears, or by coughing, sneezing or having a runny nose. Sometimes diarrhoea, abdominal pain or strongly smelling urine may indicate an infective source of the temperature.

TYPES OF FEVER

Most people are familiar with the types of fevers usually associated with common respiratory infections. They make us feel chilled to begin with, then make us feel hot and sweaty for a day or two before gradually settling down. However, not all fevers produce this type of continuous, gentle temperature. A fever that comes and goes, sometimes several times in a day, is known as a 'relapsing fever' and may indicate the presence of an abscess somewhere in the body that is sporadically releasing large numbers of micro-organisms into the circulation. Occasionally it may be a sign of an underlying malignancy. 'Intermittent fevers', on the other hand, produce spikes of temperature sometimes lasting several hours during any one day, with a complete

disappearance of the raised temperature between paroxysms. Malaria is an example of a disease producing intermittent fevers, and depending on the type of parasite responsible, the fever may be present on a daily basis (quotidian), on alternate days (tertian), or every three days (quartan).

THE CAUSES OF FEVER

Sometimes the cause of your temperature is obvious, but on other occasions it is not. If you have just come down with a raging sore throat and runny nose with earache and aching muscles, it is not too difficult to work out that you are probably suffering from an attack of influenza. On other occasions, however, a temperature may be raised in the absence of obvious clinical clues. Whatever else it does, the temperature at least proves that you really are sick. Of course, it is possible to falsify a temperature reading, and occasionally some people will attempt to do this, perhaps by placing the thermometer near a hot-water bottle, dipping it into a hot drink, or rubbing or shaking it. The difference is that despite the evidence of fever recorded by the thermometer, such people remain puzzlingly well. Usually, they soon get found out.

❷ *Have you just been exercising, are you in a hot climate, or are you half-way through your menstrual cycle?*
A physiological fever is a mild elevation of the normal resting temperature as the result of standard body metabolism. Generally, your temperature tends to be slightly higher in the evening than in the morning.

It will be slightly higher in a hot climate, and will temporarily peak after a hot bath or exercise. A spike in temperature is also seen a day or two after ovulation. Oral temperature readings can also be affected if taken too soon after having a hot drink or eating ice cream.

❷ Do you have a cough, cold, spots and/or a sore throat?

Infection undoubtedly causes the majority of fevers, and in most cases the diagnosis of the disorder producing the fever can be ascertained from the patient's clinical history and an examination. Bugs responsible for such infections include viruses, bacteria, fungi and parasites. The infection will usually produce its own characteristic symptoms to accompany the fever, but when this is not the case the sufferer is said to have a fever or 'pyrexia' of unknown origin (PUO).

In 90 per cent of cases of PUO, investigations carried out by the physician will lead to identification and appropriate treatment of the underlying cause, and the other 10 per cent will probably clear up on their own.

❷ Are there shaking chills or rigors?

Violent episodes of shaking are associated with high spikes of temperature and often signify the presence of a bacterial infection within the kidneys following a bladder infection (cystitis). Rigors are also seen with abscesses in other sites within the body, with gall-bladder inflammation through stones or infection, or with a condition called sub-acute bacterial endocarditis (SBE), an infection of a weakened heart valve that produces chronic fever. Usually, the heart valves have been damaged by rheumatic fever at some time during the patient's life, or otherwise have been deformed at birth. Bacteria that find their way into the bloodstream through something as simple as teeth descaling, through squeezing a spot on the skin, or from having a catheter inserted, can settle on the vulnerable valves, producing further growth of bacteria and in time destroying the valve itself. Anyone with a heart murmur may be prone to such infection, which before the advent of antibiotics often proved fatal. This is why some people with heart murmurs are advised to take preventative antibiotic treatment before and after certain procedures, including dental and gynaecological treatment and minor surgery.

❷ Is the temperature associated with profuse sweating at night?

This is one of the main symptoms of pulmonary tuberculosis. TB is most definitely on the increase again, despite the availability of powerful antibiotics to treat it. This is mainly because we still have a large population of poor and homeless in this country, but also because sufferers often fail to take the full 9–12 month course necessary for their treatment. The elderly in nursing homes are particularly vulnerable, and the worldwide increase in AIDS has reduced the ability of many to fight TB in the normal way.

❷ Do you work on a farm?

If you work on a farm and/or rely on unpasteurized dairy products it is possible that you could have contracted brucellosis or listeriosis. Brucellosis produces a temperature that undulates over a period of a week or so. It is an occupational hazard of veterinary surgeons, slaughterhouse workers, laboratory personnel and others. Other symptoms include sweating, weakness, headaches, loss of appetite, pain in the limbs and back, constipation, rigors, coughs, a sore throat, and joint pains.

❷ Do you eat a lot of raw vegetables or cook-chill products?

Listeriosis is an infection caused by the Listeria bacteria and is often contracted through contaminated fresh raw vegetables such as lettuce, cabbage, cauliflower, sprouts and tomatoes, and from cook-chill products. Two major types of human listeriosis are recognized. The first is found in pregnant women, where it can occur after a flu-like illness, after an abortion or following the delivery of a premature or stillborn child. The second is a different form in which meningitis or inflammation of the heart and eye can occur.

❷ Do you work with plastics?

People who work in the plastics industry can develop a temperature after inhaling fumes, and doctors, nurses and laboratory technicians are all vulnerable to contracting the diseases of their patients.

❷ Have you recently travelled abroad to the Third World?

Anybody who has travelled to a tropical country or to the Third World may have been exposed to a large number of different infections such as gastroenteritis, amoebiasis, and malaria, all of which can give rise to high temperatures.

❷ Do you inject yourself with illegal drugs?

Intravenous drug abusers are likely to introduce infection through contaminated needles, and are more vulnerable to abscesses, subacute bacterial endocarditis, hepatitis and AIDS. The effect of recreational drugs themselves can also produce fevers, amphetamines and Ecstasy perhaps being the most frequent offenders. Ecstasy, in fact, causes such a significant rise in the basic rate of the body's tick-over speed (basal metabolic rate) that the temperature can rise so uncontrollably that treatment in an intensive care unit may be necessary. In severe cases, however, this may not be sufficient to prevent death.

❷ Did the fever begin after eating?

Poor sanitation and inadequate food hygiene can produce cases of simple food poisoning, whilst meat contaminated with the parasite trichonella can lead to a worm infestation when ingested, with temperatures reaching up to 104°F (40°C). In this situation the temperature is often accompanied by swelling around the face, eyelids and conjunctivae (the delicate mucous membranes covering the eyeballs and the undersurface of the eyelids). Muscle stiffness, pain and tenderness are also common.

❷ Do you have diarrhoea, with blood, mucus or pus mixed with the motion?

This raises the possibility of a parasitic or bacterial bowel infection. Sometimes tests on the stool are necessary to identify the micro-organism responsible, although non-infective inflammation of the bowel itself as in Crohn's disease and ulcerative colitis can produce similar symptoms.

❷ Is it painful to pass water and do you need to go more frequently?

'Dysuria' and 'frequency' are the classic symptoms of a bladder infection (cystitis). There may also be rigors if the kidney itself is involved.

❷ Is there a rash?

The characteristic rashes of chickenpox, measles, scarlet fever, erysipelas and shingles are obvious clues to the cause of the underlying temperature. However, rashes don't necessarily herald an infection since allergies and autoimmune disorders such as rheumatoid arthritis can also produce them.

❷ Do you have muscle stiffness or pain?

Common virus infections, including flu, can often cause aching muscles, but so can trichinosis, a parasite found in contaminated pork, toxoplasmosis, an organism picked up by failing to wash the hands after emptying cat-litter trays, and the infections listeria and yersinia. Lyme disease is an infection contracted from tick bites in areas of Britain such as the New Forest and it too can produce a temperature associated with muscle pains.

❷ Have you had any back pain?
Back pain is a common symptom of kidney infection, and also of the rare infection of the vertebral bone known as osteomyelitis.

❷ Have you had any abdominal pain?
Pain in the upper right corner of the abdomen may be a symptom of inflammation and infection of the gall bladder, although a kidney infection could also be responsible. Appendicitis and pelvic infections will both produce quite high temperatures with abdominal pain, although in these cases localization of the pain tends to be much less precise.

❷ Are your glands swollen?
Glands can be swollen for a number of reasons, one of which may be infection. Certain medical drugs and underlying malignancies can also produce fever with swollen glands. We all know that swelling of the glands in the neck is a common result of tonsillitis or an ear infection, and if we develop an infected cut anywhere on our legs, we should not be surprised when the glands in the groin enlarge in response to the fight against infection. But generalized glandular swelling throughout the body in the groin, armpits and neck areas in particular may be a sign of nonspecific infection such as glandular fever or brucellosis.

❷ Do you have a cough or suffer shortness of breath?
Respiratory infections ranging from croup right through to pneumonia can all produce a combination of fever with breathlessness, but bear in mind that pulmonary emboli (blood clots in the lung) can also produce the same symptoms, often with associated spitting of blood.

❷ Have you had any chest pains?
Infections affecting the surface of the lung (pleurisy) or the membranes covering the outer part of the heart (pericarditis) can produce chest pain along with fever.

❷ Are there any splinter-like lines under your fingernails?
These splinter haemorrhages are characteristic of subacute bacterial endocarditis, an infection of abnormal heart valves where infected blood clots thrown into the circulation may be seen under the nails.

❷ Do you have leg pain?
When clotting or thrombosis occurs in the deeper veins of the leg it will not be visible, but may cause a high temperature as a result of infection. Pain in the calf associated with swelling of the ankle and redness is a telltale sign and should certainly be brought to the attention of your doctor as soon as possible. Those already suffering from varicose veins are particularly prone to clotting and inflammation in those veins, in which case they may become hard and tender.

❷ Do you have any chest pain?
A blood clot from the legs that finds its way to the lung will obstruct the blood flow and lead to chest pain and breathlessness. Whilst anyone can develop this problem, it is not uncommon in women, even young women, who smoke, who take the oral contraceptive pill, who are pregnant, who have had any gynaecological procedures, who have varicose veins, or who have been resting in bed without moving much for some considerable time. A blood clot that obstructs the coronary arteries will cause a heart attack by depriving that part

of the heart muscle of the blood supply so that it dies. It is the death of the cells in the heart muscle or in the lung after a pulmonary embolus that is responsible for producing the temperature indicative of these disorders.

❷ *Have you incurred any large bruises?*
After accidents or injuries sometimes quite large amounts of blood can be lost into the tissues. The various blood cells can release chemicals and toxins and these in their turn produce a raised temperature. Damaged muscle tissue can have the same effect.

❷ *Have you suffered from recent joint problems, tiredness, and breathlessness?*
In autoimmune disorders, the body, for reasons as yet unknown to the medical profession, produces antibodies against some of its own healthy tissues. These conditions, also known as 'collagen disorders', are more common in women and include rheumatoid arthritis, polyarteritis nodosa, polymyalgia rheumatica, and systemic lupus erythematosus. Along with the symptom that they all have in common, which is joint pain or arthritis, they may all produce a persistent mild or low-grade temperature. The patients are generally unwell, and may have lost weight, and there is usually tenderness, redness, swelling, and pain in many of the joints and muscles of the body.

❷ *Is the high temperature accompanied by a rash and swelling of the face, hands and ankles?*
Allergic reactions to medication such as penicillin and aspirin are not at all uncommon and often lead to skin rashes, swelling of the face, hands and ankles, and a high temperature. Certain foodstuffs may produce similar reactions in susceptible people. The cause of the raised temperature is usually evident from the above symptoms.

❷ *Has the person concerned been working or relaxing in a very hot environment for several hours with little to drink?*
Heatstroke must be the most obvious cause of a high temperature and is usually accompanied by hot, dry skin and convulsions. In severe cases it can lead to coma. It is therefore *a medical emergency* and urgent supervised cooling of the patient together with fluid replenishment is essential.

❷ *Has there been any serious weight loss, extreme fatigue and/or swollen glands?*
Many cancers can manifest themselves for the first time as a fever and may or may not be associated with other factors such as a rash, swollen glands, loss of appetite, loss of weight, localized pain, and discomfort. The temperature is the result of a number of things, including rapid cell turnover together with an acceleration of the basic tick-over speed of the body and rapid destruction of cells leading to the release of toxins into the bloodstream. Fever can, of course, also be one of the consequences of the cancer medication itself. In Hodgkin's disease and other disorders of the lymphatic system the temperature may be relapsing and remitting, something to which the temperature chart at the foot of the patient's bed would soon bear witness.

SUMMARY
FEVER

POSSIBLE CAUSE	ACTION
Physiological	No action necessary. The body will control the temperature automatically.
Infection	Symptomatic relief with aspirin or paracetamol. Identification of underlying cause and causative organism, appropriate antibiotic therapy. Surgery if necessary for large, deep-seated abscesses.
Fever of unknown origin (PUO)	Thorough medical investigations to identify causative organism or problem followed by appropriate treatment.
Blood clot	Prophylactic treatment of large varicose veins. Anticoagulants for established blood clots. Avoidance of contraceptive pill in susceptible people.
Large bruises	Fever will settle spontaneously.
Autoimmune disorder	Appropriate medical treatment, including steroids.
Allergy	With your doctor, identify and avoid responsible drug or foodstuff.
Heatstroke	Emergency fluid replacement and gradual cooling of patient.
Malignancy	Medical or surgical treatment of underlying cause.

CHANGES IN BODY WEIGHT

Any recent and relatively sudden change in body weight either upwards or downwards should be regarded critically until it has been explained. Unwanted weight gain is by far the most common complaint in my surgery, and usually is simply the result of over-eating and underexercising. Generally, the patient is aware of this. Occasionally, however, people complain of the opposite problem. No matter what they do, they just cannot gain weight and they are fed up with looking thin, gaunt or even emaciated. They want some flesh on their bones to make them look more attractive and cuddly. Generally speaking they are just constitutionally slim and there is often a family history of thinness to account for it. Having said that, there are also many patients who visit their doctor about a recent change in body weight that is not due to any deliberate change in their lifestyle and cannot immediately be accounted for. Such people have previously been entirely healthy but their loss or gain in weight has been noticed, if not by themselves, by their spouse, a relative or a friend. This is especially true if the problem is weight loss, when their appearance will be described as drawn and haggard. Often people notice that their clothes hang loosely on their frame, their belt no longer holds up their trousers, and their shirt collar is far too large. By the time this happens something like a half to one stone in weight can already have been lost.

WEIGHT LOSS

As with most symptoms, weight loss can be due to something quite trivial, or to some serious and significant disturbance. Possible causes range from an inadequate dietary intake of calories, through failure to absorb food, to a metabolic disturbance: in other words something that alters the general turnover speed of the body. To help identify the cause of any weight loss, ask yourself the following questions:

❷ *Have you also lost your appetite?*
This would certainly suggest a disease of the digestive system, and there will often be a history of heartburn, indigestion, flatulence, abdominal pain, and the regurgitation of

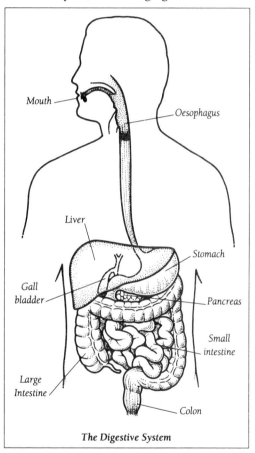

Mouth

Oesophagus

Liver

Stomach

Gall bladder

Pancreas

Small intestine

Large Intestine

Colon

The Digestive System

stomach acid into the mouth. These symptoms are suggestive of inflammation of the lining of the stomach (gastritis), inflammation of the lining of the windpipe (oesophagitis), or a peptic ulcer in the stomach or first part of the intestine. A hiatus hernia, where the top part of the stomach rolls up through the muscular, tent-like diaphragm and into the gullet with attendant regurgitation of stomach acid into the gullet, can also produce similar symptoms. Loss of appetite and weight loss in a middle-aged person who has previously enjoyed his or her food should certainly alert the doctor to the possibility of stomach cancer. That is not to say that this is a particularly likely explanation, but it is a possibility the doctor will wish to exclude right at the beginning.

❷ Is your appetite normal, or even increased?

This combination is possible as the result of an overactive thyroid (hyperthyroidism) or diabetes mellitus, or, for that matter, in anyone indulging in particularly vigorous and protracted physical exercise. Diabetes can be confirmed by examination of the urine or blood for glucose, and an overactive thyroid is often accompanied by other tell-tale symptoms. In this condition, the thyroid gland produces too much of the thyroid hormone thyroxine, and this accelerates the basic tick-over speed of the body (the basal metabolic rate). The heart rate is increased, the skin is flushed, and palpitations may be reported. There may be diarrhoea, bulging eyes, sweating, panic attacks and tremor. In short, everything within the body works faster. As a result, the appetite increases, but weight loss occurs because the dietary intake cannot keep up with the body's energy expenditure. Occasionally in particularly active young people the demands of their energy expenditure are not met by their calorie intake, and sometimes all that is required is dietary advice, with a move away from the empty calories of a junk-food diet on to more wholesome alternatives.

❸ Is there a yellow tinge to the whites of your eyes?

If your urine is also dark brown you are suffering from jaundice. This particular combination of symptoms can be the result of benign or malignant disorders. Possible benign disorders include infectious and serum hepatitis (infection of the liver), cirrhosis (inflammation of the liver), and inflammation of the pancreas or gall bladder. Where anaemia is associated with a faint, lemon-yellow tint to the skin, pernicious anaemia is another possibility. This affects women more than men, and is commonest between the ages of 45 and 65. The condition often runs in the family. The lining of the stomach fails to produce a substance required for the absorption of vitamin B12 from the gut, and weight loss and jaundice in association with intermittent soreness of the tongue and occasional diarrhoea can result. Pins and needles in the fingers and toes are another sign. When neglected, reversible early dementia may ensue.

Malignant conditions often begin with weight loss and jaundice at the same time, and consequently *this combination of symptoms should always be referred to the doctor urgently.* Virtually any form of cancer can produce these symptoms, but those that spread to the liver are the most likely. Cancers of the stomach, colon, thyroid, cervix, pancreas, gall bladder, lung, and of the liver itself head the list.

❹ Are you permanently tired and feverish?

This suggests the cause is an infection, although malignant conditions of the lymphatic system such as Hodgkin's disease and cancers of the digestive tract should not be dismissed. Any infection producing a persistent fever is likely to cause weight loss, especially gastroenteritis where there is profuse diarrhoea with loss of minerals and body fluids. But amoebic dysentery, roundworm infection and chronic inflammatory conditions of the large bowel such as Crohn's disease and ulcerative colitis can have similar effects. Deep-seated abscesses within the lung, liver, bone, sinuses or kidney may also be responsible.

❷ Have you lost weight very quickly?

In most cases weight loss is a slow, insidious process that the patient may not notice for a while. Where there is very rapid weight loss a malignancy must be excluded before any other cause. Cancers of the oesophagus or nervous system are particularly capable of producing this. *You should see your doctor about rapid weight loss immediately.*

❷ Are you running an intermittent or continuous high temperature? Are you sweating a lot, especially at night, and do you shiver as if feverish?

Tuberculosis of the lung may not always produce symptoms that indicate chest disease. Often there is no cough, just a fever and an insidious loss of weight. The same is true of cancer of the lung and lung or liver abscesses, and only further investigations including chest X-rays can lead to a diagnosis of the real problem.

AIDS (acquired immune deficiency syndrome) is another chronic infection now present worldwide. Those infected with the AIDS virus will generally develop symptoms within five to ten years, but in the early stages there are no symptoms whatsoever. Later there may be recurrent thrush in the mouth together with skin troubles, and there may be profuse sweating with severe weight loss and fever. Swollen glands and profound exhaustion generally accompany such weight loss. AIDS patients are particularly vulnerable to opportunistic infections because the very cells that normally fight infection and resist disease are themselves unhealthy. Unusual pneumonias and certain skin cancers such as Kaposi's sarcoma are common features.

❷ Do your muscles and joints ache all the time?

With autoimmune disorders, antibodies are produced that damage healthy tissues within the body. Examples are rheumatoid arthritis, polymyositis and polyarteritus. In most of these conditions the weight loss and joint and muscle pains and swelling are accompanied by a low-grade temperature.

❷ Could heavy drinking or the abuse of recreational or medicinal drugs be responsible?

Usually these are accompanied by unpredictable mood and personality changes and obvious irritability and aggression. School work, jobs and family may be neglected, and there may also be anti-social behaviour, deterioration in personal appearance, and the presence of puncture marks at the elbow and sores around the mouth. Sickness and vomiting may occur. Periods may become erratic, and constipation is common. Psychological disorders are often reported. In addition, infected sores, abscesses and boils on the skin can lead to serious blood poisoning (septicaemia), whilst injection with contaminated needles can introduce hepatitis, AIDS and other significant infections, all of which can produce fevers leading to further weight loss.

❷ Is the sufferer obsessive about his or her body weight?

Anorexia nervosa and bulimia, which are more common in young women, can lead to very severe weight loss and emaciation. Here there is a predominant and overriding fear of fatness coupled with excessive dieting and/or vomiting. Usually the problem begins between the ages of 14 and 19. Periods may be delayed or, if they have already started, may cease. Constipation is often a problem. The sufferer is more vulnerable to infections and the skin is usually pale and sallow. There may be surreptitious use of laxatives or deliberate vomiting. *Anorexia and bulimia need urgent assessment and treatment* by the doctor.

❷ *Is there also depression?*
Loss of appetite, weight loss and digestive-system upsets are also classic features of

depression and anxiety. In manic depression, the sufferer experiences mood swings ranging from the hyperexcitable state of mania through to the low, dreary, sometimes suicidal state of depression. In the manic stage, speech will be rapid and uncontrolled, there will be poor concentration, showing-off and extrovert behaviour, flights of fancy and insomnia. The physical toll frequently leads to loss of weight.

SUMMARY
WEIGHT LOSS

POSSIBLE CAUSE	ACTION
Digestive disorder (gastritis, oesphagitis, peptic ulcer, hernia)	Dietary adjustment, antacids, surgery for obstinate ulcers.
Diabetes	Control blood sugar with diet, oral medication or insulin injections.
Overactive thyroid gland	Antithyroid tablets or surgery.
Inadequate diet	Dietary adjustment.
Hepatitis	Bedrest, fluids.
Cirrhosis	Treat underlying cause. Medical and/or surgical treatment.
Inflammation of pancreas or gall bladder	Bedrest, dietary adjustment. Medical or surgical treatment.
Pernicious anaemia	Regular monthly vitamin B12 injections.
Malignancy	Identify cause and treat accordingly.
Infection	Identify organism and treat with appropriate antibiotics or antiviral agents.
Autoimmune disorder	Medical treatment, including steroids.
Alcohol or drug abuse	Education, counselling, and psychotherapy.
Anorexia nervosa, bulimia	Counselling, psychotherapy, hospital admission if necessary.
Depression	As above.

WEIGHT GAIN

Too many calories and not enough expenditure of energy through physical exercise is by far the commonest cause of weight gain, and both the problem and its solution are understood by most. What is really important is to find an explanation for weight gain where the dietary intake is unchanged, and when there are other symptoms of illness. To help this process, ask yourself the following questions:

❷ Do you feel constantly cold and sluggish and suffer from constipation?

More common in women, an underactive thyroid gland (hypothyroidism or myxoedema) arises very gradually, and with the weight gain there may be coarsening and thinning of the body hair, constipation, intolerance of cold weather, absence of sweating, dry skin, and depression. The condition is eminently treatable.

❷ Are you taking the pill or going through the menopause?

Certain hormone imbalances such as those caused by the menopause and by taking oral contraceptives can lead to fluid retention and therefore to weight gain.

❸ Are you taking any medication containing steroids?

In reasonably high doses, steroids in medications for chronic conditions such as those encountered in organ transplantation, autoimmune diseases and malignancies may produce reasonably significant gains in weight.

❸ Are you breathless, especially after any exertion, and do you have swollen ankles?

Heart failure leading to congestion of the circulation and leakage of fluid out of the blood vessels into the body tissues can produce a very rapid increase of weight over a period of days. Diuretic medication can often have a prompt and dramatic effect, and this symptom in a person with blue lips, tongue or extremities who also suffers from breathlessness and swollen ankles *should be reported urgently to a doctor for medical analysis and treatment.*

SUMMARY
WEIGHT GAIN

Possible Cause	Action
Underactive thyroid gland	Treat with thyroid hormone.
Hormonal imbalance	Restore hormonal equilibrium.
Steroid medication	With your doctor, modify dosage or use alternative therapy.
Heart failure	Drugs to act on the heart, diuretics.

LOSS OF APPETITE

A healthy appetite has always been a sign of wellbeing. Conversely, loss of appetite may go hand in hand with a number of complaints and disorders, including the psychological as well as the physical. The causes range from the short-lived and trivial right through to the protracted and serious. A common cold can take away the appetite for a short while, just as a more chronic long-term illness such as AIDS or rheumatoid arthritis can in the long run. It's almost true to say that any disorder affecting the human body can produce loss of appetite, but sometimes the associated features may give a clue to the nature of the underlying cause.

To help identify the nature of the problem causing your loss of appetite, therefore, ask yourself the following questions:

❷ *Do you have a fever?*

Infections from the common cold to AIDS can ruin a normal appetite, particularly when a fever is present. Sinusitis can also have this effect, especially in cases where the sinuses are producing a lot of mucus and catarrh that is being swallowed.

❷ *Have you had any heartburn, abdominal discomfort, diarrhoea or vomiting?*

Clearly, anything that upsets normal digestion is liable to produce loss of appetite, so inflammation of the lining of the gullet, producing heartburn (oesophagitis), inflammation of the lining of the stomach (gastritis), and any kind of peptic ulcer, whether in the stomach or the duodenum, may do the same. If the gall bladder or pancreas is malfunctioning there will be interference with normal digestion, and accompanying any loss of appetite there may be bloating, abdominal pain and wind.

Even lower down the intestine in the large bowel, inflammatory diseases such as ulcerative colitis and Crohn's disease, as well as any kind of obstruction, including constipation, may cause problems with the normal desire to eat.

❷ *Are you taking any medication?*

Most drugs used in medical practice have side effects of one kind or another and loss of appetite is one of the commonest, along with rashes, headaches and stomach irritation. If you are prescribed a course of tablets or medication and then lose your appetite, ask your doctor. It may not be the underlying illness that is causing it but the therapy itself. One common offender is digitalis, used in the control of abnormal heart rhythms such as atrial fibrillation and for heart failure, but it is always worth considering various antibiotics as well as painkillers such as codeine, morphine, aspirin and pethidine. Any of the nonsteroidal anti-inflammatory agents used in the control of arthritis can have the same effect. Even fairly innocuous potions bought over-the-counter in chemist shops may cause problems, including phenylpropanolamine, which is used in many cold preparations.

❷ *Are you particularly worried or stressed, for any reason, at the moment?*

A healthy appetite relies on, amongst other things, a healthy, happy mind. Any kind of nervous condition, for example, anxiety, stress, phobia or more serious mental illness, can affect the ability to eat, and increasingly common in the nineties are the various eating disorders, headed by anorexia nervosa and bulimia nervosa. With anorexia there is a collection of other symptoms and signs, including a false body image, an overwhelming fear of being overweight or fat, and a heavy reliance on self-induced vomiting and laxative abuse after meals.

❷ Is there also general weakness and fatigue?

When these symptoms occur in conjunction with loss of appetite, it is certainly worth thinking about hepatitis (inflammation of the liver) or glandular fever. In the former, the liver may be tender and there may even be mild jaundice with yellowing of the whites of the eyes and dark urine. With glandular fever, the classic symptoms are a long-standing sore throat and severe tiredness.

❸ Has your weight dropped dramatically?

When loss of appetite is severe and protracted enough to cause significant weight loss, a more serious underlying medical condition may be responsible. Diseases such as pneumonia, heart failure and kidney or liver disorders can all have this effect, and peptic ulcers, underactive pituitary or adrenal glands, coeliac disease and pernicious anaemia are also worth considering.

❹ Has there been any chest pain?

With this combination of symptoms, the doctor might immediately think about a lung abscess, tuberculosis, rheumatic heart disease, rheumatic fever, endocarditis, an ulcer, or inflammation of the lining of the gullet.

SUMMARY
LOSS OF APPETITE

POSSIBLE CAUSE	ACTION
Infection	Identify micro-organism responsible and treat accordingly.
Digestive disorders	Identify exact cause. Medical or surgical treatment.
Medication	With your doctor, identify and discontinue or reduce dosage of drug responsible.
Psychological	Counselling, psychotherapy, medication if necessary.
Hepatitis	Bedrest. No specific treatment.
Glandular fever	Will improve spontaneously within 3–6 months.
Heart or lung disorder	Medical or surgical treatment.
Other physical conditions	Medical or surgical treatment as appropriate.

TIREDNESS

The symptom of tiredness is one of the commonest of all encountered in the GP's surgery. So many people complain that they feel tired all the time that doctors now have a well-known abbreviation that they jot in their medical records: TATT — tired all the time. Associated complaints include: 'I just don't seem to have any energy', 'I can't be bothered to do anything', and 'I've got so much to do, but don't seem to be able to cope'.

The good news is that most doctors will at least be sympathetic even though the sufferer's relatives and friends may feel the symptoms to be all too familiar and offer rather unhelpful advice or criticism as 'Pull your socks up', or 'you're just being lazy'. In the vast majority of cases, tiredness will be due to lack of sleep or overwork. In other people, it may be caused by boredom, anxiety or depression. It is amazing, for example, how many young people complain of tiredness at work during the day but then magically find the energy for several hours of vigorous sport in the evening, or go clubbing into the early hours of the morning. The only cure for that kind of tiredness is a change of lifestyle.

However, it should always be borne in mind that fatigue can sometimes be a consequence of more serious disorders such as anaemia, an underactive thyroid gland or a virus infection.

In these cases, when lifestyle excesses are unlikely to be the source of the problem, other symptoms occurring hand in hand with the fatigue may well point to the underlying cause. To help discover the elusive cause of your chronic tiredness, ask yourself the following questions:

❶ *Are you pale and breathless? Do you feel faint at times?*

These symptoms together with general fatigue suggest anaemia, when a reduced level of haemoglobin in the blood means a reduced supply of oxygen to the various tissues of the body. This oxygen deprivation leads to a decrease in energy levels and also means that the heart and lungs have to work that much harder to pump the 'thinner' blood around the body in the attempt to make up in quantity what it lacks in quality. Other symptoms include palpitations because of the rapid pulse and breathlessness. Anyone on a diet that lacks iron, vitamin B12 or folic acid will be especially prone to developing anaemia, as will anyone with chronic blood loss, for example a woman with heavy and frequent periods. A simple blood test can check for anaemia, and when it is found dietary modification and/or investigation into the source of blood loss will be required.

❷ *Have you had a recent cold or flu? Do you have a high temperature?*

Any infection, particularly one that causes a raised temperature, can lead to tiredness. Anybody with pneumonia, a lung abscess or tuberculosis, for example, will feel absolutely exhausted. In these conditions, coughing, loss of appetite and possible chest pain on deep breathing will indicate the underlying source of the tiredness. Another condition that may be heralded by a similar collection of symptoms, although occasionally there are no such indications of the underlying problem, is glandular fever, a common condition affecting many thousands of teenagers and young adults every year. It is caused by the Epstein-Barr virus, and tiredness is a common early symptom. It too may begin with a raised temperature, together with a headache and swelling of the lymph glands in the neck, groin and armpits. A very inflamed throat that does not respond to antibiotics may well lead to the correct diagnosis, which is made from a simple blood test. Treatment consists of rest, with recovery usually taking place within 2-3 months. However, during this time sufferers certainly lack energy, feel low in spirits and sleepy during the day.

Another condition causing similar symptoms and thought to be due to a slow virus infection is ME, myalgic encephalomyelitis, otherwise known as post-virus fatigue syndrome. This often develops after a cold- or flu-like illness from which the patient appears not to make a full recovery. Characteristic associated symptoms include aching muscles, dizziness, headache, nausea and depression. There is currently no simple diagnostic test and doctors' efforts are usually aimed at excluding other conditions that could be responsible for this collection of symptoms. Treatment consists of rest, dietary modification and psychotherapy. Controversially, some specialist centres use antifungal treatments in the belief that ME may be caused by some form of allergic reaction to the fungal organism candida, which normally lives harmlessly within the bowel. ME generally clears up spontaneously within months or sometimes years.

❷ Are you very low in spirits, tearful and tense?

Approximately 15 per cent of the population will suffer from depression at some stage in their lives, and one of the commonest symptoms is fatigue. There may also be loss of appetite, problems with sleeping, lack of concentration, and headaches. Morbid thoughts, anxiety and crying are also commonplace. Hand in hand with the psychological symptoms come the physical ones, including aching muscles, indigestion, bowel upset, and chest and abdominal pain. In this situation, fatigue is generally part of the depression and tends to improve once the underlying disorder is corrected. Care should

always be exerted, however, when treating depression as many of the drugs used are capable of making the tiredness worse. Wherever possible, drugs should be avoided and psychotherapy employed instead. Nevertheless, in more serious cases antidepressant medication may be required.

❸ Could you be pregnant, or could you be approaching your menopause?

There is no doubt that fluctuating hormone levels play a very important role in causing fatigue. The tiredness associated with pregnancy is very well known and cannot be explained away purely as the result of physical changes occurring in the body such as increasing weight, slight physiological anaemia, backache, and lack of sleep. In fact, the tiredness associated with pregnancy can begin even before a positive test is made. No significant physical changes occur in the first few weeks of pregnancy other than major hormonal fluctuations in the bloodstream, and these are responsible for the fatigue. Similarly, the ovaries' failure to produce oestrogen on a monthly basis as women approach the menopause can be responsible for tiredness. Women with premenstrual syndrome also commonly report feelings of exhaustion any time in the two weeks leading up to their next period, again the result of hormonal fluctuations. Thankfully the hormone changes of pregnancy are self-limiting, but hormone replacement therapy for the menopausal woman, and progesterone supplements for women with PMS, can be very effective.

❹ Are you either bored out of your mind or incredibly stressed?

It is amazing how exhausted people can feel when they are under a lot of stress, and both too much and too little stimulation can produce stress. When we are bored, that part of the nervous system that keeps us alert and bubbly becomes underactive, making us physically and psychologically slow. Depression has a similar effect. On the other hand, excessive stress, or distress as it should be called, can saturate our body with adrenaline and other related chemical compounds, to the extent that our body can no longer respond to them. The trick is to discover a reasonable balance whereby we are able to respond to stimulation efficiently, but then be able to relax and recover afterwards. Most people suffering from tiredness due to psychological causes respond very well to rest, relaxation and simple changes in lifestyle. Occasionally people are beyond the point of no return in terms of self-treatment and are completely unable to identify the underlying problem. When this happens, or when associated physical symptoms such as insomnia, palpitations or indigestion come to the fore, cognitive behavioural therapy as part of overall counselling and psychotherapy may prove extremely useful.

❷ Do you feel cold all the time, is your hair becoming thin and dry, and have you put on weight?

These symptoms together with general fatigue point very strongly towards the possibility of an underactive thyroid gland. The thyroid gland produces the thyroid hormone thyroxine, and is the body's thermostat, controlling the speed at which it ticks over. Too much thyroxine means that everything works faster; too little, the opposite. An underactive thyroid therefore leads to a slow pulse rate, slower breathing, slower thought processes, constipation, thinner hair, intolerance of cold weather, and tiredness. Treatment is relatively simple and involves thyroid-hormone replacement in the form of thyroxine tablets.

❸ Do you have a well-balanced and adequate diet?

We all need food for energy. Without a well-balanced diet, energy levels sink as the human body can break down stored energy only very slowly.

Most people obtain immediate energy from carbohydrates and sugars in the diet, although protein, fat, minerals and vitamins, fruit and vegetables are all important too. Deficiencies of iron and vitamin B can lead to anaemia with subsequent tiredness, whilst crash diets involving high-protein formulas with little carbohydrate or sugar can lead to lethargy and fatigue. Other people who would otherwise have an adequate diet but drink alcohol in large quantities may develop a relative nutritional deficiency. In this case the tiredness will be exacerbated by additional symptoms such as bleeding from the lining of the stomach and liver disease.

❹ Are you taking any medication at the moment?

Many medications, whether in tablet, liquid or injectable forms, are capable of producing tiredness as a side effect.

Antidepressants commonly do this, and some are even used deliberately where anxiety is present together with depression in order to offset some of that anxiety. Tranquillizers, often used erroneously in the treatment of phobias and anxiety states, are now well known to produce powerful and at times overwhelming sleepiness and fatigue.

Many painkillers and drugs used in the treatment of high blood pressure are equally culpable. So, don't always assume that the condition for which you are being treated is responsible for your tiredness. The latter may well turn out to be largely due to the medication you have been given by the doctor for the original ailment.

❷ Have you recently undergone surgery under general anaesthetic?

Despite the fact that a general anaesthetic means being put to sleep, and that you're likely to have a period of convalescence in hospital after the surgery, there seems little doubt that the majority of patients suffer some reaction once they come home. A lot of this may be the result of adjusting to what has actually happened, especially if there have been inadequate explanation and unrealistic expectations in the first place. However, the effects of the anaesthetic agents themselves also play a part. On the whole these effects can be minimized by proper and thorough consultation with the doctors before such procedures, and realistic planning afterwards. Fatigue in these instances is almost always temporary, lasting 3–4 weeks maximum.

❷ Has your weight changed for no apparent reason?

Many of the functions of the body, weight control in particular, are governed by various glands. The conductor of the glandular orchestra is the pituitary gland, situated at the base of the brain. This controls the function of the adrenal glands, which in turn control the function of the reproductive organs. The pancreas and other glands work independently. Any of these glands can develop abnormalities, leading to weight changes and fatigue in the sufferer. When the adrenal gland is underactive, for example, it will cease to produce essential steroids, and severe weakness and fatigue occur. In the case of diabetes, the pancreas gland fails to secrete insulin normally, leading to abnormalities in the level of sugar in the blood with resulting weight changes and fatigue. Simple tests are available for any form of glandular problem, and the combination of tiredness with weight changes is certainly something to be brought to the attention of your GP as soon as possible.

SUMMARY
TIREDNESS

POSSIBLE CAUSE	ACTION
Anaemia	Iron or vitamin supplementation. Other medical treatment if anaemia is more serious.
Infection	If viral, bedrest and fluids. Otherwise, antibiotics if appropriate.
Depression	Reassurance and explanation, psychotherapy, counselling, and/or medication.
Hormonal	Dietary modification, Hormone replacement therapy.
Psychological	Identify problem. Psychotherapy, counselling, changes in lifestyle.
Underactive thyroid gland	Thyroid hormone.
Nutritional deficiency	Dietary modification.
Medication	With your doctor, stop medication and review.
Hospitalization	Adequate counselling. Correct levels of expectation.
Glandular problem	Medical treatment.
Tumour	Medical or surgical treatment.
Heart disease	Correct underlying problem.
Muscle disorder	Medical treatment.

2
THE DIGESTIVE SYSTEM

Essentially, the digestive system consists of a tube along which the food we eat passes. The process of digestion begins in the mouth; from there, the food and drink we consume travels down the gullet into the stomach, and from there into the small and large intestine, right down to the rectum and anus. A number of digestive juices secreted by the salivary glands, the gall bladder and the pancreas are mixed with the food to help break it down into its respective components so that efficient absorption can take place. Food and food residue are moved automatically downward through the intestine by waves of muscular contractions in the wall of the intestine itself, a process known as peristalsis.

Disorders of the digestive system can cause symptoms such as pain without interfering with the digestive process. Others, however, because they obstruct the transport of food or because they interfere with the breakdown or absorption of nutrients, can lead to digestive symptoms such as weight loss, pallor, weakness and diarrhoea. This chapter looks at the various conditions affecting the digestive system in turn.

NAUSEA AND VOMITING

Most of us will have experienced at some time the highly unpleasant sensations of wanting to be sick and actually throwing up. A colleague of mine used to reckon that nausea and vomiting in a young woman were due to pregnancy unless proved otherwise, and that the same symptoms in a young man were almost certainly the result of too much booze the night before. Unfortunately it is not quite that simple, and there are a large number of other causes that need to be considered.

Generally, however, an enquiry concerning the circumstances of the sufferer and a full examination by the doctor will pinpoint the source of the problem.

But why does vomiting occur in the first place? What actually causes it? There are two basic mechanisms that cause vomiting. The part of the brain responsible sits in a particular area in the brain stem (the base of the brain) known as the vomiting centre. It appears that when certain substances are present in the bloodstream, they can cause receptors in the vomiting centre sensitive to them to trigger the muscular contractions in the stomach and gullet that lead to vomiting. The second, apparently separate route whereby the centre can be stimulated involves certain kinds of upset in the stomach and bowel.

Nausea and vomiting can represent the body's reaction to any number of upsets and are therefore very useful in that they at least tell us that further investigation is necessary. To

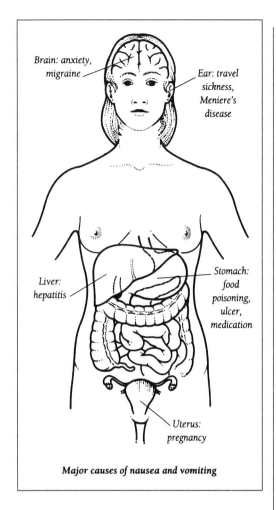

Brain: anxiety, migraine

Ear: travel sickness, Meniere's disease

Liver: hepatitis

Stomach: food poisoning, ulcer, medication

Uterus: pregnancy

Major causes of nausea and vomiting

help identify the possible underlying cause, ask yourself the following questions:

❶ *Did the symptoms start very suddenly, within hours of eating?*

Food poisoning usually, although not invariably, produces a sudden onset of sickness within a few hours of eating a contaminated meal. Depending on the bug or its toxins responsible, this may be within two to three hours or even up to 24 hours later. If a group of people who have shared a meal is affected, this diagnosis is made much more likely. There is usually intense nausea and vomiting with

occasional abdominal pain and sweating but the symptoms are usually short-lived. Vomiting is the body's natural way of getting rid of the responsible organisms, and treatment is therefore seldom prescribed. The nausea and vomiting are often accompanied by diarrhoea, again depending on the bug responsible.

❷ *Do other people close to you have the same symptoms?*

Gastroenteritis is an inflammation of the stomach and intestines, usually the result of particular viruses. Because these viruses are transmitted in much the same way as the bugs that cause the common cold, the infection can spread throughout whole communities, causing diarrhoea and vomiting.

❸ *Is the sickness brought on by motion and travelling?*

Anyone who has ever experienced seasickness or carsickness will know how awful they can be. The source of the problem lies in the body's balance mechanism, which is situated deep within the bones of the skull at the side of the head, just next to where the inner part of the ear transmits sounds to the brain. There are three semicircular-shaped canals full of fluid and every time you move your head, tiny hairs on the lining of the canal are stimulated. If these balance-conscious hairs are overstimulated, there is an overwhelming sense of nausea that can lead to vomiting.

Some people seem particularly prone to motion sickness, although there is undoubtedly a strong psychological element as well. It helps if sufferers have a clear view of what is going on around them, which is why children sitting on booster cushions in the backs of cars often feel better, and why ill passengers on cross-channel ferries are often improved if they stand on the deck where they can see the horizon.

❷ Could you be pregnant?
During the first 16 weeks of pregnancy, nausea sometimes accompanied by vomiting is a common occurrence. Usually it is mild but occasionally it can become very severe, to the extent that it can endanger both mother and baby (hyperemesis gravidarum). Dietary advice can be very helpful, and these days, with the general reluctance to prescribe any drug that could harm the baby in any way, medication is avoided if at all possible. However there are drugs available that are considered safe enough to be prescribed under supervision.

❷ Are you a heavy smoker?
Heavy smoking can itself produce vomiting by directly stimulating the vomiting centre in the brain, but it can also induce physical changes in the stomach that lead to an inflammation of the lining of the stomach and an increase in stomach acid. All of these, as well as the chronic sinusitis that can also occur, may be responsible for your nausea and vomiting.

❷ Do you also have a splitting headache?
In the classic migraine nausea and vomiting are preceded by a visual disturbance in one eye and a blinding headache on the same side. This type of nausea and vomiting may be quite severe, necessitating anti-nausea medication, with or without painkillers.

❷ Do you have a blocked nose and are you swallowing a lot of mucus?
Chronic sinusitis can produce infected mucus and catarrh that drips down the back of the throat into the stomach. This in turn leads to irritation of the stomach lining, with resulting nausea.

❷ Have you any stomach pain?
The stomach itself may be irritated by a number of things.

Excess consumption of alcohol may lead to gastritis, a generalized inflammation of the whole of the stomach lining that produces discomfort in the pit of the stomach and nausea. A stomach ulcer may produce similar symptoms but so may an infection of the liver (hepatitis), where there may be associated jaundice. If there is any kind of disorder with the gall bladder, such as infection or the presence of a stone, there will also be nausea and vomiting, often in association with pain in the upper right side of the abdomen and jaundice. In this instance, the nausea and vomiting will often be preceded by a fatty meal some two hours previously.

Any outflow obstruction from the stomach, perhaps the result of a previous ulcer with scarring, or, for that matter, any obstruction of the small bowel leading away from the stomach, where many food products are fully digested and absorbed, will also lead to sickness.

❷ Have you experienced any ringing in your ears or sudden deafness?
Ménière's disease, a disorder of the inner ear, produces episodic nausea and vomiting and characteristically causes dizziness, a progressive loss of hearing and ringing in the ears (tinnitus) as well.

❷ Have you had a recent head cold that made you feel dizzy?
Any viral infection affecting the balance-sensitive semicircular canals within the inner ear can produce the sudden onset of severe giddiness with nausea and vomiting. Patients discover that each time they move their head in any direction the dizziness and sickness become considerably worse, so much so that their eyes can be seen to be darting quickly from side to side, a phenomenon known by the medical term of nystagmus.

25

❷ *Are you taking any medication?*

In susceptible patients, two of the commonest drug side effects are nausea and/or vomiting. One drug commonly responsible for this is digitalis, used for the control of abnormal heart rhythms and which in overdose can cause significant sickness. For this reason the dosage of digitalis should always be checked, with a blood test every few months, especially when prescribed for elderly people. Drugs used in the control of asthma, for example, theophylline, and antibiotics, particularly erythromycin and metronidazole, can also be culprits. Drugs used in the treatment of inflammatory bowel disorders, for example sulphasalazine, which contains sulphonamide antibiotics, should also be considered. Anything taken for the control of arthritis, particularly aspirin and other non-steroidal anti-inflammatory agents, may produce irritation of the stomach, and strong painkillers, particularly opiates, sometimes require anti nausea tablets to control this side effect. Potassium and zinc supplements can also cause nausea and vomiting, as can the effects of chemotherapy and radiotherapy used to treat patients with cancer.

❷ *Are you taking the contraceptive pill or HRT?*

Both these can at times produce nausea, especially during the early days of taking them.

❷ *Have you lost weight and do you feel particularly tired?*

This suggests diabetes or an underactive adrenal gland producing Addison's disease. Sufferers will be thin and weak, with pigmentation of the skin and low blood pressure.

❷ *Are you paler than usual?*

Disorders of the kidney, particularly chronic renal failure which affects red blood cell production, will lead to a build-up of urea, a breakdown product of the metabolism in the blood, and this is famous for producing nausea.

❷ *Are you constantly tense and anxious?*

There is no doubt that people prone to anxiety and panic attacks may suffer from occasional bouts of nausea and/or vomiting. Acute psychological trauma, for example when bad news is broken, can also produce these symptoms.

❷ *Have you lost weight, and do you generally feel unwell and lacking in energy?*

Many illnesses but in particular cancer, hepatitis and stomach disorders, may produce nausea, as can their treatment.

SUMMARY
NAUSEA AND VOMITING

POSSIBLE CAUSE	ACTION
Food poisoning	Usually self-limiting. Antinauseants if necessary. Fluid replacement.
Gastroenteritis	As above.
Motion sickness	Simple antihistamines such as Dramamine taken before and during travel.
Pregnancy	Dietary modification. Usually ends by 16th week of pregnancy.
Heavy smoking	Give up.
Migraine	Antinauseants and painkillers.
Postnasal drip	Antibiotics.
Abdominal problems	Identify cause and treat appropriately.
Ménière's disease	Anti-histamines and referral to ENT specialist.
Acute labyrynthitis	Bedrest and antihistamines.
Medication	With your doctor, identify and then discontinue or reduce dosage of responsible drug. Antinauseants if necessary.
Contraceptive pill or hormone replacement therapy	Change formulation.
Emotional	Supportive therapy, including reassurance, counselling, individual or group psychotherapy.
Diabetes	Drugs to reduce blood sugar, including insulin. Dietary adjustment.
Addison's disease	Steroids
Kidney disorders	Dietary and fluid adjustment, blood transfusion, possibly dialysis.
Hepatitis	Bedrest, antinauseants.
Cancer or treatment for cancer	Treat underlying disorder. Antinauseants as tablets, injection or suppositories.

CONSTIPATION

As a nation, the British are somewhat obsessed with their bowels. On the one hand there are those who are far too embarrassed even to mention any word associated with them, and on the other there are those who are quite happy to describe the frequency, consistency and colour of their motions to complete strangers, even at mealtimes. But deep-seated anxiety concerning one's bowels is extremely common, and when left unresolved can lead to a great deal of concern and misery.

Constipation means different things to different people. Some people will go to the loo and open their bowels every day, year in, year out. Others will go two or three times a day. Some people, however, inherit a digestive system that is slower to turn over and they may open their bowels perhaps just once a week or every ten days. All these patterns are normal for the individuals concerned. The problem arises when your regular bowel action changes and becomes slower. Usually there is associated pain, discomfort, a feeling of being full and bloated, trapped wind and the need to strain. When these secondary symptoms occur, constipation is worth treating. In the past, however, people have all too often been led to believe that if they don't open their bowels every day their brains will become fuddled or they will get blood poisoning. Over the years these medical myths and grandmothers' tales have led people to rely heavily and unnecessarily on laxatives that artificially stimulate the contractile activity of the muscles in the large bowel. After chronic abuse of such laxatives the muscles are no longer able to respond to the normal stimuli that encourage the passage of waste products through the intestine and chronic constipation may be the direct result. Generally speaking, anyone who has been constipated for more than a week when there is no obvious cause such as dietary

changes, lying in the sun all day, or too little exercise, should seek medical advice, especially if the intake of fluid and fibre has been increased. This is especially important for people over the age of 40 as they are more likely to have a significant underlying problem than younger people.

THE NORMAL PROCESS OF DIGESTION

Whenever we eat or drink, the food and liquid are broken up into their basic components of protein, starch, and fat and are acted upon by different parts of the intestine. In the stomach strong acid initiates the process of digestion, whilst most of the absorption of essential food particles takes place in the small intestine. By the time the waste reaches the large bowel – the colon – it consists mostly of indigestible fibre, the breakdown products of the human metabolism, for example dead blood cells and other waste from the liver, and fluid. Muscular activity in the walls of the colon moves this waste along towards the rectum, but some degree of reabsorption of fluid takes place within the colon itself. If somebody is dehydrated simply because of not drinking enough or from eating particularly dry food, the body will reclaim as much water as possible from the colon, resulting in very hard pellet-like motions that are difficult to pass. So it is easy to see why a diet with adequate fibre and enough fluid is essential to the proper functioning of the digestive system. Although there is really no need to become obsessed with one's bowels, as a doctor I would have to say that those who are aware of their bowel habits will be more quickly alerted to any changes, and these are most significant when it comes to diagnosing the nature and cause of the problem, whether it is constipation or diarrhoea. In view of the fact that many people will always be embarrassed about consulting their doctor concerning their bowels, there are a number of questions you can ask yourself that may give them a clue to what is causing the problem.

❷ Does the constipation alternate with episodes of diarrhoea?

This is strongly suggestive of irritable bowel syndrome, where there is a dull aching pain in the lower left-hand corner of the belly that is often relieved by going to the loo or passing wind. There is also bloating of the stomach, cramping discomfort and nausea. Motions are passed frequently and are of small volume and there is often a feeling of incomplete emptying of the rectum.

Irritable bowel syndrome affects women more than men and certainly seems to be made worse by stress and anxiety. In the UK something like 80,000 new patients are referred to specialists each year, and for each one referred there may be ten others who put up with the problems alone. IBS is often confused for gynaecological conditions, stomach ulcers, bowel polyps and appendicitis, but all tests, including blood tests, stool specimens, barium X-ray tests and sigmoidoscopy examinations where the specialist looks directly at the lining of the bowel through a special telescope, reveal no abnormality. It is therefore usually through exclusion of other things that the common condition known as irritable bowel syndrome is diagnosed.

Diabetes can also produce alternating diarrhoea and constipation; however, if this happens in somebody over the age of 50 the possibility of a polyp or indeed a tumour, either benign or malignant, should be considered.

❷ Is the constipation very long-standing?

One of the most frequent causes of chronic constipation is a very low-fibre diet where there is also inadequate fluid intake, or where laxatives have been abused on a regular basis over a long period of time, resulting in a colon with totally paralysed muscular walls. It is also possible to see chronic constipation in irritable bowel syndrome, although usually it alternates with diarrhoea.

❷ Are you taking any medication?

A large number of drugs can produce constipation, the commonest probably being codeine-containing medications, for example cough linctuses, painkillers and stronger painkillers such as morphine. Anybody with a terminal illness taking morphine, for example, will often need a stool softener such as Dioctyl. Drugs such as verapamil, a treatment used in the control of high blood pressure, may also cause constipation, but so can calcium preparations used for the prevention of osteoporosis, or brittle-bone disease, in women who have gone through the menopause. Other drugs to consider include beta-blockers, used in the control of high blood pressure or abnormal rhythms of the heartbeat, sedatives, tran-quillizers and various antacids.

❷ Have the shape and diameter of the stool changed?

Very often sufferers with irritable bowel syndrome or some form of obstruction low in the bowel, possibly a tumour, describe their motions as being 'ribbon-like'. This can occur in the short term simply as the result of the intestine being irritated for some reason, but when it persists for more than a few days, further investigations are warranted.

❷ Has the colour of the motion changed in any way?

If there is bright red fresh blood on the outside of the motion or on the toilet paper, bleeding haemorrhoids (piles) are very likely. If there is mucus on the outside of the motion or on the toilet paper, this suggests irritable bowel syndrome, inflammatory bowel diseases such as ulcerative colitis or Crohn's disease, or, occasionally, tumours.

❷ Is there darker-coloured blood mixed with the motion?
This is more suggestive of an ulcer or tumour situated higher up in the intestine bleeding into the bowel itself.

❷ Is the stool itself completely black and tar-like?
Bleeding from the stomach from a peptic ulcer or from long-standing gastritis is a significant possibility.

❷ Is it painful to pass a motion?
Pain commonly occurs with haemorrhoids or with a fissure which is a split in the sensitive surface of the anal canal. The discomfort leads to lazy bowel habits and constipation.

❷ After passing a motion, do you feel that you have not properly emptied your bowel?
This occurs in irritable bowel syndrome, in chronic constipation where the bowel has become distended, and in the presence of various tumours.

❷ Did the constipation occur whilst on holiday?
The different bacteria in drinking water and food abroad can often produce constipation.

❷ Has there been any increase in weight?
Constipation in the presence of weight gain suggests an underactive thyroid gland which slows down all the body functions, not just the bowels. Other symptoms are intolerance of cold weather, a slow pulse, thickening of the skin and coarsening of the hair, which becomes sparser, absence of sweating, and depression.

❷ Has there been any loss of weight?
Constipation in the presence of weight loss is highly significant in that it may well indicate the onset of a cancer of the bowel, particularly in someone over the age of 50. *These two symptoms together must be investigated urgently.*

❷ Have you been on a crash diet lately?
Many people are delighted by the clockwork call of nature following a certain meal of the day. This is particularly convenient when it occurs after breakfast, but it may equally occur after lunch or dinner. This stimulation of the large bowel and rectum when the stomach becomes distended by a meal is called the gastro-colic reflex. It is strongest in children and gets more sluggish as we get older. People on crash diets often skip breakfast or other meals, relying instead on artificial low-fibre, low-calorie substitutes. These do not stimulate the gastro-colic reflex and leave very little fibre in the bowel, thereby making constipation a common problem.

❷ Have you stopped taking exercise?
Exercise is a particularly good regulator of bowel habits and few fit, healthy people complain of constipation. It is important however to drink plenty as exercise promotes fluid loss and if the fluid is not replaced, leading to dehydration, constipation can result.

❷ Have you had to empty your bladder more frequently lately?
Chronic constipation or a growth in the large bowel (colon or rectum) can enlarge the large bowel and put pressure on the base of the bladder, making you feel the need to empty it more often than usual.

❷ Have you been less aware of the need to empty your bladder lately?
This combination of symptoms suggests that a problem with the nerves controlling the function of the bladder and bowel may be responsible.

Multiple sclerosis or problems within the spinal cord itself, such as a severe slipped disc or a spinal tumour, should be also considered.

SUMMARY
CONSTIPATION

POSSIBLE CAUSE	ACTION
Dietary factors	Eat a high-fibre diet with plenty of water to prevent dehydration.
Too little exercise	Increase the level of exercise if possible; otherwise, stool softeners such as Dioctyl are useful. Adequate fluid replacement is essential.
Lazy bowel habits (discomfort from haemorrhoids)	Continuous neglect of the call of nature leads to a lazy bowel. Always go when you need to.
Holidays	Adequate fluid intake and exercise.
Medication	Discontinue medication or adjust dosage. Avoid the overuse of laxatives.
Irritable bowel syndrome	Reassurance and supportive therapy, counselling, psychotherapy and stress management together with a high-fibre diet and antispasmodics.
Underactive thyroid	Treat with thyroid hormones.
Peptic ulcer, gastritis	Medical or surgical treatment to stop bleeding.
Inflammatory bowel disease (Crohn's disease, ulcerative colitis)	Dietary adjustment, medication.
Tumours, benign and malignant	Surgery and/or radiotherapy.
Nerve disorders	Exclude multiple sclerosis and disorders of the spinal cord. Medical or surgical treatment.
Diabetes	Adequate control of blood sugar with drugs and diet.

DIARRHOEA

Just like constipation, there are a number of causes that can produce diarrhoea, whether in an acute or a chronic form. Most acute cases of diarrhoea are the result of simple food poisoning after eating out and are caused by contaminated food or drink. This is particularly so where the standard of hygiene is low, for example in the Third World and in the Tropics. Viral illnesses may also be responsible. As with cases of food poisoning where many people at a time may be affected, viral gastroenteritis tends to affect many people in the community at one time, so the diagnosis often comes to light in this way. In some people, sensitivity to excess alcohol may be enough to produce diarrhoea. In these acute cases, treatment is seldom required and in fact may do more harm than good since any agent that prevents diarrhoea where there is an infective cause will tend to incubate the germs longer within the bowel, which may in turn have damaging effects. Diarrhoea is nature's way of getting rid of the bugs, and provided the diarrhoea is neither profuse nor bloodstained, the symptom can generally be left to run its own course. In chronic diarrhoea, however, generalized weakness, dehydration and exhaustion can sometimes occur. At best it is a very inconvenient symptom; at worst it may represent the first sign of something more serious going on within the bowel.

To help establish the possible cause of any diarrhoea, ask yourself the following questions:

❶ Did the symptoms begin very suddenly, within hours of eating?

Food poisoning will usually, although not always, lead to the sudden onset of sickness and diarrhoea within hours of eating a contaminated meal. Depending on the bug responsible, this may be within two to three hours, but can sometimes be up to 24 hours later. Associated symptoms generally include intense nausea and vomiting, sometimes with abdominal pain and sweating.

❷ Do other people close to you have the same symptoms?

Gastroenteritis is an infection of the stomach and intestines that commonly produces diarrhoea and vomiting. It is usually caused by certain viruses that are transmitted in much the same way as the bugs that cause the common cold, with the result that large parts of the community may be affected.

❸ Does the diarrhoea alternate with constipation?

These are typical symptoms of irritable bowel syndrome, along with bloating, abdominal, cramp-like pain, wind, and the feeling after evacuating the bowels that the rectum is still not empty. Stools will be passed frequently, will be small in volume, and may be ribbon-like in shape. There is often a history of anxiety and the sufferer may well have had frequent attacks of abdominal pain as a child. The symptoms are often worse first thing in the morning and there may occasionally be mucus on the surface of any motions passed.

❹ Are you taking any medication?

One of the commonest listed side effects of all medications is diarrhoea. Most of us will have experienced diarrhoea at some stage from taking too high a dosage of antibiotics, but sometimes even appropriate doses sufficient to treat the infection for which they have been prescribed can cause looseness of motions, simply because the beneficial bacteria we need in our gut for proper digestion are eradicated along with the harmful bacteria causing the infection. It sometimes takes a few days after completing the course for the beneficial bacteria to reproduce themselves and

32

repopulate the lining of the gut, but generally speaking these diarrhoeal symptoms settle within a few days. However, the list of common medications that can produce diarrhoea is a long one and includes certain antacids used in the treatment of indigestion and heartburn; digitalis and quinidine use to stabilize abnormal heartbeat rhythms; cholesterol-lowering agents; anti-cancer treatments; colchicine, used in the treatment of gout; treatments for raised blood pressure; and anti-diabetic tablets. Laxative abuse and radiotherapy used for bowel cancer may produce diarrhoea due to temporary damage to the lining of the gut.

❷ Is the diarrhoea accompanied by a raised temperature?

Various infections such as dysentery, giardia and salmonella all produce a temporary inflammation of the lining of the gut along with the secretion of increased amounts of fluid, which leaks from the circulation through the wall of the intestine into its hollow cavity, with resulting diarrhoea. Any medical investigation, especially where there is diarrhoea in association with a raised temperature, should include an examination of the motions with a variety of laboratory techniques so that the causative organism or parasite may be identified and treated.

❸ Do the symptoms occur after eating a particular food?

Certain individuals may be intolerant of or allergic to one or more foodstuffs. Common culprits are shellfish and strawberries, but almost anything can, in susceptible people, trigger a reaction. Over the course of time and repeated exposure to the particular foodstuff responsible, it becomes apparent that there is an allergy or intolerance towards it and the individual simply avoids eating that food again.

However, when eating out at restaurants or dinner parties the exact ingredients of any meal are not always obvious, so that the problem remains a potential nuisance.

❹ Do you feel constantly hot and are you losing weight?

The thyroid gland is the body's thermostat, controlling the basic tick-over speed at which it works. In somebody who has an overactive thyroid gland, the heart will beat faster, there will be increased sweating, and the movement of the muscular walls of the intestine will speed up, with resulting diarrhoea. Associated symptoms include an intolerance of hot weather, weight loss, increased appetite and a fast pulse.

❺ Is there any abdominal pain and weight loss?

Chronic inflammatory conditions of the bowel such as Crohn's disease and ulcerative colitis commonly start with the symptom of diarrhoea, in association with abdominal pain and loss of weight, and occasionally pus may be seen mixed with the motions. In contrast to irritable bowl syndrome, the diarrhoea often becomes worse later in the day. These patients require further investigation and special barium X-ray tests. Sigmoidoscopy (the passage of a flexible telescope through the back passage) together with biopsy and microscopic examination of tissue samples will usually achieve a diagnosis. Treatment will then be medical and/or surgical.

❻ Have you had surgery to remove part of your intestine?

Occasionally some patients will require the removal of some part of the length of the intestine to ensure their continued good health. Such surgery may be carried out for inflammatory bowel disease, as in the case of ulcerative colitis and Crohn's disease, for cancer of the bowel itself, or for mechanical problems such as twisting of the gut with a consequent cutting-off of the blood supply. Whatever the reason, the shortening of the length of the intestine may result in a failure to absorb certain foodstuffs adequately, with resulting diarrhoea.

Similarly, in conditions such as coeliac disease, where there is an abnormality of the lining of the small bowel, there will be a degree of malabsorption in association with the common symptom of diarrhoea.

❷ *Are you over the age of 50 and noticing changes in your bowel habits?*

Any person over the age of 50 who complains that his or her bowel habits have changed recently, for example looser, more frequent motions, change in the colour of the motions, or the passage of mucus rectally for more than a week, should be suspected of having a cancer of the bowel until proved otherwise. There may indeed be a far simpler and more benign cause, but in view of the fact that in the Western world cancer of the bowel is third commonest cause of death from cancer, this diagnosis must be ruled out at an early stage, especially since early treatment can be life-saving. Symptoms may also include diarrhoea, with or without blood in the motions, but there may be alternating constipation as well. Abdominal pain is not usually an early feature of the disease and by the time the doctor can feel it as a lump through the abdomen the tumour will already be large.

❷ *Are the motions particularly foul-smelling and greasy?*

The pancreas gland, which lies across the middle part of the upper abdomen, attached to the small intestine, plays an important role in the digestion of certain foods through the action of its enzymes. When these enzymes are altered in some way by problems going on within the pancreas, there will be a failure to digest fat and protein which will then be excreted with the other waste products unchanged. When this happens the motions are greasy, particularly foul-smelling, and will tend to float on the surface of the water in the toilet pan. The stools may also be frothy and pale in colour. These symptoms are highly suggestive of pancreatic disorder and if they last for more than three or four days *should be reported to the doctor urgently* as ongoing problems in the pancreas can potentially be very serious. Common conditions include pancreatitis, an inflammation of the pancreas gland, often the result of chronic heavy drinking, and cancer at the head of the pancreas gland, a disorder more common in men than in women.

❷ *Are you diabetic?*

People with long-standing diabetes may occasionally experience episodic diarrhoea, which may be due to fluctuations in their blood sugar, or indeed to the long-term consequences of their diabetes on the arteries that supply their intestine. More commonly, however, many diabetic products such as chocolates, jam and sweets contain the sugar substitute sorbitol, which can cause diarrhoea when taken in excessive amounts.

SUMMARY
DIARRHOEA

POSSIBLE CAUSE	ACTION
Acute food poisoning	Adequate fluid replacement. Avoid antidiarrhoeals except in extreme cases.
Viral gastroenteritis	Fluid and mineral replacement. Avoid antidiarrhoeals.
Stress and irritable bowel syndrome	Reassurance and explanation together with stress management, and counselling, a high-fibre diet, antispasmodics and exercise. Avoid other medication.
Medication	Avoid laxative abuse. Identify responsible drug and either discontinue or alter dosage.
Infection	Identify responsible bug or parasite and treat accordingly.
Food allergy and intolerance	Identify and then avoid the responsible foodstuff.
Overactive thyroid gland	Medical or surgical correction.
Inflammatory bowel disease	Medical or surgical treatment.
Malabsorption	Dietary modification or enzyme replacement.
Cancer of the bowel	Surgical treatment with or without radiotherapy.
Disorders of the pancreas	Medical or surgical treatment. Enzyme replacement if necessary.
Diabetes	Adequate control of blood sugar and medical or surgical treatment. Avoid overconsumption of sorbitol.

DIFFICULTY SWALLOWING

The mechanism of swallowing is something most of us take for granted and is almost involuntary. As with breathing, we are seldom conscious of the act of swallowing, that is until something goes wrong. Swallowing requires the co-ordinated action of nerve impulses and muscular contraction. It is initiated at the back of the throat in the larynx, and then moves downwards through the oesophagus or gullet to the top of the stomach. When any part of this sequence of events is interrupted the normally smooth swallowing action will be affected.

There are a number of conditions that can make swallowing painful or difficult, most of which are short-lived, trivial and fairly easy to explain. When the throat is particularly sore, or there is a fish bone stuck in the tonsil or first part of the oesophagus, for example, the reason is fairly obvious. But when the problem has no obvious explanation and persists for more than a few days or becomes progressively worse, then it raises the possibility of a number of more serious causes, all of which require urgent investigation. Problems with swallowing should always be taken seriously and brought to the attention of the doctor *as soon as possible*. So, if you are having problems in this area, it is worth asking yourself a few questions that may give you a clue to the underlying cause.

❶ Do you have a very sore throat?
A sore throat, which can be caused by an infection or inflammation, will commonly make swallowing painful.

❷ Is there pain as well as difficulty swallowing?
This usually rules out a nervous complaint and more likely causes are a spasm in the muscles

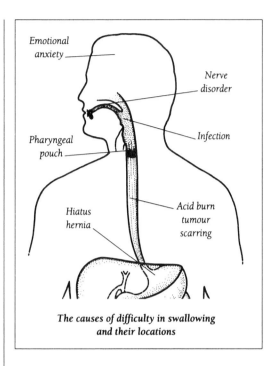

The causes of difficulty in swallowing and their locations

of the oesophagus (gullet), an ulcer, a tear caused through vomiting, or possibly a foreign body such as a fish bone lodged further down the gullet.

❸ Do you find that you can swallow, but experience pain and discomfort soon after?
This suggests an inflammation or obstruction right at the lower end of the oesophagus, such as a hiatus hernia, an ulcer or a tumour.

❹ Does the problem with swallowing, or the feeling that there is constantly a lump in the throat, always come along when you are upset or angry?
This is a common complaint called globus hystericus and is the result of a muscular spasm. It is brought on by anxiety and stress and in this respect is similar to tension headaches. It is particularly common in women.

❷ *Is the problem with swallowing associated with a hoarse voice?*

The vocal cords and the oesophagus lie next to each other, the former transmitting air from the mouth to the lungs, the latter transporting food from the mouth to the stomach. Problems occurring in one structure can therefore affect the other. Possible causes include swollen glands or blood vessels, or a tumour.

❷ *Can you swallow liquids but not solids?*

This suggests an early partial obstruction and compression of the oesophagus as the result of cancer or scarring. *It requires urgent attention.*

❷ *Do you have difficulty swallowing both liquids and solids?*

If it's impossible to swallow either, this raises the possibility of a complete obstruction in the oesophagus suggestive of a tumour, either benign or malignant. *Urgent help is essential.*

❷ *Has the problem with swallowing become progressively worse without let-up?*

All this could be due to an enlarging tumour compressing the oesophagus and *you should therefore see your doctor urgently.*

❷ *Is there any enlargement at the front of the neck?*

Very occasionally an enlarged thyroid gland can obstruct the normal function of the oesophagus as the result of compression.

❷ *Can you swallow solid food but not liquids?*

This doesn't sound like an obstruction in the oesophagus, more of a problem with the nerves controlling the first part of the swallowing reflex at the back of the throat.

❷ *Do you have any weakness or numbness?*

If you have difficulties with walking and talking, a problem with swallowing is more than likely to be related to a stroke, multiple sclerosis or other nervous condition.

❷ *Is there a tendency to painful dead fingers and toes?*

If you suffer from this in even moderately cold weather, and if there is also a tightening-up of the skin over the fingers and toes, the reason could be the auto-immune condition known as schleroderma, which can cause constriction of the oesophagus, resulting in problems with swallowing.

❷ *Can you swallow, but the food comes back later?*

This raises the possibility of a diverticulum, or pouch, in the lining of the oesophagus right at the top. This can trap food, which is then regurgitated.

SUMMARY
DIFFICULTY SWALLOWING

POSSIBLE CAUSE	ACTION
Throat infection or inflammation	Pain relief, saltwater gargles, anaesthetic lozenges, antibiotics if appropriate, removal of foreign body (fish bone).
Problems with the lining of the oesophagus (ulcer, spasm, hiatus hernia, foreign body)	Antiacids, antispasmodics; for hiatus hernia, loss of weight, with or without surgery.
Emotional complaints (globus hystericus)	Reassurance and explanation; counselling and psychotherapy; occasionally medication.
Compression of oesophagus due to glands, tumours or swollen blood vessels	Medical or surgical treatment.
Nervous disorders (stroke, tumour, polio, multiple sclerosis)	Physiotherapy and rehabilitation; surgery for tumour.
Scleroderma	Medical therapy.
Pharyngeal pouch (diverticulum)	Surgery.

EXCESSIVE THIRST

Excessive thirst is quite different from normal thirst. Where there has been increased fluid loss through sweating, perhaps from exertion on a hot summer's day, for example, then we can expect to feel thirsty afterwards. When we have eaten particularly salty food we can also expect to feel thirsty as a result. If we have suffered from an acute gastroenteritis infection with vomiting and diarrhoea we can lose sometimes quite large volumes of fluid and consequently can also expect to need increased amounts of fluid. These are all normal and predictable reasons for feeling thirsty. There are also a number of people who drink far more water than one would normally expect but not because they feel particularly thirsty. They might enjoy drinking for the sake of it, or they may be suffering from cystitis and want to dilute the germs within the bladder and flush the system through. They may be drinking more in order to help them lose weight or because they have kidney stones and are attempting to keep the urine as dilute as possible in order to prevent any further crystallization of the substances that otherwise come out of dissolved solution and form bigger stones. With excessive thirst, however, there is no obvious cause for the thirst, and no deliberate attempt to drink excessively by the individual.

NORMAL FLUID BALANCE

Normally our body constantly balances the fluid we drink with the fluid that we lose. So, if we sweat more or pass more urine, we feel thirsty and we drink more to compensate. This situation is kept in check by a series of hormones, and without them we would become either overloaded with fluid or dehydrated, either of which would within a very short space of time prove fatal. Probably the most important hormone involved is the antidiuretic hormone vasopressin, which controls the amount of fluid excreted by the kidney. A diuretic, as most people know, is something that makes you 'go'. Diuretics increase the quantity of water passed through the kidney. Vasopressin does the opposite and is one of those do-or-die life-saving hormones designed to enable survival in a drought situation. If you were stuck in the middle of the Sahara Desert, for example, with no fluid in your water bottle, vasopressin would stop any further loss of fluid from the kidney so as to preserve as much water as possible in the bloodstream. It is the feeling of thirst that produces more vasopressin in the body, resulting in the conservation of fluid. In the condition known as diabetes inspidis (totally different from the more common type of diabetes known as diabetes mellitus), there is a deficiency of vasopressin, resulting in the passing of copious amounts of urine. It is almost as if the person is on a permanent diuretic treatment. In diabetes insipidis, the sufferer frequently needs to empty his or her bladder, but this is quite different from the frequency experienced by sufferers of cystitis or by men who have an enlarged prostate gland. In both situations, although there is the frequent desire to empty the bladder, little urine is actually passed. In diabetes insipidis, large volumes of urine are passed every time. In certain stages of kidney failure, large amounts of urine will also be passed. In this case, there may be normal amounts of vasopressin in the bloodstream, but the kidney will be unable to respond to it.

In diabetes mellitus, the excessive thirst that sufferers experience is quite different. This kind of diabetes is caused by a relative or complete lack of insulin, the hormone that governs the level of blood sugar in the circulation. Too little insulin means that blood-sugar levels rise dramatically. All this sugar in the bloodstream draws fluid out of the cells in the rest of the body and makes the sufferer feel thirsty. At the same time, the kidney is unable to pass neat sugar through its system without there being large amounts of water to go with it, so that large amounts of sugary urine are passed.

This is why diabetics can have their disorder diagnosed and monitored through the testing of their urine and blood for sugar. In diabetes mellitus there is often an associated loss of weight, especially in the early stages when it is not being treated, as well as an increased susceptibility to infection, particularly in the mouth, on the skin and in the genital area, when blood-sugar levels are too high.

However, there are a number of other causes of excessive thirst that, while less common, are worth considering.

The following questions may help to throw light on the underlying cause:

❶ Has there been an increase in appetite as well as a loss of weight with the increased thirst?
This is highly suggestive of diabetes mellitus. If there have also been crops of boils on the skin or itching around the vagina or at the tip of the penis, this diagnosis is even more likely.

❷ Has the excessive thirst come on gradually?
This would suggest the possibility of diabetes insipidis due to a deficiency of vasopressin, the antidiuretic hormone, and the part of the brain that produces this hormone may be affected by the very slow-growing tumour, usually benign, that causes gradual symptoms.

❸ Has the excessive thirst come on suddenly?
A sudden onset of excessive thirst usually has some kind of psychological cause and is known as compulsive drinking. It is most commonly seen in children who drink out of habit rather than need. As such it is regarded as a form of ritualized obsessional behaviour that requires simple behavioural adjustment more than anything else.

❹ How much urine is being passed?
More than 10 pints a day is a lot and would make your doctor think about kidney disease or diabetes insipidis. Less than that could be in keeping with diabetes mellitus and certainly a simple test for sugar in the urine using a little chemical reagent pad on the end of a strip of plastic could confirm that diagnosis.

❺ Do you pass large amounts of urine even when you stop drinking?
About the only thing that can cause this is diabetes insipidis.

❻ Has there been a problem with your vision or with headaches lately?
These symptoms are commonly associated with a benign tumour of the pituitary gland, which can affect that part of the brain responsible for the production of the antidiuretic hormone.

❼ Has there been any recent paralysis, tingling sensation in the face or limbs or altered behaviour?
A recent stroke or a cancerous spread from diseases elsewhere in the body to the brain may also be responsible for an alteration in drinking habits.

SUMMARY
EXCESSIVE THIRST

POSSIBLE CAUSE	ACTION
Excessive fluid loss	Adequate fluid replacement to restore balance.
Diabetes mellitus	Control elevated blood-sugar levels with diet, oral medication or insulin injections.
Diabetes insipidus	Discover cause of inadequate antidiuretic-hormone production with the help of a neurologist. Exclude kidney failure.
Kidney failure	Medical treatment depending on the cause.
Compulsive thirst (psychological)	Counselling and psychotherapy.
Rare brain disorders (stroke, secondary spread of cancer elsewhere in the body, and benign tumours of the pituitary gland)	Medical evaluation and treatment and/or surgery and radiotherapy.

3
RESPIRATORY PROBLEMS

Breathing is all about supplying the body with oxygen for energy and removing the carbon dioxide formed when that energy is produced. When resting, human beings normally breathe about 12 to 15 times every minute, breathing in about half a litre of air per breath. Approximately quarter of a litre of oxygen enters the body per minute, and about 200 ml of carbon dioxide is exhaled. The driving force making us breathe automatically comes from centres within the brain. These send electrical signals along various nerves to the lungs and the respiratory muscles, which mainly consist of the muscles between the ribs and the diaphragm, the tent-like muscular structure that separates the chest from the abdominal cavity. As we breathe, the lungs and chest wall can be seen to expand and deflate. Breathing is also controlled automatically, becoming faster and deeper according to the levels of carbon dioxide in the blood.

For the respiratory system to work efficiently, air should be able to pass unobstructed through the windpipe and into the tubes in the lungs; oxygen should be absorbed through the very fine membranes of the little air sacs within the lungs and into the blood; and there should be adequate circulation of the aerated blood around the body so that oxygen is taken from the air sacs in the lungs to the various sites of the body that are requiring it.

Any disease process, including infections, trauma, muscular weakness, nervous diseases and circulatory disorders, among others, can impair the proper functioning of the system and lead to any number of respiratory problems.

This chapter looks at the common respiratory problems reported by patients to their doctors.

COUGHING
We have all experienced the eye-watering sensation and explosive coughing that occur when something we eat goes down the wrong way. The wrong way is, of course, downwards through the vocal cords to the larynx, or voice box and into the windpipe. Food should pass down the gullet or oesophagus and into the stomach. We are blessed with a mobile flap of tissue called the epiglottis that acts as a valve to prevent food and drink from taking the wrong turn. The larynx itself is richly endowed with sensitive nerve endings that are easily stimulated by the presence of a foreign body, whether swallowed food or noxious fumes, and these cause the coughing reflex. But coughing can also occur as the result of internal problems. A common result of infections and smoking is the build-up of the normal mucus

produced by the respiratory passageways, the bronchi, and this too can provoke coughing. Normally the glands lining the bronchi produce a small amount of clear mucus that traps tiny particles inhaled during breathing and allows them to be neutralized (rendered harmless) and removed. When the mucus becomes more copious, for example during infections or through chronic irritation from smoking tobacco, it will stimulate reflex coughing, resulting in the expectoration of obvious phlegm.

When a cough persists for more than just a few days, however, it should always be brought to the attention of a doctor. A cough that lasts more than a week suggests that the original infection has passed downwards into the bronchi and potentially into the lungs, causing bronchitis or pneumonia; longer than three weeks, and this raises the possibility of a more serious underlying condition such as asthma or even lung cancer.

To establish the possible cause of a troublesome cough, ask yourself the following questions:

❷ Did the cough start with a runny nose and sore throat?

Cold viruses are passed from person to person through the inhalation of infected droplets. These droplets pass into the atmosphere through coughing and sneezing, the very mechanisms whereby those infected strive to get rid of them. The droplets settle in the membrane lining the nose, mouth and respiratory passageways, setting up an infection that stimulates mucus production. The cough is partly a response to the irritation but also a protective device whereby germs can be neutralized and got rid of.

Happily, most people make their own effective antibodies within seven to ten days, thereby destroying the cold virus.

The cough will generally settle within a few days of the original infection but when it persists, and particularly if the mucus becomes yellowy-green in colour, suggesting a secondary bacterial infection, further medical help should be sought and antibiotics prescribed if necessary.

❷ Do you always spit up a lot of phlegm during the winter?

For chronic bronchitis to be diagnosed, there must be regular bouts of productive coughing with large amounts of phlegm on most days for at least three months every winter for more than one year. These symptoms usually occur in people who smoke, and gradually over the years they will become associated with shortness of breath, wheezing, exercise intolerance and sometimes with blueness of the lips, nose and hands. Antibiotics are required for acute infections on top of the chronic nature of the bronchitis and sufferers are always most strongly encouraged to give up smoking.

❷ Is there a sharp pain behind the breastbone when you cough?

When an infection passes downwards from the nose and throat the result may be tracheitis, where the windpipe or trachea becomes inflamed, or bronchitis, where the main tributaries of the lungs become inflamed.

❷ Do you have a pain in the chest when you cough or take a deep breath?

This suggests pleurisy, where the covering layer of the lung becomes inflamed as the result of infection spreading from within the lung.

❷ Have you lost weight and do you sweat heavily at night?

With tuberculosis, coughing may be associated with profuse sweating at night, severe weight loss and anaemia.

❷ *Do you have a high temperature and are you bringing up lots of greeny-yellow phlegm?*

Long-standing damage to the respiratory passageways caused by serious childhood pneumonia or bronchitis, for example, can lead to scarring of the lung's air passages, a condition known as bronchiectasis. Coughing, the spitting of blood and the production of large quantities of phlegm are all characteristic symptoms. A lung abscess is another possibility worth considering.

❷ *Have you become barrel-chested and constantly out of breath?*

Emphysema occurs when the walls of the little air sacs at the end of each of the lung's air passages are destroyed as a result of chronic cigarette smoking or atmospheric and/or occupational pollution. Significant shortness of breath occurs because the oxygen breathed in is inadequately absorbed into the blood. Sufferers will therefore find that they are a little blue in the face on exertion.

❷ *Is there a persistent dry cough at night (children) or wheezing when breathing out (adults)?*

Many people think of asthma primarily as a condition that causes wheezing. In fact, doctors most commonly see asthma in children in the form of a persistent dry night-time cough. So, any child who repeatedly coughs at night, but who does not appear to have a runny nose, sore throat or other cold symptom, should be considered as having asthma until proved otherwise.

In asthma, there is a reversible constriction of the muscles encircling the walls of the respiratory passages with narrowing of the internal airway. There is usually increased mucus production and inflammation of the tubes too, and the combination of these three

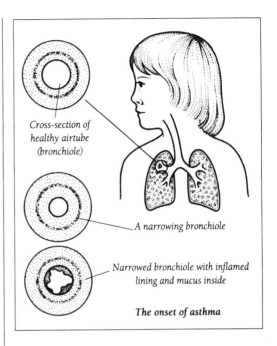

Cross-section of healthy airtube (bronchiole)

A narrowing bronchiole

Narrowed bronchiole with inflamed lining and mucus inside

The onset of asthma

things obstructs the airway, producing a high-pitched noise. This is similar to the reed in a musical instrument, which when blown through produces a noise. Although the cough is usually dry, in severe asthma the sufferer will cough up stringy phlegm, sometimes with tiny pellet-like particles called casts.

❷ *Is there a pain in the chest together with bloodstained phlegm?*

Occasionally a blood clot travelling round the circulation can lodge in the blood vessels of the lung, cutting off the blood supply to part of it. This is common in young women who take the oral contraceptive pill and who also smoke since both of these increase the stickiness of the blood and therefore also its tendency to clot. The death of part of the lung tissue produces a stabbing-type of chest pain with a slight fever and often a cough that may or may not be bloodstained.

Treatment is in the form of anticoagulants and should be carried out urgently.

❸ Are you a smoker who has had a persistent cough for more than 3 weeks?

Any person, but especially a smoker, over the age of 50 who develops a persistent cough with or without bloodstained phlegm *should be investigated for the possibility of lung cancer urgently*. Lung cancer remains one of the biggest killers in our society, although its incidence is decreasing now that the antismoking campaigns of the last few years have begun to take effect. Regrettably, there has nevertheless been an increase in the number of young girls who smoke and this fact will no doubt be reflected in 40 or 50 years by a rise in the number of cases of lung cancer in women. An early symptom of lung cancer is a persistent, irritating cough lasting for more than three weeks that is not cured by antibiotics. There may be no pain or blood in the phlegm until the very late stages of the disease, when weight loss, coughing, jaundice and shortness of breath can be seen, either individually or together. Prevention is the best policy, but early detection through X-rays will at least allow urgent treatment with surgery or radiotherapy, which in many cases can save patients' lives.

❹ Do you have any allergies?

Just as pollen can make you sneeze and detergent can make your skin itch, so dust and other airborne particles can make you cough. Allergic coughs are not at all uncommon and are in fact on the increase as more and more people have central heating in their homes. The resultant dry atmosphere produces a lot of dust and house-dust mite. This creature is present in all households and is responsible for the majority of allergic coughs. Certain forms of asthma are also allergic in origin. To help identify the possible underlying cause, the symptoms can usually be reproduced using skin-prick tests as part of an allergy challenge carried out under supervision by a doctor.

❺ Do you feel as though you can't get enough air into your lungs?

When the heart muscle ceases to pump blood around the body as effectively as it should there will be a build-up in the pressure of blood in the veins leading to the heart, resulting in congestion in the lungs. Fluid then leaks into the air spaces of the lungs, preventing the passage of oxygen into the body and leading to severe breathlessness, especially when lying flat, and a feeling of suffocation. This condition is known as pulmonary oedema and *is a medical emergency* requiring diuretics injected into a vein, which in the majority of cases is dramatically effective. Pulmonary oedema is also seen in valvular conditions of the heart or straight after a heart attack.

SUMMARY
COUGHING

POSSIBLE CAUSE	ACTION
Cold or flu	Symptomatic relief, antibiotics for secondary infection.
Chronic bronchitis	Antibiotics, both short- and long-term.
Other chest infections (tracheitis, pleurisy, tuberculosis, pneumonia, bronchiectasis, lung abscess, emphysema)	Treat with appropriate antibiotics.
Asthma	Anti-allergic preparations; broncho-dilators to stop spasms in the airways; steroids.
Chronic lung disorders	Antibiotics, steroids, oxygen therapy.
Blood clot within the lung	Anticoagulants, oxygen therapy.
Lung cancer	Surgical excision if caught early enough and if location of tumour makes surgery possible. Otherwise, or in addition, radiotherapy and/or chemotherapy.
Allergy	Try to identify and then avoid allergen, antihistamines, steroids.
Heart failure	Control high blood pressure, low salt diet, restricted fluid intake, diuretics, morphine, oxygen therapy, control of any heart-rhythm irregularity.

SHORTNESS OF BREATH

Anybody with unexplained breathlessness should take this symptom seriously as there are a large number of possible causes that need to be investigated.

Nobody who is two or three stone overweight, who smokes heavily and never takes any exercise should be surprised at being short of puff when running for the bus or walking up a three-in-one hill. If, however, there are no obvious causes, for example you suddenly become breathless whilst sitting in a chair watching TV, then this symptom is in much more urgent need of investigation.

The normal breathing process is usually completely automatic. Most of us breathe in and out around 15 times a minute, so to have to concentrate on it would be very time-consuming indeed.

We tend to become conscious of our breathing only when we are gasping for breath during physical activity or if we are particularly anxious or stressed, when hyperventilation can often be a problem. Someone who is hyperventilating will subconsciously or otherwise breathe far too quickly or deeply in a panic to get more air into his or her lungs (something known as air hunger). The result is that the body will get rid of carbon dioxide far too quickly thereby affecting the chemical balance of the blood and causing dizziness, tingling of the hands and feet and sometimes fainting. The condition is easily remedied, however, by asking the person to breathe in and out of a paper bag, which quickly allows carbon dioxide to be built up again in the bloodstream, thus correcting the chemical imbalance. It is the underlying anxiety that needs treatment rather than any respiratory condition.

It may be helpful to understand first how oxygen is transferred to the bloodstream before we look at what can go wrong.

HOW OXYGEN PASSES INTO THE BLOODSTREAM

Basically, we count on the presence of a given amount of oxygen in the air we breathe in. The oxygen is absorbed through the walls of the alveoli, the tiny air sacs found in the lung tissue itself, and is carried around in the bloodstream as part of the haemoglobin molecule in red blood cells. When there is insufficient haemoglobin, for example in conditions such as anaemia or in certain hereditary diseases such as thalassaemia, sickle-cell disease and hereditary spherocytosis, where the red blood cells themselves are faulty, the oxygen-carrying capacity of the blood is impeded. Normally, as the blood circulates around the various tissues of the body the oxygen is released from the red blood cells, thereby allowing the living cells of the body to function.

There are a number of areas in which problems can arise. For example, mountaineers know that the higher they climb, the lower the concentration of oxygen in the surrounding air, which is why they generally have supplementary oxygen supplies. In other cases, oxygen might be unable to reach the lungs because of an obstruction such as a foreign body or a swallowed tongue, leading to acute respiratory difficulties. The lungs themselves may be congested with fluid, as in heart failure, or inflamed due to an infection such as pneumonia. Anaemia effectively thins the blood so that it has less oxygen-carrying capacity. And even if the blood, heart and lungs are functioning normally, there may be situations arising in the body that put extra demands on the supply of oxygen, thereby producing breathlessness. Such conditions include high temperatures, an overactive thyroid gland, severe overweight, the use of drugs such as amphetamines, and even underlying, fast-growing cancers that are greedy for oxygen.

❷ Are you particularly pale at the moment, weak and generally tired?

You could be anaemic. Is your diet sufficient in iron from leafy green vegetables and red meat? Is there a family history of anaemia, such as is caused by hereditary spherocytosis, a condition where the red blood cells are abnormally fragile and cannot last as long as normal red blood cells. If you are anaemic the cause should be quickly identified and the levels of haemoglobin (the molecule in the red blood cell that carries oxygen) corrected as soon as possible.

❷ Do you smoke?

Any smoker can tell you that this habit makes you breathless, and the less you smoke the better. This type of breathlessness may be a short-term effect that can be reversed by giving up smoking and taking up physical activity. Unfortunately, shortness of breath due to chronic lung damage and lung cancer is not reversible and is only sometimes responsive to treatment.

❷ Do you wheeze when you are breathless and do you cough particularly at night?

These are common symptoms of asthma, especially in children. Asthma sufferers are also liable to adopt the characteristic posture of hunched-over body and arms braced against their knees as they struggle to breathe using all the muscles in their neck and chest. Again, there is often a history of asthma in other members of the family.

❷ Are your fingernails particularly convex shaped like the top of an opened umbrella?

This can gradually occur in chronic conditions of the lungs such as emphysema, where the alveoli, the terminal air sacs in the lungs, are dilated and damaged, and also in lung cancer. Additionally, there is often a blue tinge to the lips and fingernail beds in these conditions, as the lungs are unable to transmit adequate oxygen to the bloodstream.

❷ Do you suffer chest pain on exertion? Do you have a heart murmur or high blood pressure?

Anyone with a previous history of valvular heart disease, angina, heart attack or raised blood pressure could experience shortness of breath as a result of circulatory disorders and a failure to pump oxygenated blood adequately around the body. In chronic heart failure or weakness of the heart muscle itself, early symptoms include swollen ankles and breathlessness when lying flat in bed at night, the result of fluid congestion in the lungs when not standing upright.

❷ Do you feel hot all the time, or have you had a recent high temperature?

With high temperatures or in the presence of an overactive thyroid, the tissues of the body will work faster and more furiously than normal and will demand an increased amount of oxygen. The same is true with normal physical exertion, although people who are very overweight can experience breathlessness even at rest. Continual abuse of amphetamines (speed) may have similar effects, as can fast-growing tumours.

❷ Was the onset of shortness of breath sudden, with stabbing pain in the chest?

If so a spontaneous pneumothorax could have occurred, resulting in a collapsed lung. Here air escapes from the lung surface and builds up between the outer wall of the lung and the inner wall of the chest cavity. In time this forces the lung to collapse, oxygen cannot be absorbed and breathlessness occurs.

and breathlessness occurs. A pneumothorax can be small, producing only limited loss of function in the lung, or large and extensive, producing severe shortness of breath and interference with normal heart functioning. In this case, surgical treatment will be required.

❷ Has the breathlessness been preceded by pain and swelling in one of the calf muscles?

A deep-vein thrombosis or blood clot in the veins of the legs can move upwards and become lodged in the lungs. Here it produces a sharp twinge of pain together with shortness of breath and a cough that may produce bloodstained phlegm. This is common in women who take the pill and smoke.

❸ Do you work in a toxic environment?

Not so many years ago, coal miners developed pneumoconiosis, a chronic lung condition caused by the inhalation of huge amounts of coal dust. Other inhaled particles such as asbestos and wool may produce similar lung damage with resultant breathlessness.

SUMMARY
SHORTNESS OF BREATH

POSSIBLE CAUSE	ACTION
Anaemia	Identify cause, medical treatment, correction of anaemia with blood transfusion.
Smoking	Stop.
Asthma	Anti-allergic treatment, broncho-dilators, steroids.
Chronic lung conditions (emphysema, lung cancers)	Identify underlying cause and treat appropriately.
Heart disease	Medical or surgical treatment, diuretics.
Increased oxygen demand (high temparature, overactive thyroid, gland, drug abuse, fast-growing tumour)	Identify underlying problem and treat appropriately.
Foreign body	First-aid measures to remove foreign body with or without recourse to surgery.
Spontaneous pneumothorax	Surgical drainage of trapped air in worst cases.
Blood clot within the lungs	Anticoagulants.
Poor working conditions	Remove hazardous material; medical treatment.

CHRONIC HOARSENESS

Most people will lose their voice at one time or another, and in the vast majority of cases it's a short-lived problem, the result of a mild virus or an allergy. With a few steam inhalations and rest, the symptoms usually improve within a fortnight.

When they don't, however, and especially when the sufferer is over the age of 40 and also smokes, the alarm bell should start to ring as there may be a more serious underlying problem that needs to be identified. As far as doctors are concerned, any person with hoarseness whose symptoms have persisted for more than six weeks has a tumour of the vocal cords until proved otherwise. In fact this rarely turns out to be the case, but it is a policy adopted by conscientious doctors because complacency in this situation can mean the difference between life and death.

❶ Are you a heavy smoker and drinker?
This combination can produce chronic laryngitis with thickening of the vocal cords. The latter is an allergic and inflammatory response to the noxious fumes of the cigarettes and drinking can exacerbate the problem by causing a reflux of strong acid from the stomach that can chemically irritate the voice box still further.

Abstinence from smoking and drinking allows a probable reversal of the symptoms of hoarseness in time.

❷ Have you been overusing your voice?
One of the reasons why hoarseness is particularly common amongst singers, market-stall traders, racing commentators and auctioneers is that these people are always using their voices. Even Pavarotti has to take the occasional rest from opera singing, despite professional voice training having limited the risks to his voice.

❸ Did the hoarseness begin gradually in the absence of a cough or cold?
Any benign or malignant growth on the vocal cords will interfere with the spoken voice. The illustration shows the normal position of the vocal cords when breathing in and during speech. Although they are called cords, they are actually more like curtains that are drawn together for the purposes of speech. 'Singer's nodes' are small, fleshy, wart-like nobbles on the edges of the vocal cords, so-called because they are caused by the kind of overuse commonly seen in professional singers. Polyps are benign growths that can interfere with cord function. Infections such as tuberculosis and malignant infiltrations such as cancer produce similar symptoms. With these last two conditions there may also be swelling of the surrounding lymph glands in the side of the neck, as well as weight loss, fever, and bloodstained phlegm.

❹ Do you feel cold all the time, have a tendency to constipation, and have gained weight?
An underactive thyroid gland usually causes weight gain, intolerance of cold weather, constipation, coarse, thinning hair, and thickening of the skin of the lower leg. However, chronic hoarseness is sometimes also an early sign and anybody with this combination of symptoms should have a simple blood test to confirm the diagnosis.

❺ Did the hoarseness begin suddenly or following a thyroid-gland operation?
The movement of the vocal cords is controlled by the recurrent laryngeal nerve, which runs a tortuous path through the neck and chest. The nerve can be damaged anywhere along its length by a ballooned blood vessel (aneurysm) or a tumour. These possibilities should always be considered in an older patient, especially

onset of hoarseness. Accidental damage may very occasionally occur during thyroid surgery.

❷ Do you work with toxic fumes?

Even small amounts of toxic fumes can cause hoarseness. Mechanics breathing in car-exhaust fumes and workers in the rubber, plastics and smelting industries are most vulnerable.

❷ Do you suffer from severe indigestion?

In conditions of the stomach such as duodenal ulcers, gastritis, and hiatus hernias, there is a tendency for strong stomach acid to reflux upwards towards the larynx, resulting in an irritation of the vocal cords.

❷ Do your eyelid muscles tire quickly, making it hard to keep your eyes open?

In the relatively rare condition known as myasthenia gravis there is a generalized and increasing weakness of the muscles after repeated use. It particularly affects the eyelid muscles, but in severe cases the limbs too. Because of a chemical deficiency between nerve and muscle, the muscles tire very quickly and whilst speaking may be quite normal to begin with, hoarseness soon follows. The condition is treated by increasing or replacing the chemicals that are deficient or missing.

❷ Have you recently suffered a traumatic event?

Very occasionally hoarseness may arise for hysterical reasons following a traumatic event. In this case, there is no underlying physical cause and a normal cough is maintained. Speech therapy is usually effective. Hypnosis, counselling and psychotherapy are also helpful.

SUMMARY
CHRONIC HOARSENESS

POSSIBLE CAUSE	ACTION
Smoking	Give up.
Overuse	Rest; inhalation of anti-inflammatory agents.
Growths	Identify cause. Medical or surgical treatment.
Underactive thyroid	Thyroid-replacement hormone.
Damaged nerve or paralysed vocal cord	Identify cause. Surgical treatment.
Toxic fumes	Make environment safe; inhalation of anti-inflammatory agents.
Acid reflux	Treat underlying intestinal disorder.
Myasthenia gravis	Increase or replace deficient or missing chemical.
Hysterical	Speech therapy, counselling, hypnosis, psychotherapy.

4

ABNORMAL PULSE RATES AND PALPITATIONS

Pulse rates vary all the time. The average pulse rate is 72 beats per minute, but there are many factors that will accelerate or slow down the frequency at which the heart beats. Exercise, anxiety, stress, fright and certain drugs will all speed it up. Sleep, rest, cold temperature and some other drugs will slow it down.

Most of the time we are unaware of the automatic pumping action of the heart. But if the pulse rate is very rapid or very irregular, we experience what is commonly known as palpitations. Palpitations are often described as a fluttering or thumping sensation in the chest. In some cases, faintness and breathlessness may occur. The common and harmless type of palpitations are usually felt whilst resting and are abolished by exercise.

Occasionally, palpitations may bethe result of an underlying heart condition, in which case they may be brought on by exertion and should be regarded with suspicion. Irregular heartbeats, or arrhythmias, are caused by an abnormality in the electrical wiring system within the heart. They too may cause palpitations. When there is any significant irregularity, the normal pumping action of the heart may be affected, causing a reduction of the blood flow through the brain and lungs, leading to faintness, dizziness, blackouts and/or breathlessness.

ABNORMAL PULSE RATES

The pulse is the pressure wave you can feel as the blood is pushed through the body's arteries by the pumping heart. The commonest places to feel your pulse are at the wrist, just at the base of the thumb; at the front and side of the neck over the carotid artery; and at the top of the leg at the groin, over the femoral artery. The pulse gives an indication of the rate at which the heart is beating and of the pressure at which it is beating. Generally speaking, the pulse is best taken with the tips of the fingers rather than with the thumb since the latter is less sensitive and can confuse matters because it has a small pulse of its own. However, whilst the pulse rate can be reliably measured, the character and firmness of the pulse itself are more difficult to interpret. In romantic novels a weak, thready pulse often used to reflect a poor constitution or illness. Similarly, a firm, pounding pulse suggested strength and vitality. In fact, such variables as the thickness of the artery wall and the nature of the surrounding tissues, fat and muscle for example, make an interpretation of the pulse character fairly

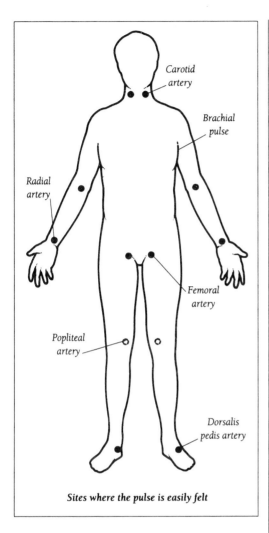

Carotid artery

Brachial pulse

Radial artery

Femoral artery

Popliteal artery

Dorsalis pedis artery

Sites where the pulse is easily felt

to 100–110 beats per minute.

NORMAL VARIATIONS IN PULSE RATES

It is important to remember that pulse rates will vary according to the demands placed upon the circulation of the body. During and after exercise, for example, the rate will increase in order to supply the exercising muscles with more blood and oxygen. After a period of time, and depending on the individual's level of fitness, the pulse rate will gradually slow to normal again. People who enjoy physical activity frequently and vigorously, however, often have a very slow resting pulse rate. Just as their limb muscles develop and enlarge, so does their heart muscle, which as a result becomes better conditioned and more efficient. Consequently, the rate at which it can perform the job of pushing the blood around the body is much slower than it would be in less fit individuals. It is not unheard-of for long-distance runners and other athletes to have normal resting pulses in the low 30s. The pulse will also increase in response to nervous signals and the release of adrenalin-like substances into the bloodstream, for example during times of psychological stress, excitement or emotion. So, outbursts of anger, frustration, elation, sexual stimulation, apprehension, and fear can all increase the frequency of your heartbeat.

A normal individual could push his or her pulse rate up to 150 or so on exercise (the younger you are the higher the figure), followed by a gradual decrease on stopping the exercise to a resting level of 65–85 (the fitter you are the faster the return to your resting level). In superfit individuals the resting pulse may remain at 30–40 beats per minute, rising to 170–180 during exercise. Usually these variations will go unnoticed, but when *symptoms* of palpitations last more than a few

unreliable. More accurate conclusions can be reached by a doctor taking your blood pressure, or listening to your heart.

NORMAL PULSE RATE

Time your pulse for 15 seconds, then multiply the number by four to give your pulse rate per minute. If you counted 20 beats during the 15 seconds, your pulse rate would therefore be 80 beats per minute. A normal pulse rate at rest will be between 65 and 85, although it tends to be higher in children and the elderly, up

If you are worried about a pulse rate that has recently and persistently become either abnormally slow or fast, consult the check list of questions in the appropriate sections below to establish the possible cause.

ABNORMALLY SLOW PULSE

There are a number of acquired medical disorders that can slow the pulse below the expected rate and which as a result may also induce palpitations.

❷ Are you taking any medication?

Anybody already taking the drug digitalis to control an irregular heartbeat – particularly atrial fibrillation, a common disorder in the elderly – may experience a slowing of the heartbeat. For this reason levels of digitalis in the blood should occasionally be monitored by the doctor and the patient should be encouraged to check his or her pulse from time to time to make sure that it isn't dropping below a critical level determined individually by the patient's doctor. Beta-blockers such as Inderal, Tenormin, Corgard, and Sectral, commonly used for a range of disorders including high blood pressure, angina, anxiety, migraine and abnormal rhythms of the heartbeat, will also slow the pulse.

❷ Do you feel constantly cold and have you gained weight?

The thyroid gland acts as the body's thermostat, controlling its basic tick-over speed. Too little thyroxine, the hormone produced by the gland, causes a pulse rate consistently below 60, although in a very fit person the rate could be as slow as 40. In addition to this, somebody with hypothyroidism will tend to gain weight, become constipated, slow down mentally and physically, and notice coarse, thinning hair and dry skin.

❷ Is your pulse rate below 60, even when you exert yourself?

If exertion also makes you feel dizzy and faint, this suggests a heart block. Despite the name, there is no actual blockage of the heart, but the messages transmitted by the electrical wiring system of the heart sometimes fail to get through from their source in the upper chambers of the heart to the lower, more powerful ventricular chambers. As a result, the powerful muscles of the latter will not contract as often as they should in any given minute. Some cases of heart block may be congenital, but it can also be secondary to other disease processes, including hardening of the arteries, immune disorders, and abnormalities of the heart muscle itself.

❷ Have you travelled abroad recently to an area of poor sanitation and hygiene?

Strangely enough, although most infections produce a more rapid pulse rate with the fever, typhoid typically produces a pulse rate slower than would be expected from the height of the temperature. Other symptoms indicating typhoid are headache, drowsiness and aching in the limbs, occasionally with a cough and nose bleeds. Any constipation in the first few days is soon succeeded by diarrhoea and generalized swelling of the abdomen. Antibiotic treatment then becomes necessary.

ABNORMALLY FAST PULSE

❷ Do you drink a lot of tea, coffee and/or cola-type drinks?

Soft drinks, tea and coffee all contain high levels of caffeine, which is a heart stimulant. So much so, in fact, that it is used in neonatal baby units to get premature babies to breathe, and to raise their heart-beat. Anyone drinking more than three or four caffeine-containing drinks, or, for that matter, more than two or three measures of alcohol, daily is quite likely to develop a faster pulse, particularly if he or she smokes, since nicotine enhances the effect.

❷ Are you pale and breathless?
Anaemia is a condition in which the oxygen-carrying capacity of the blood is reduced. Many patients refer to this as a thinning of the blood, and although academics do not like this description, it is a good one. People who are anaemic look very pale and wan, are often short of breath, particularly during and after exertion, and may suffer from angina, since the condition puts more strain on the heart. The pulse rate is also significantly increased. The reason for this is that whilst the blood is carrying less oxygen, the body's tissues still need the same amount of oxygen. The heart therefore tries to make up in quantity what the blood lacks in quality, beating faster and faster to recirculate the oxygen-thin blood more quickly so that more of it goes where it is needed. Once the anaemia is corrected, the heart rate returns to normal.

A deficiency of the B vitamins could also cause you to look pale and feel breathless, but the anaemia would be due to lack of folate or vitamin B12 rather than to lack of iron.

❷ Do you feel constantly hot and are you losing weight despite eating normally?
Just as an underactive thyroid will slow down the body's metabolism, so an overactive gland producing too much thyroxine hormone will increase it, causing a pulse rate of consistently above 100 beats per minute. Associated symptoms include diarrhoea, increased appetite, weight loss, flushed, sweaty skin, and generally high energy levels. Palpitations are also a common symptom.

❷ Do you have a high temperature?
Whilst there are a few exceptions, notably typhoid fever most infections producing a fever will also raise the pulse rate, and the general rule is ten extra heartbeats per minute for every 1°F (0.4°C) rise in the patient's temperature.

❷ Are you diabetic and on insulin?
Low blood sugar, or hypoglycaemia, is usually seen in diabetic patients with too much insulin, perhaps as the result of too high a dosage or of missing a meal. The resulting rapid pulse is associated with sweating and behavioural changes, and collapse and finally coma can follow. Rapid correction by the administration of glucose or glucagon is required.

❷ Are you taking any medication?
Because of their possible side effects, the following medications should only be taken on medical advice by anyone suffering from high blood pressure, heart problems or abnormal heart rhythms:

(i) Drugs used in asthma. Bronchodilator drugs used to relax the airways of asthma sufferers can easily stimulate the heart rate, especially if excessive doses are taken. They are prescribed in the form of tablets, injections, or spray or power inhalations. Drugs included are salbutamol, turbutaline, fenoterol and rimiterol. Other medications commonly used to treat asthma such as adrenaline, isoprenaline, and theophylline derivatives may have the same effect.

(ii) Some drugs used in cough remedies contain phenylpropanolamine, or PPA, designed to open up the air passages when you have the sniffles or a touch of bronchitis. However, just like the asthma remedies, they can produce a fast pulse and palpitations.

(iii) Antispasmodic drugs that relax the smooth muscle of the intestine produce a rapid heartbeat, and include belladonna and hyoscine medications used for conditions such as irritable bowel syndrome and diverticular

disease, as well as for simple indigestion.
(iv) Illegal drugs such as speed and Ecstasy, both of which have a powerful and at times very dangerous effect on the heart rate. Other symptoms of abuse include hyperexcitability, high temperature, dilated pupils, sweating, and heart-rhythm disorders.

❷ Are you going through your menopause?

Most women going through a turbulent menopause will recognize the hot flushes and palpitations that accompany it. These are the result of circulatory changes caused by hormone fluctuations, and may be treated with hormone replacement therapy.

❷ Do you suffer from chest pain or dizziness?

Underlying heart disease is actually a rare cause of palpitations in the great scale of things, however, when other causes have been eliminated, disorders of the heart valves themselves, of the electrical 'wiring' system or heart muscle may be responsible. Usually there are other, more significant symptoms that would alert patient and doctor to the problem, including chest pain and shortness of breath, especially when lying down, as well as dizziness, loss of consciousness and weakness or numbness in the arms or legs.

❷ Have you a cough and a temperature?

In the lungs, pneumonia, with or without pleurisy, or a blood clot in one of the major veins, can produce a fast pulse, often with chest pain, fever and shortness of breath as well. With a blood clot there will also be bloodstained phlegm.

❷ Do you suffer chest pain on exertion?

In someone suffering from angina it is not uncommon for the heart muscle to be starved of blood, resulting in chest pain and an increased pulse rate.

❷ Have you had persistent indigestion and stomach pain recently?

Sudden severe pain in the abdomen followed by collapse, however, can be the first sign of a perforated peptic ulcer in the stomach or duodenum, and would certainly be associated with the general symptoms of shock and a rapid, weak pulse.

❷ Are you suffering from any other medical conditions that you know of?

Various malignancies at certain sites of the body, including liver and kidney disorders, malignancies and inflammation of the covering layers of the heart (pericarditis), can increase the basal metabolic rate of the body and cause a fast pulse often in association with fever, jaundice and weight loss.

SUMMARY
ABNORMAL PULSE RATES

POSSIBLE CAUSE	ACTION
Abnormally slow pulse	Medication. With your doctor identify drug responsible, check blood levels if necessary, alter dosage or discontinue drug.
Underactive thyroid gland	Thyroxine tablets.
Heart block	Medical treatment, possibly with insertion of pacemaker.
Typhoid	Antibiotics.
Abnormally fast pulse	Excess caffeine, nicotine. Cut down.
Anaemia	Iron supplements or transfusion.
Vitamin B deficiency	Vitamin supplementation.
Overactive thyroid	Medical or surgical treatment.
Fever (pneumonia, pleurisy)	Treat underlying infection.
Low blood sugar	Avoid insulin overdosage, correct with glucose or glucagon.
Medication	With your doctor, identify and then discontinue or reduce dosage of drug responsible.
Menopause	Consider hormone replacement therapy.
Heart disease	Medical or surgical treatment.
Blood clot	Anticoagulants, thrombolytic agents.
Angina	Medical or surgical treatment.
Peptic ulcer	Transfusion to correct blood loss. Surgery.
Malignancy	Medical or surgical treatment.

PALPITATIONS

Palpitations are extremely common, and in most instances the problem is short-lived. The person concerned may feel slightly short of breath, sweaty and/or tense. He or she may occasionally experience a twinge of chest pain or a headache. Sometimes dizziness or faintness can accompany the symptoms, but as often as not, they cease as abruptly as they began. Usually the cause turns out to be quite trivial, perhaps a common cold or mild infection, or even an excessive consumption of caffeine, nicotine or alcohol. However, most people are aware of the importance of the normal functioning of the heart, and because palpitations can feel uncomfortable and disturbing, some people can become over-concerned about their significance, causing stress. Unfortunately, adrenaline is a mightily potent chemical that prepares the body for the 'fight or flight' reaction secondary to stress. This is all very well if you find yourself in the middle of a field being chased by a bull. Then you need the adrenaline to get your muscles moving to raise your blood pressure and heartbeat so that you can run as fast as you can. But in somebody who has cardiac neurosis, or, to put it more kindly, is 'a heart listener', the adrenaline merely serves to make the palpitations worse. The electrical wiring system of the heart muscle itself is especially sensitive to adrenaline and similar substances such as caffeine, alcohol and other stimulant drugs, for example, those used to control asthmatic wheezing, and stress and anxiety can raise the pulse from its normal resting level to about 72 beats per minute to way above 150.

Occasionally, however, especially in the case of thyroid disease, palpitations may be the first manifestation of some underlying and treatable medical condition, so if they are recent, severe and/or persistent, they should certainly be brought to the attention of your doctor.

Generally speaking, when the exact cause of the palpitations remains uncertain your doctor will carry out some simple blood tests to exclude thyroid disorders and anaemia, and may well organize an ECG (an electrical recording of the heartbeat) to pinpoint the exact abnormality. Palpitations that tend to come and go abruptly may be further investigated by the use of an ambulatory ECG machine that the sufferer carries about for a period of 24 hours and which he or she may switch on and off when the palpitations arise.

To help establish the cause of your palpitations, ask yourself the following:

❷ *Are you drinking a lot of tea, coffee and/or cola drinks?*
If you are consuming three or four cups of coffee and/or tea, and/or a lot of cola drinks, the caffeine content of all of these will stimulate your heart, causing palpitations.

❷ *Do you smoke?*
Like caffeine, nicotine stimulates the heart, leading to palpitations.

❷ *Do you suffer from stress or anxiety?*
If you are living and/or working under a huge amount of stress or anxiety, this will cause adrenaline-like substances to be released into the bloodstream, leading to palpitations.

❷ *Do you have hot flushes and irregular periods?*
Together with palpitations, these are typical symptoms of the menopause. They are the result of circulatory changes caused by hormone fluctuations and may be treated with hormone replacement therapy.

❷ *Are you pale and breathless?*
In anaemia, the blood's oxygen-carrying capacity is reduced, causing the sufferer to look

pale and feel breathless, especially on exertion. Sufferers may also be vulnerable to angina as the heart beats faster than normal in the attempt to recirculate the oxygen-poor blood more quickly. The heart returns to normal once the anaemia is corrected. Most cases of anaemia are due to a deficiency of iron; however, paleness, breathlessness and palpitations can be caused by vitamin B deficiency.

❸ Have you just eaten a heavy meal?
This can often cause harmless palpitations.

❸ Do you feel hot all the time and have you lost weight?
An overactive thyroid gland commonly causes palpitations along with diarrhoea, a fast pulse rate, increased appetite, weight loss, flushed, sweaty skin and generally high energy levels.

❸ Are you taking any medication?
Medications commonly producing palpitations include drugs used in asthma such as salbutamol and theophylline, and many painkillers and slimming pills.

❸ Are the episodes of palpitations sudden, occurring for no apparent reason?
Paroxysmal tachycardia is especially common in young women. It tends to be abolished by exercise. This is an important sign that there is no underlying heart disease. It usually improves spontaneously.

❸ Do you suffer from chest pain or dizziness?
If all other causes have been eliminated, disorders of the heart valves, of the electrical 'wiring' system or of the heart muscle (heart disease) should be considered. Usually, more significant symptoms will alert doctor and patient to the problem, including chest pain, shortness of breath, especially when lying down, dizziness, blackouts and weakness or numbness in the arms or legs.

SUMMARY
PALPITATIONS

POSSIBLE CAUSE	ACTION
Excess caffeine and/or nicotine	Cut down or stop.
Stress	Reduce stress levels through management courses and exercise.
Menopause	Consider hormone replacement therapy.
Anaemia	Iron supplements, transfusion.
Overactive thyroid gland	Medical or surgical treatment.
Medication (Paroxysmal tachycardia)	If short-lived, no treatment. If frequent and lasting more than a few seconds, anti-arrhythmic drugs.
Heart disease	Medical or surgical treatment.

IRREGULAR HEARTBEATS

Sometimes people may feel a thump or lurch in the chest, and then a disturbingly long pause before the next heartbeat. This may happen with or without the symptom of palpitations. In fact, they are experiencing early heartbeats rather than late ones, and the subsequent pause is merely the heart resting longer between beats to make up for the previous early one. They are not actually dangerous, are rarely a sign of underlying heart disease, and may simply have been induced by fatigue or stimulants in the diet.

❷ Do you very occasionally notice a single, much more obvious heartbeat?

This is an ectopic or extra beat which most people experience from time to time. It is not serious and does not require treatment, except perhaps for a little reassurance, since anything to do with the heart can understandably worry people and anxiety only makes things worse.

❷ Are you drinking a lot of coffee, tea and/or cola drinks? Do you smoke?

All these drinks contain caffeine, which, like nicotine, stimulates the heart, making it beat faster and, occasionally, irregularly.

❷ Are you taking antidepressants or thyroxine tablets?

These medications can make the heart beat faster and, sometimes, irregularly.

❷ Do you suffer chest pain on exertion?

If the arteries supplying the heart muscle become narrowed as the result of a build-up of cholesterol and other fatty deposits, chest pain and irregular heartbeats can be experienced. This is angina. The altered blood flow disrupts the normal functioning of the part of the heart that sends out electrical stimuli, resulting in abnormal heart rhythms.

❷ Have you ever been told that you have a murmur?

Any congenital or acquired valvular disorder of the heart (usually from previous rheumatic disease) can disrupt the normal cardiac rhythm. These valvular abnormalities may only become apparent during routine medical examination with a stethoscope, when a murmur is heard. However, irregular heartbeats may be the first sign of trouble.

SUMMARY
IRREGULAR HEARTBEATS

POSSIBLE CAUSE	ACTION
Simple 'ectopic' beats	Reduce caffeine intake, avoid stress, regular exercise, reassurance.
Too much caffeine and/or nicotine	Cut down or stop.
Angina	Urgent investigation. Drug or surgical treatment.
Valvular heart disease	Medical or surgical correction of underlying cause.

4
PAIN

If I had a penny for every time a patient said to me 'I'd do anything to get rid of this pain,' I'd be a rich man. Generally speaking, doctors will do whatever they can to oblige any patient suffering pain. However, in some respects patients should be grateful for the agony they sometimes suffer. I say this not because I am a sadist, but because, above all other symptoms, pain is the most useful message we can receive from our bodies.

BY TELLING us that something is wrong the unmistakable symptom of pain allows us to do something about it. Let's take the example of a silent heart attack. Most heart attacks, as you probably know, cause fairly severe and crushing chest pain, often radiating through to the back, down the left arm and/or into the tongue. Occasionally, however, a heart attack can occur without there being any pain at all. When this happens, the individual concerned continues his or her normal daily life, and this failure to rest and recover from the heart attack makes the matter far worse, with potentially fatal results.

Also, the development of cancer in various sites in the body, whether in the breasts, colon, prostate, kidneys or lungs, is in most instances free from pain in the early stages, which is one of the main reasons why early detection of cancer does not occur, making the job of the doctors more difficult and the outlook for the patient worse.

So pain is a useful symptom: veterinary surgeons, for example, do not usually give painkillers to animals because unlike us, they need the pain to remind them not to use the affected part of the body.

My advice, therefore, is to listen to your pain and ask yourself what it means.

PAIN THRESHOLDS

There are enormous differences in the way people perceive and experience pain. I once knew a midwife who could guess the cultural origin of a woman giving birth in the delivery room along the corridor of the obstetric unit merely from the scale of the screams and shouts emanating from it.

In some cultures there is no stigma in not being stoical and people make the most alarming noises as soon as pain becomes moderate to severe. In others, people may be much more likely to suffer in silence despite clearly being in intense pain.

However, much of the pain response depends on fear and ignorance on the part of the patient. It has been shown in many studies that failure to understand the cause of the pain, or a fear of its consequences, can lower the pain threshold considerably. Put people in control of their pain relief by allowing them to adjust the dosage of their painkiller or treatment, and they will handle their pain much better.

The ability to be in control of your own pain relief dissipates fear. The psychological component in pain and the reaction to it is, therefore, of vital importance in helping people to deal with it.

THE CHARACTERISTICS OF PAIN

Pain itself can have several different and characteristic features. Therefore simply informing your doctor that you have a pain in the belly, chest or shoulder will tell him or her very little. In order for a diagnosis to be reached, the doctor will first have to understand the particular characteristics of the pain and will ask the following questions:

❷ What is the main site of the pain?

It is not always easy to determine the exact source of your pain. Some parts of the body such as the fingertips contain a large number of nerve endings, making it easy to locate the pain fairly accurately, but others, such as the skin on your back and the soles of your feet, are not so well equipped so that the cause of the problem is harder to pinpoint. Therefore, whilst someone who has been kicked on the shinbone or who has a duodenal ulcer point to the spot and say with confidence that this is where the pain is coming from, it is difficult to do the same where pain in other organs of the belly is concerned.

Sometimes the pain is actually misleading. An acutely inflamed appendix, for example, will initially be felt around the bellybutton, even though the appendix is situated lower down and well to the right. Nevertheless, the main site will give the doctor some indication as to where the pain is coming from, and therefore what the underlying problem might be, allowing him or her to decide how urgently the problem should be treated. Chest and abdominal pains, for example, should always be taken seriously as they can signify critical problems in a major internal organ. Heart attacks and perforated peptic ulcers happen all the time and are potentially fatal, but nobody dies of a pain in the hand or discomfort in the left earlobe.

❷ Where does the pain travel to?

Most of us have at one time or another knocked our 'funny bone' (the area near the elbow where the ulnar nerve is close to the surface of the skin), causing a painful pins-and-needles sensation to shoot along the nerve, down the forearm to the fingertips. This is called 'referred pain'. In the same way, a heart attack with chest pain can cause referred pain down the left arm, into the left hand, or upwards into the tongue and jaw, and/or backwards through to the shoulder blades, whilst a slipped disc in the small of the back can press on the sciatic nerve, causing pain down the back of the leg as far as the foot. Less commonly, but perhaps even more dramatically, blood escaping from an abdominal organ such as a fallopian tube in an ectopic pregnancy, an infected gall bladder, or a perforated stomach ulcer, can irritate the undersurface of the diaphragm, the muscular, tent-like structure that separates the abdomen from the chest, and cause pain in the tip of the shoulder. And as I have already mentioned, an inflamed appendix may start off by causing pain around the bellybutton, but when the inflammation becomes more severe, it tends to move further down and to the right, where acute tenderness can be felt. So, experiencing pain in a certain place doesn't necessarily mean that is where the problem lies. Nevertheless, by asking where the pain travels to, good anatomical clues can be elicited, often allowing an accurate diagnosis to be made.

❷ What kind of pain is it?

Different patients describe pain in different ways. How many times have I heard such expressions as 'It's like being in a vice', 'I've got an iron band around my chest', 'The feeling is tight, heavy, crushing, like a weight'. More superficial type of pain may be referred to as sharp, shooting, or dull, and generally speaking the nature of the pain is actually quite helpful in determining its source. Sharp, shooting pains for example, are often the result of nerve irritation. Dull, achy pains that come and go are often experienced when a deeper structure such as the bowel or heart is affected.

❷ How severe is the pain?

All pain is bad, so how bad is bad? Doctors often ask the patients to describe the pain on a scale of 0–10, 0 representing mild pain, 10 the most excruciating they can imagine. On the whole, pain coming from conditions such as a kidney stone, a perforated stomach ulcer or a broken leg is usually so awful that the person is in agony. Sometimes, however, even serious conditions, including glaucoma (increased pressure in the fluid within the eye) and heart attack may not necessarily cause a great amount of pain. And any injury sustained in the heat of the moment – in a fight or during sporting activity, for example – will often be borne more easily on the playing field than it would if it occurred in the home environment. On the other hand, depression, anxiety or fear can aggravate the severity of pain and make it considerably worse. Sometimes the behaviour of the patient can be of great help. With kidney stones or gall-bladder problems, the patient is often restless, trying to adopt all sorts of different positions in the vain hope of easing the pain. Acute anxiety or hysteria can also exaggerate problems, leading to severe restlessness and groaning, but these can usually be dissipated by engaging the person in conversation and calming them. Severe pain is often associated with vomiting, sweating, an increase in blood pressure, and tremor.

❷ How long does the pain last?

This is important in determining the cause of the problem. For example, pain in the chest from angina tends to disappear within a few minutes of resting, whereas the pain from a heart attack will continue for hours. Similarly, the pain of a stitch in the abdomen or flank is liable to last a minute or two, whereas the pain from irritable bowel syndrome will usually come and go, but last several hours at a time.

❷ How often does the pain come?

Everybody who's ever had a baby knows that the pain comes at regular intervals every few minutes. So does a spasm in the intestine due to obstruction or food poisoning, whereas pain in an inflamed joint is persistent. An inflamed gall bladder with or without stones can produce pain for several hours at a time, clearing up and then returning in anything from a few months to several years.

❷ When does the pain come?

Establishing whether the pain occurs first thing in the morning, in the afternoon, or during the night will help to suggest the underlying cause. For example, migraines can for some individuals be much worse in the mornings, can occur at weekends, or can come on during periods, suggesting a hormonal trigger factor. The pain from a duodenal ulcer classically wakes the patient in the small hours of the morning, and is often relieved by meals. Pain due to bone disease is often worse when the patient is warm in bed.

❷ What makes the pain worse?

For example, if pain behind the breastbone is worse on stooping or bending, the cause is more likely to be a hiatus hernia than a heart attack. If backache is made worse by coughing and sneezing, a slipped disc becomes more likely than osteoarthritis. Pain in the shoulder on raising the arm upwards and out to the side is much more likely to be due to an inflamed tendon than to gall-bladder problems irritating the undersurface of the diaphragm.

❷ What makes the pain better?

Does abdominal pain, for example, improve after taking antacids? If so, an ulcer or inflammation of the lining of the stomach is likely. Are palpitations – the lurching sensation within the chest when heartbeats are missed – made better by exercise? If the answer is yes, the palpitations are probably benign in nature, rather than representing some serious underlying problem.

❷ Are there any associated features with the pain?

Migraines, for example, are often associated with vision problems in one eye and vomiting. Pain from a kidney stone can be accompanied by blood in the urine. Heart attacks may be accompanied by shortness of breath, nausea, sweating and faintness.

All pain should be analysed in relation to these ten cardinal features. By asking yourself these questions first, you will be able to give your doctor information that will be very useful in helping him to help you to find the source of the pain. Let's look at pain coming from the various parts of the body in turn.

HEADACHE

Headaches can represent something fleeting and quite trivial, or be the first sign of some serious underlying disorder. In fact, it is relatively rare for a headache to be caused by anything sinister, whilst the common migrainous or tension-type headaches are experienced by most of us.

Simple, short-lived headaches are usually easily explained. Most of us almost expect a headache when we are tired, hungry, stressed, anxious, worried or dehydrated. Anyone who has driven a long distance, especially at night, or who has sat in front of a VDU for too long will know the headache of eyestrain. A recent

visit to the dentist, an overvigorous work-out in the gym, or a few too many drinks the night before are also trigger factors. When we can readily explain our symptoms, most of us do not worry, and in fact headaches by themselves account for only a small percentage of reasons for visiting a GP. However, when the symptoms become particularly annoying, recurrent or chronic, that is when we take the problem to the doctor.

When people become concerned about the persistence of their headaches, they often worry about a brain tumour, but in fact less than 1 per cent of all severe and persistent headaches are caused by major disease processes, and even these by no means always defy definitive treatment. Paradoxically, the brain itself, that mass of nerve tissue that controls all of human life, is incapable of feeling any pain. The structures within the skull that transmit pain are the coverings lining the brain and spinal cord (the meninges), the blood vessels, and the fibrous partitions separating the different compartments of the brain. Nevertheless, headaches can be the first sign of a serious illness, and any unexplained persistent headache should be brought to the attention of your doctor, especially in the following circumstances:

• The headache is not improved by sleep, but instead produces sleep disturbance
• The headache is paroxysmal, coming and going in violent waves
• The headache is made worse by coughing, sneezing or movements of the head
• The headache is in the temple area and is accompanied by visual disturbances in the eye on the same side
• A migraine headache occurs for the first time after the age of 35

In order to help you and your doctor reach a conclusion about the true origin of your headache, ask yourself the following questions:

❶ Are you suffering from stress or anxiety?

Tension headaches are probably the most common type of all. The pain is usually felt at the back of the head and in the neck, and unlike some headaches is usually on both sides. It can persist for weeks or months, with only short periods of let-up, but the severity of the pain can vary in intensity from day to day. This type of headache does not generally interfere with sleep, and may well be improved by a good night's rest. It may be experienced at any time of day, and is usually described by the patient as crushing, pressing, or like having a tight band round the head. Most people who suffer from this type of headache will admit to having a fair degree of stress and anxiety in their lives, and if they are frank about it, will be able to identify a number of unresolved personal problems. Tension headaches are also often associated with prolonged contraction of the muscles at the back of the head and neck, for example as the result of sitting or sleeping awkwardly or driving. The solution often lies in simple changes to the patient's lifestyle, along with adequate rest and relaxation, aided perhaps by simple massage of the muscles at the back of the neck. Physical manipulation by a physiotherapist, osteopath or chiropractor could also be considered.

❷ Is the headache accompanied by visual disturbances and nausea?

These symptoms are particularly characteristic of migraines. Migraine sufferers will often be aware that an attack is impending. They may feel weary, depressed or short-tempered, and find it difficult to tolerate normal intensities of light and noise. The pain itself, which is usually described as 'throbbing', generally starts above or behind the eyes, and is almost always on one side of the head only, with sufferers finding that it tends to be the same side each time.

There will commonly be visual disturbances consisting of fading or wavering vision accompanied by an arc of flickering brilliance that affects one half of the field of vision. This may develop later into temporary blindness on that side and occasionally even the ability to speak normally can be temporarily affected. Nausea and vomiting may follow. Attacks can occur from 2–3 times a week to 2–3 times in a lifetime and seldom last longer than 4–12 hours. They are often improved by sleep.

Migraines usually begin in adolescence or at least before the age of 30. A family history of migraine is common, as is a tendency to travel-sickness during childhood. Migraines beginning after the age of 35 should be brought to the attention of your doctor *as soon as possible* because more serious disorders need to be excluded.

Attacks are often brought about by certain trigger factors, including stress, physical and mental fatigue, menstruation, fluorescent lights, eyestrain, certain foods such as cheese and chocolate, and alcohol, particularly red wine (the rougher it is, the more likely it is to be a trigger factor). Strangely enough, they often occur the day *after* some stressful event, annoyingly just when you are ready to relax. For this reason the first day of a holiday or the beginning of a weekend may be ruined. The solution lies in establishing and then avoiding the precipitating factors, plus relaxation therapy and the prescription of long-term preventative or short-term therapeutic medications.

❸ Are the headaches short-lived and frequent?

Cluster headaches are a type of migraine that tend to occur more commonly in men, and are so-called because they can occur as frequently as several times a day for some weeks. The pain often begins behind the eyes, comes on very quickly and without warning, and reaches its peak within a few minutes. The good news is that it has often disappeared within the hour. Like a migraine a cluster headache may be triggered by alcohol, but unlike a migraine, it is not necessarily relieved by sleep. In fact, it is not unusual for sufferers to be woken up by one. Cluster headaches subside spontaneously.

❷ Do you have a fever?

Viral and bacterial infections, including the common cold, can cause headaches for a variety of reasons. An elevated temperature, for example, can by itself produce a headache, as can the resulting dehydration. If the toxins produced by the micro-organisms also dilate the blood vessels both within and on the outside of the skull, it can result in the same sort of throbbing headache experienced during a hangover. This vascular type of headache is made worse by shaking the head or by stooping, and in this respect is similar to a migraine.

The solution depends on adequate fluid intake, appropriate treatment of the infection, cooling of the temperature, and if necessary the prescription of antipyretics such as paracetamol.

❷ Have you drunk too much alcohol?

Alcohol-induced headaches are often accompanied by nausea and an upset stomach, and are largely the result of dehydration stretching the sensitive blood vessels coursing over the brain (it is the pulsation of blood through the sensitive blood vessels that produces the throbbing pain), plus the direct effect of the toxins within the alcohol on the blood vessels themselves. Alcohol also tends to reduce the level of glucose circulating in the blood, leading to weakness and lethargy. The solution, therefore, for an established hangover

is to correct the dehydration with adequate fluid intake, and to restore blood glucose levels by eating something rich in starch or carbohydrates.

Mild painkillers can be taken if necessary.

❷ Are you suffering from depression or anxiety?

Depression, anxiety, hunger, stress, fatigue, worry, tension and eyestrain can all contribute to the kind of headache that sufferers usually describe as a band around the head or pressure on top of the head. Constant headaches are commonly associated with true clinical depression, and are often only corrected following appropriate and effective treatment of the underlying depression. Other solutions include the encouragement of a positive attitude, relaxation therapy, psychotherapy, and medications to treat mixed anxiety and depression.

❷ Have you had a heavy cold?

Headaches caused by acute or chronic sinusitis (inflammation of the air spaces within the bony structure of the face) usually begin during or following a cold or flu. The pain will be experienced in the forehead and behind the eyes. There is usually nasal congestion with discharge, and the resulting discomfort, which is aggravated by bending forwards, is often localized to a specific area of the forehead or cheekbones. The discomfort is generally worse in the morning, as drainage of the sinuses is not possible when lying flat in bed, and is exacerbated by vigorous movement of the head, coughing and sneezing, temperature changes in the surrounding environment, drinking and smoking. Treatment consists of antibiotics, but if that fails to clear the problem and there is persisting fluid within the sinuses, surgical drainage of the sinuses will be necessary.

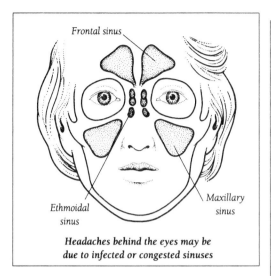

Frontal sinus

Ethmoidal sinus

Maxillary sinus

Headaches behind the eyes may be due to infected or congested sinuses

❷ Is the eye painful to the touch?

In chronic and acute glaucoma, increased pressure of the fluid in the eyeball caused by the buildup of fluid can lead to pain in the eye itself and significant headaches. Measurement of the fluid pressure in the eye (tonometry) can be carried out by a doctor or optician to confirm the diagnosis. Treatment requires the application of eye drops, or, in severe and acute cases, surgery.

❷ Is your neck movement restricted?

Even mild degeneration in the small joints between the neck vertebrae – cervical spondylosis – can produce irritation of the nerves and muscles in this area. The resulting headache often grows worse as the day goes on, and is prominent at the back of the head, the top of the skull and in the neck itself. There is often associated restriction of movement in the neck, a previous history of whiplash injury or neck damage, or tension and discomfort in the neck muscles.

❷ Do you have any problems with your teeth or gums?

Gum disease (gingivitis) and dental decay with abscess formation can produce referred pain experienced by the patient as a headache. Appropriate dental treatment with or without antibiotics is required.

❷ Do you have earache?

Infections of the middle ear (otitis media) and occasionally of the outer ear canal can sometimes produce headaches localized to the side of the problem. Treatment with antibiotics and painkillers is usually satisfactory.

❷ Is the headache accompanied by a sore throat?

Severe tonsillitis, tonsillar abscesses (quinsy) and the very rare cancer of the back of the nose and throat (nasopharyngeal carcinoma) may all occasionally cause headaches. The throat is usually the main source of discomfort, but an associated temperature or referred pain occasionally result in the sufferer complaining of a headache first.

❷ Do you have a throbbing pain in the temple?

One particular type of headache is characteristically localized to the temples, generally on one side of the head only, and occurs mostly in older people. It is caused by temporal arteritis, a chronic inflammation of the arteries in this area, and usually lasts for days or even weeks. Patients often find they can touch the tender spot, and that chewing or talking make the pain worse. If clotting of the blood within the temporal arteries occurs, the sufferer's vision may also be impaired. This symptom is most important because it can represent the first manifestation of an obstruction of the blood flow to the eye, which if left untreated may result in blindness. Temporal arteritis is often accompanied by generalized aches and pains in the body. There may be a temperature and weight loss too. If these symptoms sound familiar, *see your doctor immediately* as a simple blood test followed by a biopsy of the artery can confirm the diagnosis. Urgent treatment with steroids will if used in time prevent blindness in one or both eyes, or, even worse, a stroke.

❸ Have you suffered a head injury?

Superficial injuries to the head can produce headaches simply because the scalp is very tender. Sometimes, however, and especially in the elderly, trivial knocks can cause bleeding beneath the skull, and when this happens blood can gradually collect between the skull and the brain, compressing vital structures. In this case, headaches may be accompanied by drowsiness or confusion. A special X-ray or brain scan can make the diagnosis, allowing curative treatment to be carried out.

❸ Is the headache accompanied by neck stiffness and vomiting?

Any irritation of the membranes covering the brain or spinal cord will produce a persistent, non-throbbing headache that can be severe. Often there is accompanying neck stiffness, nausea with vomiting, and discomfort on looking at bright lights (photophobia). The irritation may be due to the presence of an infection, as in meningitis and encephalitis (inflammation of the brain), or to the presence of blood that has leaked from a blood vessel, either spontaneously through congenital weakness or uncontrolled high blood pressure, or after external trauma. *These symptoms should be reported to a doctor without delay.*

❸ Are you taking any medication?

Although only a few drugs are ever used to treat headaches, there are an enormous number with the potential to produce them. Perhaps the most obvious are the nitrate-type drugs prescribed for angina such as glyceryl trinitrate, isosorbide dinitrate and their analogues. These are designed to dilate the arteries of the heart, but in doing so they also widen the blood vessels in the scalp, causing a sudden, intense, flushing-type headache when the head suddenly feels full and throbs. However, other drugs can also produce headaches in more subtle ways. So, if your headaches began soon after the prescription of any drug, whether an anti-arthritic, an antibiotic, a hormone, an antidepressant, a hypnotic, or whatever, check with your doctor to see if the drug itself could be responsible.

❸ Is the pain dull, worse in the mornings and affected by your posture?

When headaches are particularly persistent and severe, sufferers tend to worry about the possibility of a brain tumour proving responsible. In fact, in the great scale of things, tumours account for very few of the commonly reported persistent headaches. Nevertheless, headaches due to brain tumours have typical features. The pain is dull in nature, poorly localized, non-throbbing, and tends to become more severe with time. It can disturb your sleep, is often worse in the morning, and is exacerbated by exertion, coughing, sneezing, straining, lifting or bending. It may also be accompanied by nausea and vomiting.

A doctor confronted by a patient with these symptoms will try to detect signs of raised pressure within the skull as a result of the tumour simply by looking at the back of the eye with a special torch (an ophthalmoscope) for swelling of the optic-nerve head (papilloedema). Whether or not this is present, if these symptoms persist for more than a few days, the patient should be referred to a neurologist for further investigations.

❷ *Is there throbbing pain at the back of the neck, and is it worse in the mornings?*
The problem could be high blood pressure. Though many patients ask to have their blood pressure checked when they have regular headaches, it is only in the very late stages of drastically neglected high blood pressure that headaches result. Should this be the case, the answer lies in *urgent* reduction of blood pressure through weight loss, diet, and drugs.

SUMMARY
HEADACHE

POSSIBLE CAUSE	ACTION
Tension headache	Lifestyle changes. Rest, relaxation, massage, physiotherapy, osteopathy.
Migraine	Preventative or acute medical treatment.
Cluster headache	Pain relief.
Infection	Antibiotics if appropriate.
Hangover	Fluid replacement, sugar and mineral replacement, starchy foods, pain relief.
Depression or anxiety	Counselling, psychotherapy, medication.
Sinusitis	Antibiotics, antihistamines, surgery.
Glaucoma	Eye drops, possibly surgery.
Cervical spondylosis	Physiotherapy, osteopathy, neck collar, anti-inflammatory medications, surgery.
Dental problems	Dental treatment.
Ear problems	Antibiotics, painkillers.
Throat infection	Antibiotics.
Temporal arteritis	Steroids urgently.
Head injury	Medical or surgical treatment.
Meningial irritation	Appropriate antibiotics.
Medication	With your doctor, identify and then discontinue or reduce dosage of drug.
Brain tumour	Surgery or radiotherapy.
High blood pressure	Medical treatment.

A PAINFUL EYE

I've always been fond of the expression 'It's better than a poke in the eye with a sharp stick'. Few things can be worse, because the surface of the eye is extremely sensitive. The commonest cause is a simple foreign body in the eye, for example an eyelash or a bit of flying grit but there are a range of other problems that can give rise to trouble. The important question that distinguishes the more trivial problems from the more serious is whether there is any disturbance of vision linked with the pain. Visual disturbance can signify a penetrating injury to the eye or inflammation within the internal structure of the eye itself, either of which can, if left untreated, lead to some degree of permanent loss of vision.

❷ Is the eye red and producing a sticky discharge?

This is simple conjunctivitis, which is due either to an infection or to an allergy. Infectious conjunctivitis tends to cause watering, soreness and discharge in the eye and there is marked redness, particularly under the lids. There is blurring of vision when the pusy matter collects over the surface of the eye but this is usually restored by blinking. This type of conjunctivitis often goes hand in hand with colds, especially in children, in whom the condition is extremely contagious. Allergic conjunctivitis, on the other hand, occurs as a reaction to dust, fumes, sprays, make-up, pollen or moulds, in fact to a whole host of possible foreign substances. The eye tends to be extremely itchy and red, and in severe cases there is obvious lumpiness, especially under the lower lid. The greeny-yellow discharge seen in infectious conjunctivitis only occurs if there is a secondary infection. Treatment of the two conditions is quite different, with antibiotics prescribed for infectious conjunctivitis, and

anti-allergic or steroid drops for allergic conjunctivitis.

❷ Is there a distinct lump on or in the eyelid?

A stye is a bacterial infection in the gland that secretes oil to lubricate the eyelashes. When the gland becomes blocked, a red, painful swelling like a small boil occurs, and sometimes these can be quite sizable. There is often an associated inflammation of the eyelid (blepharitis) with lids that are generally red, dry and sore. Rubbing the eyes can spread the infection, enabling another stye to begin. Treatment consists of antibiotic therapy and occasionally, if it is very large, surgical evacuation of the stye under local anaesthetic.

❷ Is there something in your eye or could you have scratched it?

Any foreign material that gets into the eye is liable to cause intense watering and discomfort. The odd wayward eyelash can irritate, but a scratch on the surface of the cornea (the clear, front part of the eye) from a stray branch or stick may cause intense pain. Another injury commonly seen in doctors' surgeries is a fleck of dirt that has been blown into the eye from the road, or a speck of rust that has fallen into the eye of a mechanic working underneath his car. Young mothers are prone to having their eyes scratched by the sharp fingernails of their babies.

The foreign body may scratch the surface of the eye, leading to pain and discomfort for a few hours, or it may lodge on the surface of the eye, causing increasing discomfort every time you blink. Whatever the problem is, a thorough examination of the surface of the eye, including a look underneath the lid, is essential and sometimes the doctor will use a special fluorescent stain called fluorescein to help identify any deeper injury to the eye. Finally, if the foreign body is still stuck or embedded in the eye, local anaesthetic drops can be applied to allow the removal of the foreign body with the help of a fine needle.

❷ Do you suffer from migraines?

The classic migraine produces a one-sided but intense headache with nausea and sometimes vomiting, often preceded by partial blindness in one half of the field of vision and flashing arcs of light known in the medical profession as teichopsia. Migraines may also cause numbness or weakness in one half of the body, resembling a temporary stroke, but the headache itself is often experienced within the eye. The combination of other symptoms in conjunction with the eye pain usually clinches the diagnosis.

❸ Did your eye suddenly become red and painful? Is your vision foggy and do you see haloes around lights at night?

Glaucoma is an increase in the pressure of fluid in the eye itself. It is the commonest treatable cause of blindness in this country and accounts for a very large proportion of all blind registrations. There are two types of glaucoma, the commonest being chronic glaucoma, which has no telltale symptoms such as pain, but a gradual build-up of the fluid pressure produces an ever-decreasing field of vision with multiple blind spots and, after many years, complete tunnel vision. In the other form, known as acute glaucoma, the pressure increase is very sudden and there is severe redness of the eye, tenderness of the eyeball and a serious threat to vision. In the former condition, simple application of drops is usually sufficient to control the problem, but *acute glaucoma usually requires urgent hospitalization* and surgical reduction of the fluid pressure with the help of drugs. Glaucoma is far more commonly seen in people who have close relatives with this condition. These individuals and anybody over the age of 40 should be checked for glaucoma every 2–3 years.

❹ Is there a rash on your face?

The characteristic rash of the shingles virus infection can appear anywhere on the body, including on the face and forehead and around the eye. In this case, however, there may be infection of the surface of the eye itself, which if left untreated may cause permanent scarring with reduction in vision. Consequently, anyone with facial shingles, particularly if it affects the forehead, who also experiences eye pain should consult his or her doctor *immediately*. Antiviral drops and ointment can be very effective.

❺ Do you need glasses or contact lenses?

Occasionally, high degrees of long- or short-sightedness or an irregularity of the surface of the cornea (astigmatism) can lead to eyestrain. This happens when the ciliary muscles that control the shape of the lens within the eye are made to work extra hard as, like any other muscle, they can ache when overused. Correction of the visual problem with contact lenses or glasses will normally remedy the situation.

❻ Is the pain worse when stooping or bending forward?

The problem is probably sinusitis.

The sinuses are a widespread collection of air spaces in the bony structure of the face, most of which surround the eye on three sides. When they become inflamed as the result of an infection or an allergy, referred pain may be felt in the eye itself. The pain is typically worse when stooping or bending forward. Thus a recent cold or flu virus or severe nasal obstruction caused by an allergy are all highly significant if eye pain is experienced on one or both sides.

SUMMARY
A PAINFUL EYE

POSSIBLE CAUSE	ACTION
Conjunctivitis	If infective, antibiotics in drops or ointment. If allergic, decongestant drops, steroid or allergy-preventing drops or ointment.
Stye	Antibiotic ointment. Occasionally, surgical excision.
Foreign body	Removal under local or general anaesthetic.
Migraine	Tablets, injections or suppositories.
Glaucoma	Drops for chronic glaucoma. Urgent medical (drops and tablets) treatment or surgical treatment for acute glaucoma.
Shingles	Antiviral drops and/or ointment.
Eye strain	Glasses or contact lenses from optician. Laser sculpting to reshape the front of the eye may in future become fashionable.
Sinusitis	If infective, antibiotics, surgical drainage if chronic. If allergic, steroid nasal drops or spray.

PAIN IN THE EAR

Pain in the ear has many potential sources, but the patient suffering from this symptom most commonly seen in doctors' surgeries is the child with a streaming cold, a sore throat and a raging earache, usually on one side. In these cases, examination of the eardrum with a special telescope called an auriscope will show a red, inflamed, sometimes bulging eardrum, allowing the diagnosis of ear infection to be made. Sometimes there is no redness or inflammation but the eardrum is shown to be either bulging outwards or pulled inwards, indicating either increased or decreased air pressure in the cavity behind the eardrum known as the middle ear. The cavity is connected to the back of the nose by the Eustachian tube which allows the transmission of air, enabling the air pressures within the middle-ear cavity to equate with atmospheric air pressure. It is the movement of air along this tube that makes our ears pop or click when we take off or land in an aircraft or go through a tunnel on a train. When the Eustachian tube is blocked because of mucus or catarrh, or by enlarged adenoid glands at the back of the throat, the air pressure cannot equalize and the result is pressure on the eardrum. This can cause quite severe pain at times, and no amount of air hostesses' boiled sweets or chewing gum will relieve the discomfort. However, there are a number of other causes of ear pain, so ask yourself the following questions:

❷ *Do you have or have you recently had a cold?*

Nasal congestion, sinusitis, catarrh and enlarged tonsils or adenoids will all block up the Eustachian tube, leading to pressure differences in the middle-ear cavity and eardrum discomfort. This happens often in children, but can also happen in adults.

❷ *Is your hearing temporarily affected?*

Virus and bacterial infections can occur in the middle-ear cavity, causing redness, swelling and inflammation of the eardrum, all of which the doctor will be able to see with an auriscope. Middle-ear infections are particularly common in children, some of whom suffer from recurrent attacks, especially between the ages of two and ten, but antibiotics and pain relief are usually effective. Sometimes, in recurrent infections where there is also recurrent tonsillitis and/or adenoiditis, surgical removal of these glandular structures with the fitting of grommets into the eardrum to drain the contained fluid is performed. Grommets are hollow, dumbbell-shaped devices that allow the collected fluid to drain from the middle-ear cavity to the outside.

❷ *Does it hurt if you pull your ear gently?*

As with any area of the skin, the outer ear canal can be affected by eczema or local infections such as boils. Because the skin in the ear canal is stretched tightly over the bony structure surrounding it, any inflammation can produce intense pain and antibiotics are often required.

❷ *Has your hearing been affected suddenly, following a trauma or loud noise?*

Very loud and very sudden noises, severe middle-ear infections and trauma can all rupture the eardrum. One example is the case of 'yuppy's ear' where the yuppy concerned was so intent on answering his mobile telephone whilst driving his car that he accidentally rammed the aerial into his ear, perforating his eardrum in the process. The condition is intensely painful and although it often repairs itself spontaneously, surgery is sometimes required to fix it.

❷ Are there any dental problems?
Anybody with impacted wisdom teeth may well have experienced pain in the ear before being told by the dentist the real source of the problem. Similarly, teething children seen rubbing their ears on the affected side are suffering from referred ear pain caused by the emerging teeth cutting their gums.

❷ Has there been any recent infection?
When infected or inflamed, the hollow air spaces in the bony structure of the face known as the sinuses can cause referred pain in the ear. When this occurs in the air space in the bone directly behind the ear (mastoiditis), the hearing itself may be threatened, in which case surgical intervention may be required.

❷ Is the pain made worse by opening your mouth wide?
The temporo-mandibular joint is the little joint just in front of the ear, between the skull and the lower jaw, which allows the lower jaw to move up and down. Inflammation here can cause a clicking sensation or even a locked jaw, and can occasionally produce pain felt in the ear. Usually the absence of any other symptoms and signs in the ear itself and the fact that the pain becomes worse when the mouth is opened wide will suggest the real source of the problem.

SUMMARY
PAIN IN THE EAR

POSSIBLE CAUSE	ACTION
Cold	Symptomatic relief with decongestants.
Middle-ear infection	Antibiotics, antihistamines, surgical insertion of grommets in chronic cases.
Outer-ear infection	Antibiotic/steroid combination cream or drops.
Ruptured eardrum	Heals spontaneously, otherwise surgery.
Dental problems	Dental treatment.
Sinusitis	Antibiotics, antihistamines, steroids, decongestants, occasionally surgical drainage.
Inflammation of tempero-mandibular joint	Cortisone injection, hypnotherapy.

PAIN IN THE TONGUE

Soreness or discomfort of the tongue is quite common, but very occasionally more intense pain can be felt as the result of rather less common conditions.

If you are experiencing pain in the tongue, ask yourself the following questions to help determine the underlying cause.

❷ *Has there been any injury?*

Accidental biting of the tongue during eating and chewing, and injuries to the tongue from the teeth sustained during an epileptic fit will obviously give rise to pain. Luckily, the tongue has a tremendous ability to heal itself without infection taking place and usually this is the case. However, any injury will produce some swelling and if you are not careful, this localized enlargement of the tongue can lead to further accidental damage. Saltwater gargles and antiseptic mouthwashes are useful.

❷ *Can you see or feel any ulcers inside the mouth?*

Shallow but tender ulcers on the tongue, gums or inside cheek are often associated with minor viral illness. They may be brought on particularly by stress and anxiety and respond well to local application of iodine-containing lotions or tiny pellets of cortisone held against the ulcer by the tongue.

❷ *Do your dentures fit properly?*

Ill-fitting dentures can irritate the tongue and lead to inflammation. It is always worth checking with your dentist to make sure that your dentures are not the source of your tongue discomfort. Sometimes all that is required to solve the problem is the scaling-down of a rough surface on the denture.

❷ *Do you look pale and feel tired?*

Anaemia, commonly known to the layman as 'thin blood', is well known for causing a smooth, painful tongue (glossitis), and there may also be red cracks at the corner of the lips (angular stomatitis). The good news is that establishing an adequate intake of iron with extra tablets and/or injections soon remedies the problem.

❷ *Are you a heavy smoker?*

There is no doubt that heavy smokers can develop inflammation of the tongue as a result of altered bacterial coating on the tongue together with nicotine staining and build-up of 'fur'. Cutting down or stopping smoking is important and usually does the trick. Antiseptic mouthwashes may speed up recovery.

❷ *Do you have any facial pain as well?*

Any irritation of the nerves (neuralgia) running into the tongue can result in pain in the tongue itself. The pain is usually knife-like and there may be other tell-tale signs of irritation of the nerves elsewhere in the face, such as discomfort when shaving, chewing or talking.

❷ *Are cold sores present?*

Cold sores generally affect the lips and adjacent part of the face, but the characteristic blisters can also be apparent on the surface of the tongue, usually the tip. In severe infections, acyclovir antiviral tablets can be used.

❷ *Is there any associated chest pain?*

If the heart muscle is starved of oxygen because of a blood clot in one of the main arteries supplying the heart, the result will be a heart attack, or angina if the obstruction is only partial. Often the pain of these conditions is referred to sites other than the chest, and pain radiating down the left arm or upwards into the jaw and tongue is common. *The combination of chest and tongue pain therefore requires the urgent attention of a doctor.*

❸ *Are there any painless white patches on the tongue?*

Like cancer elsewhere in the body, cancer of the tongue is commonly not uncomfortable or painful until the late stages. However, if you have a pearly white or grey-coloured lump on the surface of your tongue, and particularly if you are a cigarette or pipe smoker, you should get it checked by a doctor. Needless to say, this is an uncommon condition.

SUMMARY
PAIN IN THE TONGUE

POSSIBLE CAUSE	ACTION
Injury	Self-healing, sometimes stitching.
Aphthous ulcers	Iodine-containing paint. Application of cortisone pellets.
Dentures	Possible adjustment.
Anaemia	Iron supplements or injections.
Smoking	Stop or cut down.
Neuralgia	Identify cause. Painkillers or nerve stabilizers.
Cold sore	Acyclovir tablets if necessary.
Angina	Medical or surgical treatment.
Cancer	Surgical excision, with or without radiotherapy.

PAIN IN THE THROAT

Contrary to popular belief, sore throats are not always due to simple cold infections, and certainly will not always respond to antibiotics. It is therefore worth asking yourself the following questions about your symptoms:

❷ Is your sore throat accompanied by a cold?

The vast majority of throat infections are caused by the viruses responsible for the common cold. When an infection comes in from the outside, the tonsils, which are really just glands on the surface of the back of the throat, enlarge and become tender, leading to the characteristic sore throat of tonsillitis. The infection is mild and self-limiting, with the body's antibodies becoming effective against the virus within five to six days and reaching their peak at ten days. Antibiotics have no effect whatsoever against viruses but are often prescribed at the request of patients, who believe that this will shorten the illness. However, the body's own defence mechanisms can deal with virus infections naturally, and if antibiotics do appear to do the trick, it is simply that the final days of the prescribed course of antibiotics have coincided with the peak in the effectiveness of the antibodies.

Bacterial tonsillitis, on the other hand, is more severe. Often there is a marked collection of white spots on the surface of the tonsils, representing the presence of pus, and there may also be a high temperature and more significant generalized illness. In these cases antibiotics certainly are of benefit but unfortunately the only real way to tell the difference between a viral and a bacterial sore throat is for a doctor to swab the throat with some cotton wool on the end of a long stick and then grow any organisms found in a special culture medium in a hospital laboratory. Because this takes time, the practice

is seldom pursued, the doctor making the decision as to whether or not to prescribe antibiotics on the basis of his or her experience and the statistical chances of the infection being bacterial. There are, however, a special group of patients for whom antibiotics provide necessary extra protection. People with diabetes, heart murmurs, or underlying kidney disease should perhaps be given antibiotics just in case, as infection getting into the body by way of the tonsils can sometimes produce more serious consequences elsewhere. Usually doctors will make it very clear in a patient's records that they should always have antibiotics for throat infections, and the sufferers themselves should certainly be aware of it.

Tonsils tend to be surgically removed in children who have more than half a dozen serious cases of tonsillitis each year, or in whom the enlargement causes obstruction to swallowing or speech difficulties. In recent years, surgical removal of the tonsils (tonsillectomy) seems to have fallen out of favour somewhat, but once again this operation is making a comeback and there is no doubt that carefully selected patients benefit greatly from it.

❷ Has your sore throat persisted much longer than usual?

Glandular fever is caused by a special type of virus known as the Epstein-Barr virus, and produces a more prolonged tonsillitis along with a number of other symptoms. To begin with, there is often an acute sore throat that refuses to settle on its own within a few days, or respond to antibiotics. There is also intense tiredness, muscular weakness and, occasionally enlargement of the spleen and mild jaundice. Particularly common in adolescents, it is not highly contagious and is only transmitted by close contact with other sufferers, hence its other name of the 'kissing disease'. It runs a variable course, often lasting a good 3–4 weeks but not uncommonly causing symptoms of tiredness and exhaustion for up to several months. Antibiotics are not effective, and some such as ampicillin and amoxycillin should definitely be avoided, as they can commonly cause a skin rash when taken during an attack of glandular fever.

❷ *Have you swallowed a fish bone?*
Occasionally, sharp fish bones can lodge at the back of the throat. Removal under adequate light with a special elongated pair of forceps is necessary.

❸ *Is your nose blocked up? Do you have a dry cough?*
I have seen many patients suffering from a dry, painful throat that is made worse by swallowing who turn out to have no infection of any kind when investigated. This type of throat inflammation (pharyngitis) is almost certainly allergic in origin or associated with dry air as a result of modern central heating and dust. It is made worse by nasal congestion and breathing through the mouth when asleep, so paying attention to these factors and a trial of anti-allergic medication are well worthwhile.

❹ *Do you suffer from heartburn as well?*
Acid reflux, or the constant bringing-up of powerful stomach acid as a result of indigestion or wind can produce inflammation at the back of the throat and intense soreness. Treatment of the underlying stomach condition is required. Milk is no longer thought to be terribly effective at reducing stomach acid, but it does at least coat the back of the throat.

SUMMARY
PAIN IN THE THROAT

POSSIBLE CAUSE	ACTION
Tonsillitis	If viral: symptomatic relief only; if bacterial: appropriate antibiotics.
Glandular fever	Rest, symptomatic treatment.
Fish bone	Surgical removal.
Allergy	Avoid causative factors; anti-allergic medication.
Acid reflux	Treat stomach condition.

PAIN IN THE NECK

Patients suffering from aches and pains arising from the neck are not at all uncommon in general practice. The part of the spine that forms the neck – the cervical spine – allows a very wide range of movement, but as a consequence is also very prone to injury. The worst of these is a broken neck, caused by the fracture or dislocation of the delicate vertebrae in this area, with the outside possibility of bruising, severance or compression of the extremely sensitive spinal cord that runs through the middle of the cervical spine. Fortunately, this is relatively rare, but because of the risk of further injury to a damaged neck, no victim should ever be moved until experienced first-aiders or health-care professionals are on the scene. For other possible causes of a painful neck, ask yourself the following questions:

❷ Have you been in an accident, especially in a car?

Whiplash injuries are often sustained in car accidents, particularly when the car is shunted from the rear, although the headrests supplied in more modern cars have helped. Sporting injuries can also be to blame, for example in contact sports, skiing or boxing. Whiplash is caused by a sudden thrusting forwards and then snapping back of the head, and produces intense and sometimes long-standing pain. It is possible that in the heat of the moment no pain is experienced, but the sufferer can wake up the next morning with severe pain, discomfort and limited movement in the muscles of the neck. With any kind of whiplash injury, an X-ray is usually advisable and some kind of surgical collar should be supplied to limit any further irritation to the stretched muscles. In most cases muscle-relaxant medication or anti-inflammatory tablets will be sufficient to tide the patient over the few days for which the

pain lasts. In some instances, however, the pain becomes persistent and chronic, and long-term physiotherapy will also be necessary.

❷ Are the muscles at the back of the neck very tender?

Even without any history of trauma the powerful muscles at the back of the neck can go into a spasm. Sometimes this can be caused by stress, or by sitting at a desk for long periods of time or sleeping with your head in an awkward position. Occasionally, as the result of an awkward movement or from allowing your neck to remain fixed in a certain position, for example falling asleep in front of the TV with your neck unsupported, the nerve supplying those muscles can be nipped between the vertebrae of the neck, causing the muscles to bunch up tightly and painfully. In this basically protective mechanism, the contracted muscles prevent any further movement in the vertebrae, thereby stopping the nerve from being pinched further.

❷ Is moving your neck painful?

People often underestimate just how heavy their head can be. The neck has to take the full brunt of this weight for several decades, so it is little wonder that osteoarthritis, or wear-and-tear arthritis, begins to occur in the neck from the age of about 25. This form of arthritis, which is called cervical spondylosis, leads to further inflammation involving ligaments, muscles and joints, which over the course of time produces bony outgrowths at the edges of the vertebrae. These may be seen on X-ray and as time goes on are increasingly likely to impinge on the nerves emerging from the spinal cord in this area. Pressure on these nerves produces pain (neuralgia), which can radiate along the full length of the nerve into the shoulder, down the arm and into the fingers (brachial neuralgia). Patients with this condition often experience a grating or gristly sound when they move their neck, and are prone to tension headaches or occipital neuralgia headaches felt at the top of the head, sometimes accompanied by a tingling or cold sensation.

❷ Does turning your neck or looking up make you feel dizzy?

Cervical spondylosis as osteoarthritis in the neck is called, is part of the normal aging process and when severe results in restricted movement, dizziness, vertigo, muscle spasms and neck pain. It is common over the age of 65.

Two important arteries run up the side of the cervical spine, supplying the back of the brain, the bit responsible for balance, with blood. Pressure on these arteries from osteo-arthritis in this area can therefore bring on the sensation of dizziness with a resulting lack of balance and sometimes a tendency to fall over, especially when looking up to the ceiling or over the shoulder.

To test for this, make sure you have someone with you, just in case you fall, and then stand with your feet together and your eyes closed. Open your eyes and look up at the ceiling. If you have advanced cervical spondylosis, you will feel quite disorientated and could easily lose your balance.

❸ Are your glands swollen?

Swollen glands anywhere in the body can cause pain and discomfort.

In the neck, the glands are situated either side of the windpipe at the front, and slightly to the side, and are most commonly enlarged secondary to acute tonsillitis, an ear infection or a scalp injury. The glands are particularly painful when they swell quickly, as they do in the above conditions, but may be larger and less tender in the chronic swelling that occurs in more serious disorders of the blood such as leukaemia and lymphoma.

❹ Is there any swelling over the base of your windpipe?

A thyroid swelling (goitre) due to either an under- or an overactive thyroid gland is common and not usually painful. The gland changes size as it attempts to compensate for the amount of thyroid hormone it is producing.

Thyroiditis is an inflammation of the thyroid gland generally caused by an autoimmune phenomenon in which the body produces antibodies to its own thyroid gland. It is not serious, just uncomfortable.

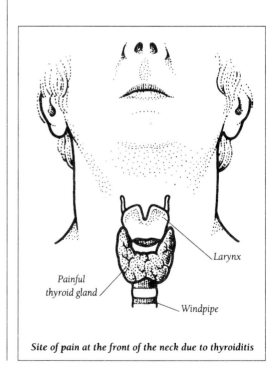

Larynx

Painful thyroid gland

Windpipe

Site of pain at the front of the neck due to thyroiditis

SUMMARY
PAIN IN THE NECK

POSSIBLE CAUSE	ACTION
Whiplash injury	X-ray, neck collar, muscle relaxants, anti-inflammatory tablets.
Muscle spasm	Rest, muscle relaxants, painkillers.
Osteoarthritis (cervical spondylosis)	Physiotherapy, painkillers, anti-inflammatories, heat, manipulation, osteopathy (unless there is associated vertigo).
Swollen glands	Antibiotics for infection, medical treatment for blood disorders.
Thyroiditis	Medical treatment.

PAIN IN THE SHOULDER

Generally speaking, pain in the shoulder will be caused by acute or long-standing injuries that have in some way affected the structures of the shoulder joint, particularly the bone, tendons or muscles. Because the shoulder joint is extremely mobile and allows movement in every plane, it is also more prone to damage. This is why dislocation of the shoulder joint is so common, and why any kind of discomfort in this area can severely limit simple daily activities such as dressing, hair washing, and carrying shopping. Occasionally, however, shoulder pain may be referred from other structures and areas, and it is therefore worth asking yourself the following questions, so that any kind of shoulder pain can be correctly identified:

❶ Has there been any recent injury?

An awkward fall on an outstretched hand, for example, can easily dislocate the shoulder joint, causing immediate and severe pain. The patient will be unable to move the shoulder joint normally, and the arm will usually be held with the elbow flexed and the forearm supported by the other hand. However, the problem could also be that the humerus, the bone at the top of the arm, has been dislocated, coming to rest in front of or behind the socket in which it normally sits.

It's not always easy to tell which of these problems has occurred, so X-rays are always required for the doctor to be able to manipulate the dislocation back into its correct position, and in order to ascertain the likelihood of any damage to surrounding blood vessels or nerves.

Where shoulder injuries are less severe there may be no dislocation, just bruising, stretching and tearing of the muscles and tendons of the shoulder joint, in which case pain and stiffness are the predominant symptoms experienced.

❷ Have you put your shoulder to vigorous and unaccustomed use lately?

This is probably tendinitis, or inflammation of the tendons. A number of important tendons run around the shoulder joint, any one of which can become inflamed through overuse or as the result of a heavy strain. Perhaps the commonest is injury to the supraspinatus tendon, which gives the typical symptom of 'painful arc'. Someone with this problem, standing upright, arms by his or her side, will be able to lift an arm out to the side several degrees before the pain begins. Then, because the inflamed part of the tendon is irritated by the bony contours of the shoulder joint, the pain will increase as the arms are raised further. Once the arm is raised sufficiently high to 'free' the inflamed part, the pain will promptly disappear. Because of the poor blood supply to tendons, the pain and discomfort of tendinitis can persist for weeks or months, and one of the more effective forms of treatment consists of a cortisone injection in or around the specific tendon.

❸ Is there a 'creaking' sensation when you move your shoulder?

This suggests bursitis. Bursa is the medical name given to the little pocket of fluid that enables free and easy movement of tendons and muscles around bones and joints. Occasionally, due to overuse, injury, infection or generalized rheumatic disease such as rheumatoid arthritis, these bursae can become inflamed and swollen so that movement produces pain. Effective treatment consists of eradicating any infection of the bursa, or cortisone injection if the bursitis is purely inflammatory.

❹ Are other joints also affected?

Like most joints, the shoulder joint can be affected by inflammatory forms of arthritis, including rheumatoid arthritis, or, more commonly, by osteoarthritis ('wear-and-tear' arthritis).

Swelling, pain and stiffness are the commonest symptoms, and the shoulder joint must be looked at in conjunction with all the other joints in the body in order to establish whether there is any generalized disorder demanding treatment.

❷ Is moving your shoulder both difficult and painful?

With a frozen shoulder, movement is severely limited and is associated with pain and discomfort. The condition is due to an inflammation of the capsule or covering envelope around the joint, which may occur as the result of a minor injury or overuse, but often for no known reason. Intense physiotherapy and manipulation are required to free it. Occasionally, cortisone injections can be dramatically effective very quickly.

❷ Is there any restriction of movement in the neck?

A slipped disc in the neck region is quite capable of pressing on a nerve emanating from the spinal cord in that area and produce referred pain in the shoulder joint. There are usually enough associated signs and symptoms such as restricted neck movement and pain to absolve the shoulder from blame. Sufferers of a slipped disc in the neck will have full and free movement of the shoulder.

❷ Is there a skin rash over the shoulder?

Shingles can affect any area of the body, including the shoulder, initially causing a burning or itching feeling that develops into severe pain. Usually it is only with the appearance of the characteristic shingles rash

several days later that the diagnosis can be made.

❷ Have there been any symptoms in the chest or abdomen?

Sometimes pain in the shoulder can be referred from distant sites, including from the heart during an angina attack or a full-blown heart attack, when it tends to be felt in the left shoulder.

Pain may also be referred from the surface of the lung in pleurisy, from a blood clot on the lung, heartburn, inflammation of the gall bladder, perforation of a stomach ulcer, an abscess under the diaphragm, inflammation of the 'envelope' surrounding the heart (pericarditis), or a rupture in a major artery in the chest or abdomen. Other rare disorders, including benign and malignant tumours, can also be to blame, but these are only rarely seen. Shoulder pain, however, can sometimes be the first symptom, with other symptoms developing as the problem becomes more severe.

If you experience this combination of symptoms, *you must see a doctor as soon as possible*, if only for your peace of mind, so as to rule out some of the more serious possibilities.

❷ Is there pain anywhere in your arm?

Occasionally, problems in the extremities of the body may be responsible for shoulder pain. Pressure on the nerve in your wrist (carpal tunnel syndrome), 'tennis elbow' (inflammation of the muscle and tendon fibres of the forearm where they attach to the bone in that area, usually the result of unaccustomed overuse), and a trapped nerve at the back of the elbow joint can all cause pain to be referred to the shoulder.

SUMMARY
PAIN IN THE SHOULDER

POSSIBLE CAUSE	ACTION
Injury	Rest, ice initially, heat later, physiotherapy, painkillers or anti-inflammatories.
Tendinitis	Rest, laser treatment, cortisone injections.
Bursitis	Antibiotics if caused by infection; cortisone injection if inflammation.
Arthritis	Physiotherapy, anti-inflammatories, cortisone injection.
Frozen shoulder	Intense physiotherapy, anti-inflammatories, cortisone injection.
Prolapsed disc	Medical or surgical treatment.
Pain from internal organs	Medical treatment as appropriate.
Pain from the extremities (carpal tunnel syndrome, 'tennis elbow', a trapped nerve)	Appropriate medical or surgical treatment for areas concerned.

PAIN IN THE ELBOW

Pain in the elbow joint is most often the result of an injury caused by overuse, for example, 'tennis elbow'. In this condition, excessive use of the forearm muscles attached to the bony protuberance on the outside of the elbow joint leads to chronic inflammation and pain. Tennis can certainly be a cause, but in fact it more often than not affects people who have never played tennis, and other occupations such as using a screwdriver and indulging in a good session of DIY can produce identical symptoms. Tennis elbow is thus a general term used to describe this form of tendinitis. However, because there are a number of other conditions that can cause pain in the elbow, examining the nature of your symptoms will help to establish the underlying problem.

❷ *Have you been overdoing it lately?*
Acute discomfort on the outer part of the elbow joint where the forearm muscles are attached to the lower part of the humerus (the bone in the upper arm) is known as tennis elbow. Only a few fibres of the tendon are affected, but the pain and discomfort experienced is disproportionate to this, and sometimes even carrying a shopping bag or holding a pen is impossible. Golfer's elbow is a similar problem but affects the inner part of the elbow, where different tendons are attached.

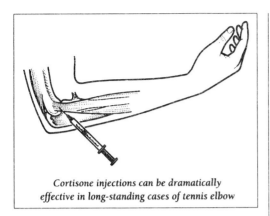

Cortisone injections can be dramatically effective in long-standing cases of tennis elbow

❸ *Are other joints affected and do you feel unwell generally?*

The elbow, like all other joints, can be affected by osteoarthritis (also known as 'wear-and-tear' arthritis), by rheumatoid arthritis, or by acute inflammation, as in rheumatic fever. Only by looking at the joint individually and then comparing it to other joints can the cause be discovered, so it is worth considering any associated symptoms, such as whether or not you feel unwell generally, which might suggest an autoimmune disease such as rheumatoid arthritis; whether or not other parts of the body are affected, suggesting perhaps rheumatoid arthritis, or any other kind of autoimmune or inflammatory disease such as lupus erythematosus or gout; and whether any kind of overuse of the elbow joint has recently occurred, suggesting an acute reaction to unaccustomed exercise for example.

❹ *Is the elbow red, hot, swollen and stiff?*

Infections affecting the elbow joint arise when the skin over the point of the elbow is contaminated by bacteria that migrate under the skin to the fluid-filled pocket (the bursa) and from there into the joint itself. However, very occasionally organisms producing gonorrhoea and tuberculosis can be responsible, and therefore any painful elbow joint with redness and swelling accompanied by temperature should be examined and treated by a doctor.

SUMMARY
PAIN IN THE ELBOW

POSSIBLE CAUSE	ACTION
Tendinitis	*Rest, anti-inflammatory medication, cortisone injection into the tendon sheath, or surgery if extremely persistent and resistant.*
Arthritis	*Identify type. Appropriate medical or surgical treatment.*
Infection	*Identify causative organism. Antibiotic therapy.*

PAINFUL JOINTS

The function of joints is to give the skeleton flexibility and movement. All joints enable at least two different bones to move against another, but clearly some joints are more mobile than others. The shoulder joint is perhaps the most mobile of all, allowing an enormous range of movements in every plane. Being a ball-and-socket joint, it allows forward and backward movement of the arm, movement towards and away from the body, and rotation internally and externally of the arm. However, this also means that it is fairly easy to dislocate. By contrast, the sacroiliac joint between the sacrum, the very base of the spine, and the back of the pelvis is hardly capable of movement at all.

Most of us are only conscious of our joints when they play up or become painful. We take for granted the ability to lift and rotate our shoulders so that we can comb our hair or get dressed in the morning, but when a shoulder joint becomes inflamed, or a knee joint becomes stiff and painful, the consequences can be very harsh indeed.

There are many possible causes of painful joints, but there are a number of questions you can ask yourself that may give some good clues to the diagnosis.

❷ *Have you had any recent injuries?*

Any acute strain or stress to any joint in the body can start up an inflammatory process. Bone ends are usually coated with a layer of cartilage, and this cartilage is bathed in synovial fluid, which is secreted by the synovial membrane lining the capsule that holds the joint together. When a joint is injured or traumatized in any way, whether through nipping the synovial membrane or chipping a piece of bone or cartilage from the surface of the joint, the synovial membrane is irritated and produces a great deal more fluid. This fluid

and the chemicals within it are responsible for the swelling and the resulting pain. Occasionally pain in a joint can occur a day or two after a trivial injury that may not have been noticed at the time. Generally speaking, this kind of swelling tends to resolve spontaneously through internal absorption within a few days.

❷ *Have you sustained any significant injuries in the past?*

Occasionally an acute injury to a joint can render that joint particularly prone to problems in the future. Slipped discs are a typical example, as anybody with a weak back will tell you. Any kind of fracture involving a bone within a joint or dislocation of a joint is also liable to produce secondary arthritis, which may occur weeks or years after the original injury. In the days when a torn knee cartilage was removed by open operation instead of the keyhole surgery favoured today, patients were always warned to expect some degree of arthritis in years to come.

❷ *Are your joints most painful when being used?*

If you have pain in your knees or hips in particular, and if they stiffen up when resting and get more painful during the day, you probably have osteoarthritis, also known as 'wear-and-tear' arthritis. Whilst it's convenient to consider it in this way, rheumatologists know there are other factors at work that need to be borne in mind, including heredity and congenital structural irregularities. Nevertheless, it is still true to say that overuse of and excessive strain on a joint, particularly over a period of many years, will make you far more liable to developing osteoarthritis. That's why boxers often complain of arthritic wrists and hands, and footballers of gammy knees. Weight-bearing joints are particularly severely affected, especially the knees and hips. In fact, hip replacements, and increasingly knee-replacement surgery, account for a very high proportion of orthopaedic operations carried out today.

❷ Do you feel generally unwell?

This is a characteristic symptom of rheumatoid arthritis, a totally different disease from osteoarthritis in that it is not so much a degeneration of the structures within a joint, but a generalized illness affecting the whole body, the joints included. It affects about 3 per cent of the population, and for some reason women, especially young women, more than men. A common way for the symptoms to start would be with symmetrical swelling of both ankles or wrists together with pain and discomfort, often accompanied by a general feeling of tiredness, especially in the morning, weakness and possibly anaemia. Most

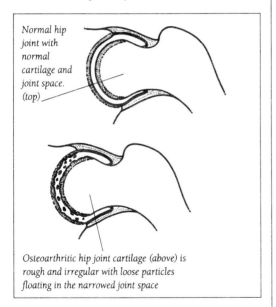

Normal hip joint with normal cartilage and joint space. (top)

Osteoarthritic hip joint cartilage (above) is rough and irregular with loose particles floating in the narrowed joint space

structures in the body can be affected by rheumatoid arthritis, including the eyes, lungs, heart, spleen and bone marrow. It is what we call an autoimmune disease, where, for reasons

as yet unknown to the medical profession, some external factor triggers our own antibodies to recognize certain tissues in our body as foreign. The result is an inflammatory reaction in these issues, and the symptoms outlined above. The disorder is a progressive one and is characterized by a series of relapses and remission. It varies in severity from person to person, but by and large it is one of the most serious forms of arthritis and generally requires frequent GP or hospital care. Treatment involves a combination of physiotherapy, drugs and surgery, although a range of complementary therapies such as acupuncture, exclusion diets and homeopathy have also proved useful.

❸ Do you have a high temperature?

Joints are just as vulnerable to infection as any other part of the body. Occasionally simple cold viruses can produce a temporary swelling of the joints, but two well-known culprits are German measles in an adult and hepatitis. Pains in the smaller joints of the body that flit from one area to another in a person under the age of 20 could well indicate rheumatic fever, and this is often preceded by a nasty bacterial sore throat, which is the initiating factor in the disorder. Bacteria can also find their way into the joints through infections of abnormal heart valves (bacterial endocarditis) in susceptible individuals, or from the outside when a deep boil or abscess penetrates through to a joint. Even gonorrhoea, the sexually transmitted disease better known for its ability to produce a genital discharge, can be carried by the bloodstream to the joints, resulting in a particularly nasty and destructive arthritis if left untreated.

❹ Do you have a painful, red, swollen big-toe joint?

Anybody who has ever had gout, or seen somebody with it, will know that the symptoms are usually pretty unmistakable. A classic case will produce a red-hot throbbing inflammation of the big-toe joint so excruciating that it cannot bear weight or be touched. Usually this is the only joint affected, although occasionally gout occurs in the smaller joints of the body, including the wrists and elbows. It is caused by an acute accumulation in the blood of uric acid, a breakdown product of certain types of protein in the body. Some people seem to make too much uric acid, or are unable to excrete it adequately through the kidneys, and their tendency to develop gout is partly inherited. Having said that, a diet rich in purine-type proteins, for example fish roe and red meat, and heavy alcohol consumption can also precipitate an attack of gout. Treatment consists of either dealing with the very occasional acute attack, or preventing the build-up of uric acid in the bloodstream by daily therapy with tablets.

❷ Do you have a scaly skin rash?
Most people who have heard of psoriasis know it as a skin disorder producing characteristic reddened circles overlain with thick silvery scales. However, in a proportion of sufferers a form of arthritis also develops, resulting in painful joints. The skin rash is usually the giveaway sign, making diagnosis straightforward, but occasionally the skin problems may be restricted to one or two areas of the body, or affect only the fingernails.

❷ Have you badly twisted or injured a joint accidentally?
Bleeding into a joint for any reason, whether it is spontaneous or secondary to trauma, will result in a painful inflammation with swelling and restriction of movement. Evacuation of

the irritant blood from the joint space and treatment of any coagulation defect are essential.

❷ Are you taking any medication?
All drugs have side effects. Amongst the unwanted consequences of drug therapy, the commonest of which are skin rashes, nausea, tummy upset and diarrhoea, are painful joints. Obviously some medications are more likely to do this than others, so it is always worth checking with your doctor if you are taking any form of medication and your joints become painful.

❷ Has there been any genital discharge?
Reiter's syndrome involves three separate components. There is genital discharge, an inflammation in the eyes, which look red and feel uncomfortable, and arthritis. The syndrome occurs in individuals who have a hereditary predisposition to react to the germ that in other people merely produces a nonspecific-urethritis type of infection. The disease is sexually transmitted but tends to run a self-limiting course, clearing up on its own within a matter of weeks after an initial course of antibiotics for the discharge.

❷ Have you noticed any recent changes in your bowel habits?
Joints can be affected by inflammation occurring in the bowel. This is probably an example of an autoimmune disorder, but painful joints may also go hand-in-hand with such conditions as ulcerative colitis and Crohn's disease. So, if there is any alteration in your usual bowel habits, for example recent constipation or diarrhoea, together with joint symptoms, inflammatory bowel arthritis may be the reason.

SUMMARY
PAINFUL JOINTS

POSSIBLE CAUSE	ACTION
New injury	Ice packs, elevation, rest, strapping, anti-inflammatory medicines.
Old injury	Heat, building-up of the muscles on either side of the joint, physiotherapy, sometimes steroid injections into the joint, anti-inflammatory medication.
Osteoarthritis	Heat, exercise, physiotherapy, hydrotherapy, acupuncture, cortisone, anti-inflammatories.
Rheumatoid arthritis	Rest, heat, splinting when the disease is active, cortisone, anti-inflammatories, surgery.
Infection	Antibiotics where appropriate.
Gout	Anti-inflammatory medication for acute attacks, or long-term medication to reduce uric-acid levels in the blood.
Psoriasis	Anti-inflammatory medication.
Bleeding	Treat coagulation defects, or remove blood from within a joint by a needle.
Medication	With your doctor, identify and then discontinue causative drug.
Reiter's syndrome	Antibiotics initially, then reassurance.
Inflammatory bowel disease	Steroids, anti-inflammatories.

PAIN IN THE BREAST

Painful breasts are felt by most women at some time in their lives and for many women the problem is a cyclical one, occurring premenstrually throughout their reproductive life. Generally speaking, this type of discomfort is hormonal and is not associated with any more serious, underlying condition. Contrary to popular belief, cancer of the breast, which most women are afraid of when they notice symptoms in their breasts, seldom manifests itself through pain or discomfort. In fact, doctors will often be able to reassure women who have a single breast lump that is painful and tender that it is most likely to represent a cyst or an area of simple mastitis. On the other hand, a painless breast lump that is firm to the touch and solid-feeling, which tends to be non-mobile and fixed to the deeper tissues, and which may be overlaid by puckered skin resembling orange peel, is highly suggestive of a malignancy and should be investigated by the doctor *as a matter of great urgency*. It is another example of how the absence of pain can lead to delayed diagnosis of a serious underlying disease. So, to help identify the nature of the problem, ask yourself the following questions:

❷ *Does it come on every month, in the few days before a period?*

Premenstrual mastitis, that is breast discomfort with or without generalized lumpiness of the breast tissue, is very common. Some women come to live with it from the start of their periods right through to the menopause. The problem is almost always on both sides and occurs particularly in the week leading up to the period. The fluid retention caused by the increased level of female sex hormones in the blood at this time can also lead to lumpiness and occasional cyst formation that the doctor or the patient herself, may be able to feel. It may be worth avoiding caffeine-containing drinks such as tea, coffee and colas during this stage of the cycle, and some women have reported that taking evening primrose oil or increasing their intake of starchy foods during these few days improves their symptoms.

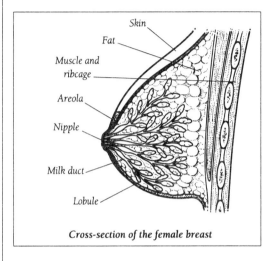

Skin

Fat

Muscle and ribcage

Areola

Nipple

Milk duct

Lobule

Cross-section of the female breast

❷ *Are you pregnant or breast-feeding?*

One of the first symptoms of pregnancy is tingling in the breasts. As pregnancy continues the milk ducts in the breasts develop, and engorgement and congestion of the surrounding tissues can cause discomfort. The same situation applies during breast-feeding and even more so when breast-feeding is avoided as then the breasts can become massively congested and distended until the hormones sort themselves out and decrease in amount again. Supportive bras, the application of heat to the breasts, the expression of milk and the avoidance of infection are of paramount importance.

❸ *Are you taking the contraceptive pill or hormone replacement therapy?*

The additional sex hormones contained in both the contraceptive pill and in hormone replacement therapy are capable of stimulating the breast tissue and producing discomfort.

These are common side effects, which every patient taking them should be made aware of. Generally they settle within a month or two of the medication starting.

❸ Are you taking any other medication?
A number of drugs can produce discomfort in the breast tissue, including digitalis, which is used to correct irregularities of the heartbeat and Aldomet, Inderal and Aldactone, used in the treatment of high blood pressure and heart failure (a weak heart). However, a number of other miscellaneous drugs, including certain long-acting tranquillizers and drugs used in the treatment of cancer of the prostate in men, can also produce breast discomfort.

❸ Are you drinking excessively?
Excess alcohol can damage the liver, leading to a failure to excrete excess oestrogen from the body. In men particularly this can lead to breast stimulation and discomfort, a condition known as gynaecomastia.

❸ Do you jog regularly?
'Jogger's nipple' occurs when the nipple is chafed by a running vest. A small coating of Vaseline is all that is required.

SUMMARY
PAIN IN THE BREAST

POSSIBLE CAUSE	ACTION
Mastitis	Supportive bra, hot baths, painkillers, oil of evening primrose. Avoid caffeine and increase intake of starchy foods.
Pregnancy and lactation	Supportive bra, local heat application, painkillers if necessary. Expression of excess breast milk, or suppression of lactation by medical means if necessary.
Hormonal treatments	Consider other treatment for condition if side effects don't settle within 2–3 months.
Other medications	With your doctor, identify and then discontinue or reduce dosage of drug responsible.
Alcoholism	Abstinence and medical treatment.
Jogger's nipple	Apply Vaseline.

CHEST PAIN

Chest pain usually gives rise to considerable alarm, with most people's main concern being the possibility of a heart attack. In fact, there are a large number of other causes of chest pain that generally speaking are more likely to be the problem, but chest pain should always be regarded as critical until proved otherwise as the price of ignoring even a mild heart attack can be extreme. In particular, anyone with one or more of the following positive risk factors should take the symptom of chest pain very seriously indeed:

• Being over the age of 40 (men) or 50 (women)
• Having high blood pressure
• Having high levels of cholesterol or other fats in the blood
• Having a family history of heart disease
• Being diabetic
• Smoking and taking too little exercise
• Being under high levels of stress or anxiety

A conscientious doctor will always visit a patient with chest pain at any hour of the day or night to exclude the possibility of a heart attack. He or she will know full well that it could turn out to be just another false alarm, but if the diagnosis is proved correct, prompt attention could save a life, especially as coronary heart disease is now the single biggest killer in Britain.

However, there are a number of other important structures within the chest, all of which are supplied by sensitive nerve endings, and all of which are therefore capable of transmitting the sensation of pain. On either side of the heart are the lungs, and behind it, running down the middle of the chest and through the muscular, tent-like structure of the diaphragm into the stomach is the gullet or oesophagus. The rib-cage, bones, muscles and nerves can also be responsible for chest pain, whilst less frequent causes are the gall bladder

(actually lying within the abdomen, but quite capable of producing referred pain into the chest) and arthritis in the vertebrae of the spine.

❷ Is the pain severe, associated with nausea and breathlessness?

Heart attack is the most significant cause of chest pain and the one that always needs to be ruled out. Strangely enough, a heart attack is not always described as painful. In fact, it's quite possible to suffer a heart attack with no pain whatsoever, in which case doctors describe it as a 'silent myocardial infarction'. Usually, however, the sufferer complains of severe pressure on or behind the breastbone, or a tight band around the chest. The pain is often associated with shortness of breath, sweating and palpitations. There may be nausea, vomiting, faintness and dizziness. The pain is usually in the middle, below the breastbone, and often radiates through to the back, up to the neck and ears, into the jaw and tongue, into the shoulders and down the arms, most commonly on the left side. Most patients look and feel ghastly. In the majority of cases they are obviously seriously unwell, and anybody with these symptoms over the age of 40 should contact his or her doctor urgently.

Generally speaking, women suffer heart attacks later in life than men. It is rare for a woman to have a heart attack before she goes through the menopause, a time when the protective female sex hormone oestrogen begins to decline in the bloodstream. Exceptions to the rule include younger women who smoke, who take the oral contraceptive pill, who are diabetic, who have high blood pressure, who have raised cholesterol levels, or who have had a hysterectomy with simultaneous removal of the ovaries anytime before their expected natural menopause. Men who smoke, take too little exercise, have raised blood pressure, high cholesterol levels, and family history of heart disease are equally vulnerable to heart attack.

❷ Does the pain come on during exertion of any kind?

The pain of angina is similar to that of a heart attack, and going on the symptoms alone, it can sometimes be impossible to distinguish the two. In angina, the pain is caused by a partial obstruction in the blood vessels that supply the heart muscle with oxygen, the result of a gradual 'furring up' with fatty deposits and cholesterol. Just as a muscle in your leg will start to ache when you walk up a hill because it isn't getting enough oxygen, so the heart muscle will ache when hardening of the arteries occurs, blocking the oxygen supply. This is because emotion, stress and anxiety as well as exercise all raise the pulse rate and blood pressure, making the heart muscle work harder. Because the heart is working harder, it needs more oxygen, but the supply is restricted, and so the crushing, pressing pain occurs. The pain is often alleviated when physical activity ceases. It may be accompanied by shortness of breath and weakness, and typically occurs after a meal in cold weather. The pain may last from just a few minutes up to 30 to 40 minutes, and the longer it lasts, the more difficult it is to distinguish it from a heart attack. Angina is a symptom of significant and serious heart disease. It may precede a heart attack and can be regarded as a sign that preventative treatment against a heart attack is required. *Anybody with this type of chest pain should seek medical attention urgently.* Glyceryl trinitrate, which can be dissolved under the tongue, swallowed, or taken in the form of a special skin patch, can rapidly alleviate the pain of angina, and therefore represents an extremely good therapeutic test for this diagnosis.

❷ Do you suffer from indigestion?

Heartburn, as I think everybody knows, is actually nothing to do with the heart at all, but has gained its name because the discomfort of indigestion is felt in the chest. Stomach acid regurgitates up from the stomach into the gullet, where it burns the sensitive lining and produces pain. There is not always a clear-out association between heartburn and meals, and the symptoms may be slow to respond to the usual treatment with antacids. As a result heartburn is sometimes difficult to distinguish from angina or a heart attack, and many a patient has been admitted to a hospital's coronary care unit for investigation only to be returned home a day or two later with the all-clear on the heart and a bottleful of antacid.

❷ Has there been any recent viral illness or general fatigue?

The heart itself is wrapped up in a special thin membrane called the pericardium. If this becomes inflamed, irritated or infected, and the commonest cause would be a viral infection, chest pain can result. The quality of the pain is similar to that of angina, except that it may be made worse by taking a deep breath. Whilst symptoms and an examination will suggest the cause, diagnosis will be confirmed by an ECG tracing, a mechanical recording of the electrical activity of the heart. Pericarditis sometimes results from a heart attack, and in very rare incidences may develop in association with auto-immune disorders or from malignancy.

❷ Is the pain sudden and excruciating and is the sufferer over 60 years of age?

This suggests an aneurysm, a rare condition mainly seen in patients over the age of 60. *Chest pain arising from this disorder is an acute medical emergency.* Aneurysms occur when the major arteries emanating from the heart become diseased. Ballooning of the artery occurs together with hardening of the artery walls and clot formation, and as time goes on the brittle artery walls can begin to split. Normally, as the heart beats, blood is pumped in pressure waves through the arteries. In an aneurysm, however, where there is a split in the artery-wall lining, these waves of pressure open the split further, causing severe, knife-like pain. Often the pain is also or only felt in the back, either between the shoulder blades or in the lumbar area, and emergency surgery is necessary.

❷ Is there a cough, wheeze or fever?

Pneumonia itself may make a patient cough, feel short of breath, feverish and weak, but when the covering surface of the lung becomes inflamed, pain may result as well. Both lungs are covered by a double-layered envelope of membrane that has a rich supply of nerve endings. These membranes are called the pleura, and when inflamed, infected or irritated pleurisy results. Pleuritic pain is easily identifiable and occurs on deep breathing, and is particularly bad when sneezing or coughing. Pneumonia and pleurisy often go hand in hand.

❸ Are you a smoker and/or are you on the contraceptive pill?

If so, and you experience chest pain, *a pulmonary embolus should be considered urgently*. This is a blood clot in one of the major blood vessels within the lungs. Where there is a complete obstruction of the blood vessel, tissue death in the area of the lung supplied by the artery will occur, causing sudden chest pain, perhaps with blood being coughed up. In severe cases, severe shortness of breath, clinical shock and sometimes death may result. There are a number of predisposing factors, particularly for women, that ought to be borne in mind. These include any kind of

inflammation of the veins in the leg due to varicosities or injury, and prolonged bedrest where there is stagnation of the blood flow through the veins in the legs, especially following operations in the pelvic area. Women who smoke and take the pill already have an increased risk of blood clotting, and are more vulnerable. Once a blood clot has formed it can travel through the system to the blood vessels of the lungs.

❹ Is there significant breathlessness with sharp chest pain?

This suggests a pneumothorax, a condition where the surface of the lung bursts open through a weak area, allowing air to escape into the surrounding space between the lung and the chest wall. The lung tissue collapses and pain, usually of a sharp, sudden nature, is experienced. Pneumothorax can happen spontaneously in otherwise healthy individuals through a little blister on the surface of the lung, or it can occur when there has been asthma or bronchitis with emphysema. Occasionally the cause is more obvious, for example where the lung is punctured by a fractured rib.

❺ Are the ribs very tender to touch?

Any movement, however minor, including coughing, bending and twisting, can cause severe pain as the broken bone ends of a cracked or fractured rib rub together and irritate the nerve. Fractures can even occur quite spontaneously in conditions such as osteoporosis or malignancy. In osteoporosis (brittle-bone disease) the bones become less solid and therefore much more fragile. The process occurs very gradually from the age of 35, particularly in women, with women who have had an early menopause, who cannot take physical exercise, or who are tall and thin being especially prone. Very occasionally certain conditions can spread to the bones of the rib-cage, allowing spontaneous fracture and/or pain to occur. The types of cancer most likely to do this are prostate, breast, lungs, stomach and liver cancers. Bone scans are used when the source of the pain is not obvious.

Pain from the ribcage can be the result of a viral infection of the intercostal muscles (the muscles between the ribs), or of an inflam-mation of the little joints between the front ribs and the breastbone. Pain caused by these conditions will be reduced by direct pressure from the fingers over the affected joints.

Shingles, a virus infection that gets into the nerves after chickenpox and lies dormant for many years, can often produce an intense, sharp, pain around one side of the chest before the characteristic clusters of blisters appear.

SUMMARY
CHEST PAIN

POSSIBLE CAUSE	ACTION
Heart attack	Admission to hospital. Cardiac monitoring. Medical treatment.
Angina	Weight loss. Stop smoking. Supervised exercises. Medical treatment. Surgery.
Heartburn	Dietary modification, antacids.
Pericarditis	Medical or surgical treatment for underlying cause.
Aneurysm	Emergency surgical treatment.
Pneumonia or pleurisy	Antibiotics and pain relief.
Pulmonary embolus	Medical treatment with anticoagulants.
Pneumothorax	If small, bedrest; if large, surgical drainage of chest.
Fractured rib	If fractured through injury, rest. If fractured through osteoporosis, exercises calcium, vitamin D, fluoride, HRT and other medical treatment. If fractured secondary to malignancy, radiotherapy.
Viral infection of rib muscles	Rest, pain relief.
Shingles	Acyclovir antiviral cream or tablets.
Heartburn	Antacids, dietary modification.

BACK PAIN

Back problems today have reached almost epidemic proportions. There are very few people who can honestly say they have never experienced back pain, and most people will experience it at some time or another during their life. It is the commonest reason for taking time off work, and millions of days are lost to industry every year as a result. The cost in human terms of the pain, misery and suffering that accompany back problems is mirrored only by the enormous cost to the NHS of trying to put such people back on their feet.

Many doctors simply attribute the reason for all these problems to a basic design fault in the human spine, arguing that we were really designed to walk on all fours as our ancestors did, and that the make-up of our vertebrae is such that the ravages of gravity and upright posture will inevitably take their toll. The answer is far from being so simple. People who are aware of the importance of good posture and of maintaining strong and healthy back muscles have certainly proved that it is possible to have a trouble-free existence. Unfortunately, however, very few of us ever put our back muscles to their proper use, which is, of course, to support the spine. Despite recent technological advances, furniture and office designers have still not ironed out all the problems associated with sitting at desks for long periods of time, whilst even the more physically active are at risk because they rarely learn the correct and safe lifting techniques. As a consequence heavy and awkward objects are lifted and carried with a bent back and straight legs, thus putting enormous strain on the vertebrae and the cartilage discs between them. It is little wonder that back pain is so common.

THE ANATOMY OF THE SPINE

The spine consists of a stack of roughly cylindrical bones called vertebrae and the disc-like cartilages between them. It runs from the base of the skull down to the pelvis, supports the head and trunk, and allows a good degree of mobility. Depending on the part of the spine in question, there will be more or less movement, with more rotation and forward flexion in the neck than in the lower lumbar spine, for example, but more stability and strength in the latter regions. Along most of its length it encloses and protects the spinal cord, which is formed by a bundle of nerves that transmit messages from the brain to the various parts of the body through the individual nerve roots that emerge on each side between the vertebrae. The spine is also responsible for the production of blood cells in its bone marrow.

SOURCES OF PAIN

Back pain can come from any of the structures in or around the spine, which makes precise diagnosis extremely difficult for patient and doctor alike. Not only that, but pain arising from inflammation in one area can be transmitted along a nerve to an entirely different area, so that the actual site of the pain can be extremely misleading. A good example of this is sciatica. Typical sciatica is caused by pressure on the sciatic nerve, which is formed by several nerve roots merging outside the spinal column to run down the back of the leg, allowing movement and also transmitting sensation from the limb. It is extremely common in association with back problems, but the affected individual may in fact only complain to the doctor of a sharp, knife-like pain or burning sensation down the back of the leg and into the bottom of the foot. In this case, sciatica can be the only sign that there is a spinal problem. This is a good example of 'referred pain' – pain experienced away from the site of the real problem – and highlights just how problematical it can be to locate the precise source of back trouble.

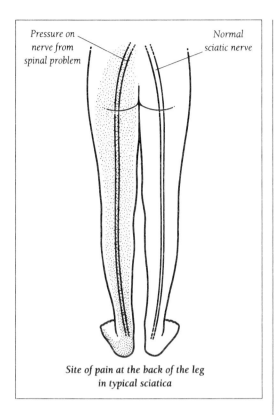

Pressure on nerve from spinal problem

Normal sciatic nerve

Site of pain at the back of the leg in typical sciatica

BASIC CAUSES OF BACKACHE

Eighty-five per cent of all back pain is the result of injury, inflammation or arthritis in the various structures that make up the spine. A further 10 per cent of problems are due to a true 'slipped disc', or prolapsed intervertebral disc (PID), resulting from damage to the cartilaginous disc between the vertebrae. The gelatinous centre of the spongy ring of cartilage that forms the disc is pushed backwards against the spinal cord itself, or the nerves emerging from it, and is usually caused by bad lifting technique or by a sudden awkward movement.

A very small proportion of back pain will represent a serious disease occurring elsewhere in the body. Rheumatoid arthritis and cancer spreading from other sites such as the breast or prostate can erode vertebral bone and cause

severe, boring pain to be felt in the back area.

Occasionally, people will experience back pain that turns out not to be connected to the spine at all, for example with some gynaecological and kidney problems. Back pain, because it is so common and often tedious for the doctor to sort out, is often poorly investigated and treated. However, with thorough examination, a precise diagnosis can be reached and appropriate therapy instigated. Despite popular belief, X-rays are rarely very useful, as soft-tissue injuries – the majority of all back problems – are not shown up on X-ray films. A special X-ray that uses a radiopaque dye injected into the space around the spinal cord is more useful, as are magnetic nuclear resonance scans and diagnostic epidural anaesthetics.

An epidural involves a combination of local anaesthetic and an anti-inflammatory substance being injected through a fine needle into the space surrounding the inflamed nerves in the back. Because it is sometimes difficult to pinpoint the cause of back pain, the epidural can be used to diagnose as well as to treat. Thus, generally speaking, pain relief following this procedure favours the diagnosis of pressure on nerves from a slipped disc rather than inflammation of the joints between the vertebrae. Treatment of the latter consists purely of pain relief or muscle-relaxant tablets, although various forms of physiotherapy, including ultrasound treatment, exercises and traction, are very valuable. Supportive corsets can help, and the increasing use of acupuncture may also provide clinical benefits. In fact, the world of alternative medicine can offer useful additional remedies, in particular osteopathy, chiropractic and shiatsu massage.

❷ *Did the pain come on suddenly?*

Acute back pain brought on by lifting a heavy object or by twisting awkwardly is generally the result of trauma to the structures in or around the spine itself. Muscles may be torn or strained, a disc may prolapse and press on the nerves, or the nerve may be stretched over a bony outgrowth where there is wear-and-tear arthritis. Similarly an underlying weakness in the bone due to osteoporosis (brittle-bone disease) or secondary cancer that has spread to the vertebrae from elsewhere can also cause problems following sudden movement.

❷ Is the pain long-standing?
Regrettably, most back pain is long-standing. Although muscles tend to heal fairly quickly, ligaments and inflamed joints, both of which

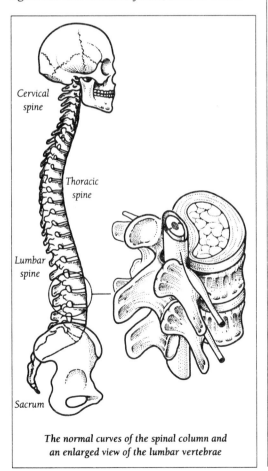

Cervical spine

Thoracic spine

Lumbar spine

Sacrum

The normal curves of the spinal column and an enlarged view of the lumbar vertebrae

have a relatively poor blood supply, will take several weeks or months to settle. In fact, inflammation and arthritis in the joints tends to be chronic, and it is wiser to think in terms of prevention of deterioration rather than cure. However, even long-standing backache can be improved through physiotherapy, exercise and correct posture, whilst changes in your mattress together with modern drug treatment can work wonders.

❷ Has there been any previous back injury?
Previous trauma to the back causing bruised or fractured vertebrae may later lead to secondary arthritis with resulting stiffness and pain.

❷ Are the normal curves of the back present?
When you stand sideways on to a mirror, you should be able to see the four basic curves of the spine. In your neck the spine should curve inwards, towards the throat, and there is a similarly shaped curve in the small of the back. Conversely, between the shoulder blades and at the back of the pelvis (the sacrum), the spine should curve outwards, away from the body. This curvature is altered in certain conditions. For example, in a prolapsed disc with attendant muscle spasm in the small of the back, there is loss of the forward curvature in this area, and the spine here looks extremely flat and rigid. In osteoporosis or ankylosing spondylitis (bamboo-spine arthritis), there is marked forward curvature of the thoracic spine (the part between the shoulder blades), with hunching of the back and a stoop. Shortening and forward bending of the spine is also seen in osteoporosis (dowager's hump).

❷ Is the back pain worse on movement?
Acute stabbing pain brought on by movement suggests entrapment of one of the sensitive

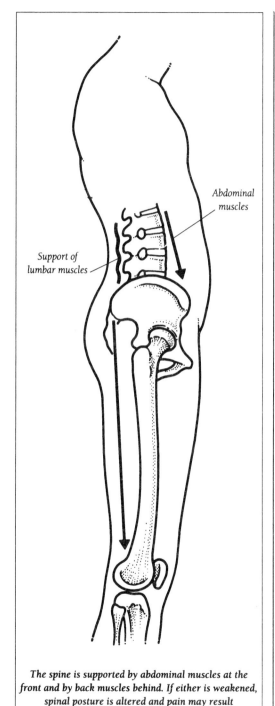

Abdominal muscles

Support of lumbar muscles

The spine is supported by abdominal muscles at the front and by back muscles behind. If either is weakened, spinal posture is altered and pain may result

nerves within or emerging from the spine, a painful but necessary reminder from your body that you should be resting. See your doctor if the pain persists for more than three days or so (by this time most trivial muscle strains and spasms will have settled on their own).

❷ *Is there pain on coughing or sneezing?*
This suggests movement of a freshly prolapsed disc pressing on a nerve and is a reminder to rest. Again, see your doctor if the pain persists for more than three or so days.

❷ *Do you feel generally unwell?*
Fever, weight loss and fatigue could represent disorders affecting other parts of the body as well as the spine. Rheumatoid arthritis, for example, could produce all these symptoms, as well as pain, stiffness and swelling in other joints, especially hand joints, some time previously.

❷ *Is there any weakness or pins and needles in the legs?*
If so, there might be pressure on the nerves from above, creating potentially serious consequences in the future for mobility and muscle strength in the legs. The commonest reason for this would be a slipped disc.

❷ *Has there been any difficulty controlling the bladder or bowels?*
This is the most urgent symptom of all with back pain as neglect can lead to permanent problems. *Urgent surgical correction is usually necessary.* Usually the cause will be a severely slipped disc in the lowest part of the spine.

❷ *Is the backache worse at period times?*
Women with a retroverted uterus may experience low back pain, especially during periods. This can be confirmed through an internal examination.

❷ Is there any significant vaginal looseness accompanied by a bulge or waterworks problems?

Prolapse occurs when the uterus or vagina drops downwards in the pelvis from its normal place. This happens when the muscles of the pelvic floor that support the uterus become weak. It may occur in women who are overweight or who have experienced childbirth where there has been significant stretching of the pelvic-floor muscles, which have not subsequently been able to tone up properly again. Very mild prolapse may not cause any symptoms, but if serious, the neck of the womb, or at times some of the womb itself, can emerge from the vagina to become visible on the outside. More common than uterine prolapse, however, is prolapse of the vaginal walls, when the walls of the vagina become weakened allowing the bladder and the rectum to push inwards into the vagina, producing a distinct bulge. This causes a constant discharge, and there may be alteration of bladder and bowel function, with possible constipation, regular urinary infections and even stress incontinence. Symptoms include a feeling of bearing down, particularly when standing or exercising, and a dragging feeling in the lower abdomen. This may be accompanied by backache and generalized tiredness and fatigue.

❷ Does the pain coincide with your periods?

Sufferers of endometriosis may experience low back pain as the cells that normally line the uterus and produce monthly bleeding migrate to other areas of the pelvis causing irritation and bleeding there.

❷ Are you emptying your bladder more often or passing bloodstained urine?

Kidney infections and kidney stones are notoriously capable of producing pain in the loin, because they are situated so near to the spine.

❷ Are there any associated abdominal symptoms?

Structures within the abdomen, such as the appendix, the large colon or gall bladder, can also produce backache when they become inflamed.

❷ Has there been any general weight loss?

Generalized weight loss accompanying a chronic, boring pain in the back could indicate a serious disorder within the body. Possible causes include chronic infections like osteomyelitis (inflammation of the bone marrow) and tuberculosis, blood disorders such as leukaemia and multiple myeloma, and cancer spreading from elsewhere.

Urgent referral to your doctor for full investigation is required.

❷ Is there a pulsating lump that can be felt in the abdomen?

Occasionally, someone suffering from an aortic aneurysm will feel pain in his or her back. The aorta is the body's major artery, beginning in the chest, in the heart's left ventricle, and then curving down and into the abdomen. It is very vulnerable to arteriosclerosis (hardening of the arteries), which if left untreated can lead to an aneurysm developing, when the artery wall balloons out and a pulsatile swelling can be felt in the abdomen. If the artery begins to split, intense pain may be felt in the back as well as the abdomen. *This constitutes a surgical emergency requiring immediate transferral to hospital.*

SUMMARY
BACK PAIN

POSSIBLE CAUSE	ACTION
Injury	Application of ice first, heat later, complete bedrest if necessary, simple painkillers for 3–4 days. If symptoms persist, consult your GP.
Wear-and-tear arthritis (osteoarthritis, spondylosis)	Exercise, painkillers, antiinflammatory medication, physiotherapy, hydrotherapy, chiropractic, osteopathy.
Osteoporosis	Exercise, hormone replacement therapy, calcium supplements.
Slipped disc (prolapsed invertebral disc)	Initially rest. If recovery is slow or incomplete, traction, physiotherapy, acupuncture. In more serious cases, epidural anaesthetics, surgery.
Trapped nerve	As above.
Rheumatoid arthritis	Physiotherapy, antiinflammatory drugs, gold and other drugs.
Retroverted uterus	May be corrected by a 'ring' or pessary.
Prolapse	Surgical correction or, in older women, a pessary.
Endometriosis	Hormonal treatment or surgery.
Kidney infection	Antibiotics.
Kidney stone	Lithotrypsy or surgery.
Inflammation of appendix, large colon or gall bladder	Medical or surgical treatment as appropriate.
Chronic infection (osteomyelitis, tuberculosis)	Identify cause. Medical or surgical treatment.
Blood disorder (leukaemia, multiple myeloma)	Chemotherapy, blood transfusion, bone-marrow transplantation, radiotherapy.
Cancer	Medical or surgical treatment of initial cancer, hormone treatment, radiotherapy.

ABDOMINAL PAIN

Abdominal pain should always be taken seriously. Usually the pain will be due to something common and trivial such as wind, overeating, indigestion, minor food poisoning, or constipation. However, there are a large number of different structures in the abdomen and one of the main problems in diagnosis is that it is not always easy to identify the exact source of the pain.

For example, inflammation in any of the abdominal organs is generally felt around about the bellybutton, and it's only when the inflammation becomes extreme that the pain will be felt in a specific area of the abdomen, usually because the more sensitive structures lying over the inflamed abdominal organs become inflamed themselves (peritonitis).

It is for this reason that all doctors will regard abdominal pain as serious until proved otherwise, and whilst cramp-like pains with sickness or diarrhoea following a suspicious meal can reasonably be left to run their course for 12 hours or so, pain that doubles the patient up, brings him or her to tears, or comes in ever-increasing waves needs professional observation.

In fact, any unexplained moderate to severe abdominal pain that has persisted for more than a few hours warrants a doctor's opinion.

THE ANATOMY OF ABDOMINAL PAIN

It can be difficult even for qualified doctors to discover the exact source and significance of abdominal pain, so careful consideration of the nature of the pain, its site and any associated features is essential. It also helps to know the exact positions of the various structures with in the abdomen.

Let's look at the belly in the same way that doctors do, and divide it into quarters, describing each in turn.

PAIN IN THE RIGHT UPPER QUADRANT

Here are the liver, behind and below it the gall bladder, the top right-hand section of the large bowel, and the pancreas gland. Anything affecting these structures can lead to pain predominantly in the top right-hand corner of the belly and under the ribcage. To help identify the possible cause of pain in this area, consult the check list of questions below.

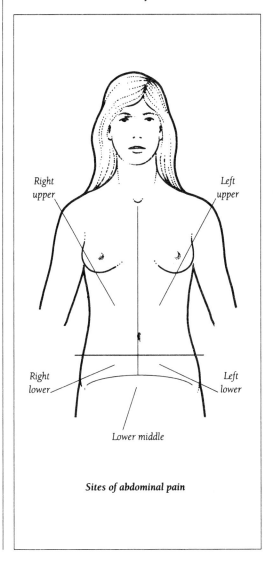

Sites of abdominal pain

THE LIVER

The liver is the largest organ in the abdominal cavity and one of the most important. Cone-shaped, it sits neatly under the ribcage on the right-hand side, below the diaphragm. It regulates the levels of most of the chemicals and molecules in the blood, manufacturing some and getting rid of others. Amongst those it makes are proteins to form blood plasma, others to help with immunity, coagulation factors, which allow blood to clot, and molecules that act in the transportation of oxygen and cholesterol in the circulation. The liver can also store glucose, which it releases back into the bloodstream when required, and filter out unwanted or poisonous substances from the blood, including many medicines, altering them so that they can be got rid of through the gall bladder or urine. It is relatively hardy in that it can still function when much of it is has been damaged by injury or disease. However, there are many disorders that can befall it, some of which produce the symptom of pain. Amongst the commonest of these problems are infections, toxic poisoning and heart failure, which can often produce the additional symptoms of jaundice, pale-coloured motions, dark urine and severe listlessness and fatigue.

❷ *Have you eaten anything suspicious lately, especially whilst travelling abroad?*
Infectious hepatitis, otherwise known as hepatitis A, is contracted through contaminated food or drink. It can certainly occur in this country, but is more commonly picked up when travelling in foreign parts with poor standards of hygiene. The illness tends to last about six weeks in all, causing lassitude, weakness, intolerance towards cigarette smoke and alcohol, and profound loss of appetite. The liver can swell and become tender but recovery is usually guaranteed.

❷ *Have you shared potentially contaminated needles with a drug abuser or had a blood transfusion outside the UK or in the Third World?*
Hepatitis B or serum hepatitis is a much more significant illness than hepatitis A, and in a small percentage of sufferers can have very serious or even fatal consequences. This blood-borne virus can be transmitted directly from person to person, and is particularly prevalent amongst intravenous drug abusers who share contaminated needles, and in homosexuals. Another type of viral hepatitis is called 'non-A non-B'. This produces similar symptoms to those mentioned above, and also tends to be transmitted through contaminated blood transfusion and dirty needles.

❸ *Have you recently had a long-standing very sore throat and swollen glands?*
Glandular fever can also affect the liver, producing some swelling and tenderness along with the above symptoms.

❸ *Is your alcohol consumption excessive?*
You could be suffering from cirrhosis of the liver. One of the functions of the liver is to remove poisons and toxins from the bloodstream. Regrettably, some of these are self-inflicted and liver damage that may or may not be reversible can be the result of excessive consumption of paracetamol or alcohol. The recommended safe levels of alcohol consumption are 21 units per week for men, and 14 units per week for women. (One unit is half a pint of beer or one glass of wine or one pub measure of spirit.) More than 50 units for a man or 30 units for a woman over any length of time is considered dangerous for physical, psychological and social reasons. As far as the liver is concerned, chronic alcoholics do not allow it enough time to recover from the onslaught of large quantities of alcohol, leading

to liver-cell damage with swelling of the entire liver. In this case, the telltale symptom is discomfort or pain under the ribcage on the right-hand side.

❷ Are you taking any medication?
Because medicinal drugs are mostly broken down by the liver, the liver is susceptible to the possible side effects of these medications. Some damage the liver cells by a process similar to allergy called 'sensitization', which is not dose related. Others damage the liver in much the same way alcohol does, that is the chemicals in the drugs directly interfere with liver-cell functions. These are all 'toxic' reactions. Some antibiotics, blood-pressure tablets and certain long-acting tranquillizers are all capable of producing a painful liver.

❷ Do you suffer from shortness of breath and swollen ankles?
If so, your abdominal pain may in fact be caused by heart problems. Like all muscles, the heart becomes weaker and less efficient with age and lack of exercise. When it is unable to contract as forcefully and efficiently as it used to, blood returning to the heart from the rest of the body cannot flow through it as rapidly as it should, causing pressure to build up in the veins travelling to the heart. The liver is the first organ to be affected by this increased pressure, and becomes congested, like a sponge full of water. When this happens quickly, tenderness and a dull aching kind of pain can result.

❷ Have your skin and eyes developed a yellowish tinge?
If your urine is a darker colour than normal, your liver could be inflamed as a result of any of the causes already mentioned, but also by infection or stones in the gall bladder and secondary cancers in the liver from other sites.

THE GALL BLADDER

Just behind and below the liver sits the gall bladder, a saggy, pear-shaped structure whose main function is to get rid of unwanted products passing through the liver into the gut. It makes special fluids called enzymes, and these enable our bodies to digest and absorb fatty substances in our diet. When the gall bladder becomes inflamed common symptoms include indigestion, bloating and wind, especially after eating a fatty meal, and in acute inflammations there may be nausea and vomiting with sweating and a high temperature. Because it is situated behind the liver, the gall bladder can cause pain not only in the front, but also right through to the back, especially on the right side. If you suspect the problem lies with the gall bladder, ask yourself the following questions:

❷ Do you have a fever?
Infections of the gall bladder (cholecystitis) can be acute, beginning suddenly or chronic, i.e. long-standing. In both cases there will be interference to the normal digestion of fatty foods, as well as pain in the right-hand upper quarter of the abdomen, which will be tender to the touch. With a chronic infection, the basic function of the gall bladder can be curtailed, leading to a permanent inability to tolerate fat in the diet and a functionally useless gall bladder that nevertheless is still capable of causing problems in the future. Sufferers pass foul-smelling, pale and frothy motions due to the presence of undigested fat, and a fatty meal will bring on pain in the right upper quadrant.

❷ Does the pain come and go?
Although anybody can develop gallstones, and a very large number of people have gallstones without suffering any symptoms, the people most likely to be affected are women in their forties who are fat, fair and fertile. No one is

sure why this is so, but women of this age group who are overweight and on the pill certainly do seem to be more prone. Gallstones form when too much cholesterol is produced compared to the amount of detergent-like substances in the bile, which keeps cholesterol in solution.

Most gallstones consist of crystallized cholesterol. A stone forming in the gall bladder moves continuously but only causes trouble when it obstructs the out flow of bile from the gall bladder. In fact, a large number of people have gallstones without suffering any symptoms. However, if an obstruction does occur, the result is biliary colic, with a very severe coming-and-going type of pain, often accompanied by jaundice, dark urine and fever.

THE PANCREAS

The pancreas is a gland with two main functions, firstly the digestion of foods through special enzymes, in which function it is similar to the gall bladder, and secondly the production of insulin, which controls blood-sugar levels. The enzymes in the pancreas that digest food are extremely powerful, and if they escape from the cells that make them into the surrounding tissues, for example as the result of inflammation, alcoholism (which causes long-term damage to the pancreas) or cancer, they produce severe inflammation and pain. The pain is usually accompanied by nausea, vomiting and sweating, tends to be worse when lying down, and is often felt in the back.

❷ Can you feel the pain go through to the back?

Inflammation of the pancreas (pancreatitis) characteristically produces abdominal pain that goes through to the back.

❷ Are you a heavy drinker and/or smoker?

Excessive consumption of alcohol and/or tobacco over long periods can commonly trigger inflammation of the pancreas (pancreatitis).

❷ Do fatty foods bring on the pain?

Gall-bladder disease and gallstones can trigger pancreatitis, and this link may be exposed if fatty foods frequently bring on the symptoms.

❷ Have you lost a lot of weight and has you skin become yellow?

Although these symptoms may be caused by relatively common conditions such as hepatitis, the possibility of a tumour within the pancreas should be excluded and your doctor should be consulted without delay.

THE BOWEL

The bowel does, of course, run through the entire abdomen, but here we are concerned with the top right-hand corner of it. Its function is to digest and absorb food, retain water and expel to the outside any remaining wastes and residues through the squeezing action of its muscular walls. Trouble here tends to cause a dull, colicky type of pain that comes and goes in waves.

❷ Do you have diarrhoea or constipation?

The excess efforts of the muscular walls of the colon in these situations frequently cause abdominal pain.

❷ Do you suffer from stress together with alternating diarrhoea and constipation?

Together with cramp-like abdominal pain, bloating, wind, and the feeling after evacuating the bowels that the rectum is still not empty, these are characteristic of irritable bowel syndrome.

❷ Have you lost weight and also noticed blood in your motions?
This suggests colitis (inflammation in the lining of the bowel), including ulcerative colitis and Crohn's disease, a peptic ulcer or a tumour.

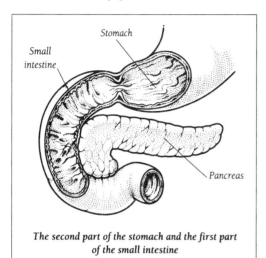

The second part of the stomach and the first part of the small intestine

❷ Are you over 60 and prone to constipation?
A likely explanation is diverticulitis, when small pouches in the lining of the bowel become blocked by intestinal contents, leading to local inflammation.

THE KIDNEY
The kidneys lie on either side of the spinal column. They filter out waste products from the blood, which are then carried away by the ureters to the bladder and on to the outside.

The right kidney can cause pain that is occasionally mistaken for pain arising from the other structures in this part of the abdomen. Most kidney pain is felt in the flank or the back, but infections, abscesses, blood clots or kidney stones ought to be considered.

❷ Do you have a temperature and feel you need to empty your bladder more often than normal?
A kidney infection is likely, especially if there is also loin pain and a hint of blood in the urine.

❷ Do you have a blistery rash on the right side of your chest or abdomen?
The characteristic rash of shingles will often explain the cause of pain in this area. The pain can precede the onset of the rash by several days.

❷ Is the pain excruciatingly sharp?
This is the classic symptom of a kidney stone. The pain is acute and severe, travelling from the loin down through the flank and into the groin.

❷ Is there any blood in your urine?
A stone from the kidney, infection in the bladder or kidney, or a blood clot in the blood vessels feeding the kidney can all produce this symptom.

❷ Do you feel sick, have a high temperature that comes and goes, and have you recently lost weight?
An abscess in the kidney is a possibility, especially if you need to empty your bladder more frequently than usual.

❷ Have you got a cough and a high temperature?
Very occasionally pneumonia in the lowest part of the right lung can produce pain in the right upper quadrant.

Finally, it's worth saying that occasionally patients are rushed to hospital by doctors who have diagnosed a problem in the right upper quadrant, but they turn out to have something quite different. For example, and especially in older people, pneumonia forming at the very bottom of the right lung can mimic the symptoms of gall-bladder problems, particularly if there is no temperature or cough. Also, the pain caused by the onset of shingles can be felt before the rash develops, leading to the suspicion of a liver or gall-bladder problem. All is made clear, however, after a few days when the characteristic blisters on the skin appear.

SUMMARY
ABDOMINAL PAIN IN THE RIGHT UPPER QUADRANT

POSSIBLE CAUSE	ACTION
The Liver	
Hepatitis	*Bed-rest, fluids, dietary modification, hygiene precautions.*
Glandular fever	*Rest, symptomatic treatment.*
Cirrhosis of the liver	*Medical and/or surgical treatment.*
Medication	*With your doctor, identify and then discontinue drug responsible.*
Heart failure	*Medication to improve heart function and diuretics to reduce blood volume.*
Liver cancer	*Medical and/or surgical treatment.*
Gall-bladder infection (cholecystitis)	*Antibiotics and painkillers.*
Gallstones	*Break up the stones with lithotrypter (high frequency ultrasound), dissolve with drugs, or remove using flexible telescope passed through mouth and stomach, or surgery.*
The Pancreas	
Pancreatitis	*Emergency medical treatment. Avoid alcohol and smoking.*
Pancreatic cancer	*Currently incurable. Supportive therapy only.*
The Bowel	
Diarrhoea or constipation	*Symptomatic relief.*

Continued . . .

SUMMARY
ABDOMINAL PAIN IN THE RIGHT UPPER QUADRANT

POSSIBLE CAUSE	ACTION
Irritable bowel syndrome	High-fibre diet, antispasmodics, stress management.
Colitis (ulcerative colitis, Crohn's disease)	Medication. Occasionally surgery.
Peptic ulcer	Antacids and/or surgery.
Diverticulitis	High-fibre diet, antibiotics, antispasmodics, occasionally surgery.
Bowel cancer	Surgery.
The Kidney	
Kidney infection	Antibiotics.
Shingles	Acyclovir medication in cream or tablets.
Kidney stone	Lithotryptor or surgery.
Kidney abscess	Antibiotics and/or surgical drainage.
Blood clot	Medical treatment, including anticoagulants.
Pneumonia	Antibiotics.

PAIN IN THE LEFT UPPER QUADRANT

This part of the abdomen contains the spleen, the stomach, the pancreas, the bowel and the diaphragm itself.

THE SPLEEN

The spleen lies beneath the ribcage on the left-hand side of the body and is responsible for processing and organizing the various blood cells in the circulation. One of its major functions is to filter out old red blood cells that have had their allotted time of approximately 120 days in the circulation, and then get rid of them. These red blood cells are then broken down into their various components, with some being returned to the circulation for reprocessing, and others excreted from the body. The spleen also harbours and manufactures many of the white blood cells vital for fighting infections and inflammations such as blood disorders and glandular fever, and is thus an essential part of the immune system. It responds to these conditions by swelling, so that its covering envelope or 'capsule' as it is called, stretches and causes pain. A doctor will be able to feel the enlargement with his or her hands when the spleen emerges from behind the ribcage. When the capsule of the spleen breaks, as it does sometimes in glandular fever or through direct injury in a car accident for example, there will not only be pain, but circulatory collapse of the patient, sometimes with blue discoloration in and around the navel.

❷ *Have you had a prolonged sore throat recently?*
Glandular fever is a distinct possibility, especially if you are between the ages of 12 and 25. The commonest symptoms are fatigue and weakness, which can last several weeks or months. In severe cases there may be temporary enlargement of the liver, spleen and lymph glands.

❷ *Do you feel excessively tired and weak?*
You may well be anaemic as a result of a blood disorder such as glandular fever, certain hereditary conditions, for example sickle cell disease and thalassaemia, or even leukaemia.

❷ *Have you suffered any blunt injury to your left side?*
Pain below the ribcage in the left upper quadrant could represent a bruised or ruptured spleen. This is a not uncommon injury in car accidents or contact sports such as rugby. The pain will be followed by the circulatory collapse of the patient, sometimes with blue discoloration in and around the navel. *This condition requires urgent diagnosis and immediate surgery.*

The Stomach

The stomach is a distensible, bag-like organ that stores food for up to several hours at a time. It is involved in the continual process of digestion that begins at the mouth with the salivary glands and ends in the colon with water retention. The stomach's powerful acid content breaks food down into manageable particles and allows the efficient action of protein-digesting enzymes. Most people think their stomach is bang in the middle of their belly, but in fact it is more to the left side.

❷ *Do you suffer from indigestion due to overindulgence?*
One of the commonest causes of pain in this area is inflammation of the lining of the stomach (gastritis), which can be caused by the consumption of too much alcohol and/or rich, fatty or spicy foods.

❷ *Are you a heavy smoker?*
Smoking is another common cause of gastritis (see above).

❷ *Is the pain worse when you bend forward, lift something or lie flat in bed?*
This is characteristic of a hiatus hernia, when the upper part of the stomach pushes up into the gullet through the muscular, tent-like structure called the diaphragm that separates the abdomen from the chest. When this happens it interferes with the valve at the lower end of the gullet so that strong stomach acid regurgitates up into the gullet, causing heartburn. The problem is particularly common in people who overeat, who are overweight, or who are physically active. Stooping and bending forwards can often make the pain worse.

❷ *Is the pain severe enough to wake you at night?*
If it is also localized enough for you to be able to point to it with your fingertip, an ulcer is a possibility. Pain caused by an ulcer is often worse at night when the stomach acid is not neutralized by food.

❷ *Have you lost weight quickly and do you feel generally unwell?*
Stomach cancer can cause pain, but unfortunately by the time it does, the cancer is already fairly advanced. Weight loss, anaemia and loss of appetite are usually much more in evidence than pain.

THE PANCREAS
The pancreas lies across the centre of the upper abdomen and can therefore cause pain in the left as well as in the right upper quadrant. If you suspect the problem lies with your pancreas, consult the check list of questions on page 104.

THE BOWEL
The top left-hand corner of the large bowel is quite capable of causing pain in the left upper quarter of the abdomen. To establish whether this is the cause of your problem, see pages 104–105.

THE DIAPHRAGM
The diaphragm is the muscular, tent-like structure that separates the chest from the abdomen. It can be injured through lifting heavy objects or twisting awkwardly since muscle fibres here can tear just as they can anywhere else. Occasionally a severe blow to the ribs may be responsible. The diaphragm can also be irritated by disorders in any of the structures above or below it.

❷ *Does it hurt whenever you bend or twist?*
This suggests muscular strain or rib damage, which is always made worse by movement and which may well reach a peak two or three days after the original injury.

❷ *Do you have a cough and a high temperature?*
Pneumonia or pleurisy can impinge on the diaphragm, causing pain on coughing or breathing deeply.

❷ *Was sharp abdominal pain followed by collapse?*
Disorders of many abdominal organs can lead to the presence of blood or air below the diaphragm, causing pain. A ruptured ectopic pregnancy or a perforated stomach, for example, can do this.

Early symptoms can be surprisingly mild, but once perforation occurs, *urgent investigation and surgery is needed.*

SUMMARY
ABDOMINAL PAIN IN THE LEFT UPPER QUADRANT

POSSIBLE CAUSE	ACTION
The Spleen	
Glandular fever	Rest, symptomatic relief.
Congenital or acquired blood disorder	Removal of spleen or anti-cancer treatment.
Ruptured spleen	Surgery.
The Stomach	
Gastritis	Antacids, stop smoking and drinking alcohol, dietary advice, medication.
Hiatus hernia	Weight loss, diet, antacids, no smoking or alcohol. Occasionally surgery.
Stomach ulcer	Antacids, H2 antagonists to block acid production, drugs to protect stomach lining.
Stomach cancer	Surgery.
The Diaphragm	
Damaged rib or chest muscles	Rest.
Pneumonia or pleurisy	Antibiotics.
Perforated abdominal organ	Urgent surgery.

PAIN IN THE RIGHT LOWER QUADRANT

Anatomically, the most significant organ in this area is the appendix. Also present are the bowel, the right ureter, right ovary and right fallopian tube.

THE APPENDIX

The appendix is a short, hollow, tube-like structure attached to the first part of the large bowel, the caecum. In humans it has no function and probably represents a part of the digestive system made obsolete through evolution. However, distributed along its length are small lymph glands and if these become enlarged due to infection within the body, or if the lumen of the organ becomes blocked, inflammation can quickly occur.

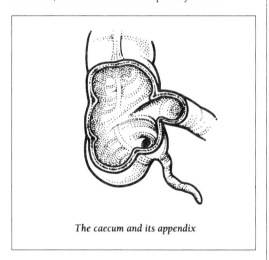

The caecum and its appendix

❷ *Did your stomach ache start in the middle and then shift to the right-hand side?*

An inflamed appendix that requires surgical removal is experienced by one in six people. Patients with appendicitis are usually young, below the age of 25, and generally complain first of a dull ache around the bellybutton. After a matter of hours this may clear up spontaneously in which case there is no need to consult a doctor. Alternatively, the pain may shift to a position to the right and below the bellybutton, exactly where the appendix sits, and become much more severe. The position of the appendix itself may vary in different people and occasionally pain in the back or in the back passage may be experienced. In true appendicitis the patient is usually totally off his or her food, may have a temperature, a little bit of diarrhoea or constipation, and may vomit. In the later stages the belly becomes extremely tender over the area of the appendix, and sufferers characteristically draw their knees up to the chin so that the abdominal wall is not stretched over the appendix. By this time the problem is a surgical emergency and urgent help is required.

THE BOWEL

The part of the bowel adjacent to the appendix can be affected by a number of disorders. Problems here tend to bring on a dull, colicky type of pain that comes and goes in waves. If you suspect this could be the source of your abdominal pain, consult the check list of questions on pages 104–105.

THE URETER

The ureter is the tube that drains urine from the kidney above it to the bladder below it. It is very richly supplied with nerve endings so any abnormality affecting the ureter will cause intense and severe pain.

❷ *Is the pain excruciating and accompanied by blood in the urine?*

Most commonly the problem is due to a stone passing down from the kidney towards the bladder, resulting in classic renal colic. Renal colic causes pain of the utmost severity that comes and goes in waves and is enough to reduce grown men to tears, parading around the bedroom on all fours. The pain may arise anywhere from the flank, down into the right- and left-hand corner of the abdomen and further towards the groin or testicle on the same side. An associated symptom is the presence of blood in the urine, which clinches the diagnosis. If in doubt, however, an X-ray of the abdomen can identify the presence of the stone. Occasionally, the ureter can be compressed by the enlargement of surrounding organs where tumours or bands of fibrous tissue can be responsible.

THE OVARIES

The ovaries are almond-shaped glands situated on either side of the uterus, just below the opening of the fallopian tubes. They contain unfertilized eggs and are responsible for the production of female sex hormones.

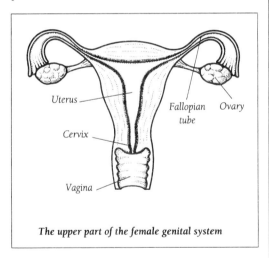

The upper part of the female genital system

❷ Is there pain on intercourse?
Ovaries can be enlarged by cysts, either benign or malignant, or by solid tumours, which may or may not give rise to swellings as well as pain. In fact, pain may be present only with the deep penetration of intercourse and may not necessarily be present in the abdomen at all, although it usually is.

❷ Does the pain recur on a cyclical basis, coinciding with your periods?
Endometriosis is a condition that may affect the ovary, producing pain, and is caused by the migration of cells that normally line the uterus to structures outside the gynaecological organs. The cells respond in the same way as they did when lining the uterus in that they produce monthly bleeding, and this in turn leads to scarring and adhesions in and around the area of the ovary and fallopian tubes, causing pain either spontaneously or during intercourse. The pain may also be felt in the lower back.

THE FALLOPIAN TUBE

The fallopian tubes connect the uterus to the ovaries on each side and permit the transportation of egg and sperm so that fertilization can take place.

❷ Are you or could you be in the early stages of pregnancy?
Normally, the egg passes from the ovary, along the fallopian tube to the uterus where it is fertilized. It then embeds itself in the lining of the uterus, where a normal pregnancy occurs. However, if the fertilized egg stops in the fallopian tube, it may implant and begin to grow. The fallopian tube is a very narrow structure with weak walls, and as the fast-growing embryo enlarges it may cause a rupture and profuse bleeding from the blood vessels in this site. Because it is initially fairly painless, the bleeding may continue unabated, collecting in the lower part of the abdomen and eventually leading to low blood pressure, fainting and collapse. *This is a ruptured ectopic pregnancy and should be treated as a surgical emergency.* Anybody in the early stages of pregnancy, usually at about six weeks, with unexplained lower abdominal pain and who feels faint should always bear this possibility in mind *and see their doctor immediately.*

❸ Is the pain accompanied by abnormal vaginal discharge and a temperature?
Pelvic inflammatory disease is the second condition commonly affecting the fallopian tubes, and refers to inflammation as a result of infection, often of a sexually transmitted nature. Diseases such as chlamydia and gonorrhoea are the main culprits, but bacterial infection introduced accidentally as a result of

inserting a coil (intra-uterine device) can cause the same problem. Any woman experiencing discharge from the genital area coupled with the presence of a dull aching pain in the lower abdomen should therefore investigate the problem urgently, as, if neglected, pelvic inflammatory disease can sometimes result in long-standing infertility.

SUMMARY
ABDOMINAL PAIN IN THE RIGHT LOWER QUADRANT

POSSIBLE CAUSE	ACTION
The Appendix	
Appendicitis	Observation in hospital until spontaneous resolution, surgery if worsens.
The Ureter	
Stone in ureter	Wait for spontaneous passage of stone, lithotryptor (high-frequency ultrasound) to shatter stone, or surgery.
Compression by surrounding organs	Surgery, radiotherapy or chemotherapy.
The Ovaries	
Ovarian cysts	May resolve spontaneously, otherwise surgery.
Ovarian tumours	Surgery and/or anti-cancer treatment.
Endometriosis	Hormonal treatment and/or surgery.
The Fallopian Tube	
Ruptured ectopic pregnancy	Urgent surgery.
Pelvic inflammatory disease	Antibiotics and surgery for any long-term complications.

PAIN IN THE LEFT LOWER QUADRANT

Generally speaking, pain in the left lower quarter of the abdomen may arise from exactly the same structures as in the right, except that there is no appendix here to cause problems. One of the commonest culprits is irritable bowel syndrome, or spastic colon, where the muscular walls of the large bowel frequently go into painful spasms for reasons not yet clear to the medical profession.

With pain in the lower left-hand side of the abdomen, it is particularly important to exclude cancers, benign tumours, diverticulitis and other inflammatory bowel conditions.

If you suffer pain in the left lower quadrant of your abdomen, consult the check list of questions on pages 112–114.

PAIN IN THE LOWER-MIDDLE ABDOMEN

The structures here include the lymph glands, which run up the side of the spinal column, the bladder, the rectum, the bowel, and in women the uterus. There is also the aorta, the body's major artery. This takes blood from the heart to the legs, and here separates into two major arteries the common iliac arteries on either side of the pelvis.

THE BLADDER

The bladder lies in the middle of the lower part of the abdomen. It collects urine excreted by the kidneys and running down the ureters and is emptied by the opening of the muscular valve at its lower end. When the bladder walls are stretched, the sensation comes to our notice by way of nervous signals transmitted along the spinal cord. The bladder is most often affected by infections, irritation, and the presence of blood in the urine.

❷ *Are you peeing more often than usual?*
The feeling that you need to empty your bladder more often than usual accompanied by burning or stinging when you do go is highly suggestive of a bladder infection (cystitis).

❷ *Is there blood in the urine?*
The passage of urinary stones usually produces a sharp and severe pain, often with bloodstaining of the urine.

❷ *In a man, is there difficulty starting or stopping peeing?*
This suggests an obstruction to the outflow of urine from the bladder as a result of an enlarged prostate gland. With this condition, there may have been a history of difficulty in passing water, of getting up at night to pass water, or having to go during the day every 20–30 minutes, as well as poor stream and problems starting.

The Rectum and Large Bowel

Any of the problems associated with the bowel as listed on pages ??-?? can cause pain in the lower-middle part of the abdomen. However, two other possible conditions should also be borne in mind.

❷ *Do you ever pass blood and mucus with the motions?*
Inflammation of the lining of the rectum, often a form of colitis, can cause pain in this area. The persistent appearance of mucus and blood with the motions in a person over 55 requires examination to exclude the possibility of rectal cancer.

❷ *Have you suffered in the past with penile discharge?*
Chronic inflammation of the prostate gland in men can cause pain in this area, as this gland sits just in front of the rectum.

THE UTERUS

The uterus is a hollow, muscular organ that sheds its lining in response to hormonal fluctuations each month if pregnancy does not occur. The uterus is connected to the vagina below and to the two fallopian tubes on either side at the top and is located in front of the rectum and behind the bladder in women.

❷ *Is there swelling of the lower abdomen accompanied by irregular periods and/or a need to empty your bladder more often?*
Enlargement and discomfort of the uterus occurs quite commonly in normal pregnancy, but the presence of muscular lumps in the wall of the uterus (fibroids) will cause a similar enlargement. Fibroids are less common in women who have had more than two children, and indeed an ancient medical adage once said 'good girls have fibroids, and bad girls have babies'.

Fibroids may be felt through the wall of the abdomen or during an internal examination carried out by a doctor. There may be associated urinary problems due to pressure on the bladder or bloating and discomfort of the pelvis as a result of the congestion of blood vessels.

❷ *Do you suffer pain inside on intercourse?*
Pain felt in the lower-middle abdomen can be the result of endometriosis which is discussed in more detail on page 156. Sexually transmitted diseases such as gonorrhoea or chlamydial infection causing pelvic inflammatory disease or even the presence of an intra-uterine contraceptive device (the coil) will also produce discomfort here. Swelling of the ovaries due to cysts or growths may also produce pain in the abdominal midline as the ovaries lie just to the side of the uterus.

THE BLOOD VESSELS

The large blood vessels in the lower abdomen may be affected by hardening of the arteries and by splitting of the wall of the blood vessel, with consequent ballooning (aneurysm) and severe haemorrhage.

❷ *Is the pain cramp-like and do you pass blood through the rectum after a meal?*
Just as angina affects the heart, hardening of the arteries supplying the intestines with blood may produce so-called mesenteric angina. Symptoms of this include cramp-like pain and blood being passed through the back passage soon after eating a meal.

❷ *Is the pain excruciatingly sharp, radiating through to the back?*
If you also have high blood pressure and/or high blood cholesterol levels, this may be a sign of a ruptured aortic aneurysm, which is *a surgical emergency*.

SUMMARY
PAIN IN THE
LOWER-MIDDLE ABDOMEN

POSSIBLE CAUSE	ACTION
The Bladder	
Cystitis	Antibiotics.
Kidney or bladder stone	Spontaneous passage, lithotryptor (high frequency ultrasound) to shatter stone, or surgery.
Enlarged prostate gland	Medical or surgical treatment.
The Rectum and Large Bowel	
Colitis	Medical or surgical treatment.
Rectal cancer	Surgery.
The Uterus	
Fibroids	Leave if found incidentally and not causing any symptoms, otherwise surgical removal if interfering with fertility or causing symptoms, or hysterectomy if large and interfering with periods.
Endometriosis	Hormonal treatment and/or surgery.
Pelvic inflammatory disease	Antibiotics.
Ovarian cysts or tumours	Surgical treatment.
The Blood Vessels	
Aortic aneurysm	Urgent surgical grafting.
Mesenteric angina	Surgical treatment.

PAIN IN THE SIDE

Pain in the side or flank is a little more unusual and when compared with discomfort in the front of the belly there are relatively few causes to choose from. The kidneys are probably the most significant source of problems in this area, most often causing discomfort in the loin and the part of the back between the shoulder blades and the top of the pelvis, but also in the sides. To help determine the underlying cause of your pain, ask yourself the following questions:

❷ Could you have strained a muscle?

It's quite possible through bending or lifting a heavy object to pull the muscles in one or both sides. The pain may come on immediately, so that cause and effect are clear, but minor injuries may not become apparent for a day or two after the exertion, in which case the diagnosis may not be so obvious. However, the pain is usually aggravated by such movements as stretching, and can be eased by rest and the application of heat.

Sudden, sharp contractions of the abdominal muscles generally make the pain worse, and coughing and sneezing agony can become genuine agony.

❷ Is there any blood in the urine?

If there is a pinkish tinge to the urine or even obvious blood, this raises the possibility of a stone either within or moving down from the kidney, or an infection in the 'waterworks' system such as cystitis or a kidney infection. Pain caused by a stone will be sharp and come in waves.

Less commonly, this combination of symptoms can be seen in people who develop blood clots that travel through the circulation to lodge in the kidney, especially those who take too high dosages of the anticoagulants used to treat the clot.

❷ Does the pain come in severe waves and move downwards to the lower abdomen and groin?

This suggests a stone passing from the kidney down the very sensitive ureter towards the bladder.

❷ Do you feel the need to empty your bladder more often?

This as well as burning or stinging is a common symptom of an infection in the genitourinary system such as cystitis.

❷ Is there nausea and vomiting?

Deep-seated kidney infections (pyelonephritis) can cause both nausea and vomiting, and if there is also intense shivering and alarming shaking fits, known as rigors, this diagnosis is even more likely.

❷ Do you have a dull aching sensation in the flank?

Occasionally, even in adulthood, this can be the result of a congenital kidney abnormality that has taken many years to manifest itself. In fact, congenital abnormalities affecting the kidney and its draining tubes are amongst the commonest. A shrunken, scarred kidney that doesn't function properly and is more prone to infection, and a kidney that has more than one drainage tube or drainage tubes with abnormal valves obstructing the flow of urine are quite commonly seen, and can cause enlargement of the kidney substance itself with collection of urine and cyst formation.

❷ Is the pain accompanied by recurring urinary infections?

Fairly large benign cysts can also develop during the course of life, causing a dull, aching sensation in the flank. These cysts produce stagnation of urine, which makes frequent infection more likely.

❸ Do you have a high temperature that comes and goes accompanied by progressive weight loss?

A kidney abscess could very well be the cause as abscesses release infective organisms into the bloodstream in large numbers sporadically.

❸ Is there a sudden knife-like pain when you bend or twist?

Between each of the spine's vertebrae is a spinal nerve. These nerves run to every part of the body, sending signals to the muscles to initiate movement and transmitting the sensation of pain, temperature and position back to the brain. Injury or any form of arthritis in the spine can impinge on these nerves, causing pain to be transferred along the nerve to distant sites, including the side.

❸ Has there been any tingling or irritation in the skin, followed by a blistery rash?

With shingles there will be a painful rash in one area on one side of the body. It is caused by a chickenpox infection lying dormant in the tissues, often for many years, becoming active and inflaming the nerves in one part of the body. However, some days before the characteristic blistering rash appears, there is often itching and irritation in the skin of the affected area, accompanied by sharp, stabbing pains.

SUMMARY
PAIN IN THE SIDE

POSSIBLE CAUSE	ACTION
Muscle strain	Rest, heat, painkillers.
Kidney or bladder infection	Antibiotics.
Kidney abscess	Antibiotics.
Kidney stone	Lithotryptor (high-frequency ultrasound) or surgery.
Congenital abnormalities	Surgery if necessary.
Cysts	Surgery if sizable and interfering with kidney function.
Blood clot or haemorrhage	Assess coagulability of blood with blood tests. If excessive, treat cause and take anticoagulants. Anticoagulant dosage should be monitored as excess also produces bleeding into the urine.
Spinal problems	Identify cause and treat.
Shingles	Acyclovir or famcyclovir antiviral treatment.

PAIN IN THE BACK PASSAGE

Judging by the number of commonly used expletives synonymous with this diagnosis, it is obvious just how uncomfortable and irritating pain here can be. Not only is this area richly supplied with sensitive nerve endings, but we spend much of our daily lives sitting down, so that if something is wrong, we are reminded of it almost every minute of the day. In addition, problems here are capable of causing enormous embarrassment. Whilst it is fine to show off one's war wound or an injury sustained in the heat of the battle on the sports field, it is not so wonderful to have to report a pain in the back passage, even to your doctor.

As you will see, most causes are fairly trivial and benign as well as remediable, but just occasionally the symptom of pain in this area can herald the onset of more significant problems.

❷ Do you suffer from constipation?

Although during my medical career I have treated hundreds of patients for thousands of different problems, the most grateful are usually those who have been given treatments by the district nurse to relieve extremely hard impacted motions in the back passage. With a high-fibre diet, plenty of fluid intake, and if necessary lubricating suppositories, sufferers can avoid the problem.

❷ Is there bleeding when you go to the loo?

This suggests haemorrhoids or piles, which basically are varicose veins in an awkward place. Arteries are blood vessels that carry oxygenated blood under pressure to various sites of the body to keep the tissues alive, whilst veins are the blood vessels that carry deoxygenated blood away from the tissues and back to the heart and lungs. Veins have thinner walls than arteries and when pressure builds up the walls expand and become vulnerable to rupture and bleeding. When this happens in the rectal area there may be discomfort and pain, as well as itching, and often an obvious lump can be felt emerging from the anus. If such enlarged veins persist, or if they are irritated by constipation or even frequent diarrhoea, rupture and heavy bleeding can occur. The important thing is that the blood is fresh and bright red and seen on the outside of the motion or in the toilet pan rather than mixed with the stool itself. This is an important point because blood mixed in with the motion or blood that is dark in colour tends to signify bleeding from higher up the bowel, a more ominous sign.

❷ Is there a split in the skin that isn't healing?

A deep split or fissure in the surface of the lining of the back passage to the outside, the result of constipation or infection, is similar to the painful splits that can develop in the hard skin of the hands or fingertips. It can be repaired by using healing creams, and suppositories and avoiding constipation, but occasionally surgery is necessary.

❷ Has any injury been incurred?

People with severe constipation, those who indulge in anal intercourse or who have inserted any kind of object into the back passage can tear the sensitive lining within the anus and rectum and experience pain as a result. Such tears are usually self-healing, but in view of the difficulty of maintaining perfect hygiene in this area, abscess formation is always a possibility.

❷ Is any tender boil present?

A perianal abscess is a painful and not uncommon occurrence. Like a deep-seated boil, it is a very tender swelling just next to the back passage. If very small, it may respond to antibiotics, but usually surgical drainage to evacuate the material within it is necessary.

❷ Has there been persistent diarrhoea?

Frequent diarrhoea from whatever cause can inflame the internal surface of the back passage, producing pain. The diarrhoea may be the result of simple food poisoning, of inflammatory colitis, of laxative abuse or of bowel tumours, all of which require appropriate correction.

❷ Does the pain come and go?

Diverticulitis is one of the commonest benign abnormalities of the large bowel. It develops as we grow older, and describes little pouches that form in the lining of the colon and push through to the muscular coat surrounding the bowel. These pouches can trap waste products, causing infection and inflammation, which in turn result in spasms of the muscle. Depending on the site of the diverticulitis, pain may be felt in the abdomen or lower down in the back passage.

❷ Is there occasional rectal bleeding without piles?

This suggests the presence of polyps, pear-shaped stalks of tissue arising from any hollow organ of the body. When they occur in the lower part of the bowel, they can twist at the base of the stalk, cutting off the blood supply and becoming infected. Simple removal is all that is required.

❷ Is there persistent or recurrent rectal bleeding?

If it persists, nobody should ever assume that rectal bleeding is due to simple haemorrhoids because cancer in this area and the last part of the large intestine is by no means a rarity. A simple test in which the doctor examines the rectum with a gloved finger to test for the presence of a growth is all that is required, and can certainly make the difference between life and death. So, if you have rectal bleeding that persists unabated for more than a few days, or which returns soon after settling down, always consult your doctor.

❷ Are there any irregularities with your periods, or do you suffer deep-seated pain on intercourse?

In women there may be a number of other causes of pain in the back passage, including an ovarian cyst or pelvic inflammatory disease. The site and radiation of the pain from either of these conditions can vary and it is not all that unusual for the pain and discomfort to be felt rectally as well as or instead of in other areas.

❷ Is there fever accompanied by loss of appetite and nausea?

The position of the appendix can vary, and if situated behind the colon on the right side it can certainly cause pain towards the back of the bowel. If your doctor suspects appendicitis, he or she will examine the back passage with a gloved finger and detect significant tenderness in this area confirming the diagnosis.

❷ Is the pain fleeting and occasional, and are you under a lot of stress?

Proctalgia fugax is the name that describes an intense but short-lived pain in the back passage that is quite sufficient in severity to wake the sufferer at night. The pain is caused by muscle spasms brought on by emotional tension and has no serious significance.

❷ Has there been any significant penile discharge?

The pain of chronic inflammation of the prostate is often said to be like sitting on a golf ball. Often there is also a history of discomfort passing water, of needing to go more often, of discharge from the penis, and sometimes of a

mild temperature. So if you have pain in the back passage and any of these symptoms, you should consider the possibility of prostatitis.

SUMMARY
PAIN IN THE BACK PASSAGE

POSSIBLE CAUSE	ACTION
Constipation	High-fibre diet, exercise, plenty of fluids, laxatives.
Haemorrhoids	Cream, ointment, suppositories, sclerosing injections or surgery.
Fissure	Healing creams and ointments, surgery if necessary.
Injury	Avoid causative factors; treat constipation.
Abscess	Antibiotics, surgical drainage.
Diarrhoea	Medical treatment for underlying reason.
Diverticulitis	High-fibre diet, antibiotics, antispasmodics, surgery.
Polyp	Surgical removal.
Bowel cancer	Surgery and/or radiotherapy.
Gynaecological problems	Medical or surgical treatment of underlying problem.
Appendicitis	Surgery.
Proctalgia fugax	Reassurance.
Prostatitis	Antibiotics.

PAIN IN THE GROIN

Contrary to popular belief, the groin is nothing whatsoever to do with the genitalia, but is rather the area where the top of the leg meets the lower part of the abdomen. In the deep crease across this junction lies the inguinal ligament, a strong, cord-like structure that tethers down the various tissues beneath it. Pain in the groin can emanate from a number of sources, some of which may be more obvious than others.

❷ Can you feel a single, soft lump?
A hernia can form in various sites in the body, but most commonly occurs at the groin, when it is called an inguinal hernia. In this case, a weakness in the muscular wall of the abdomen allows a loop of intestine to push into the groin. Pain is caused as the weak muscle fibres are pushed open and stretched still further, and there is also a distinct bulge that can vary in size from quite tiny to several inches in diameter. The bulge itself is generally not tender, although the muscle fibres at the edges are, and it will only become tender if the blood supply to the underlying intestine is obstructed by the surrounding muscle constricting the base of the lump, thereby allowing strangulation and gangrene to occur. The bulge may come and go, being most noticeable when the sufferer is standing, and sneezing and coughing, which increase the pressure of the abdominal contents, will often produce a sudden increase in the size of the hernia.

❷ Can you feel a lot of hard lumps?
Just as the lymph glands at the front and sides of the neck become enlarged as a result of tonsillitis, so any type of infection affecting the lower leg, back passage or lower abdomen can produce enlarged glands in the groin. The glands' function is to deal with inflammation and infection from these sites, and swelling is their normal response. They can also be affected by more generalized disorders such as brucellosis and glandular fever, as well as by much rarer blood diseases such as leukaemia and lymphoma. Enlargement of the groin glands alone usually suggests a local problem, for example an infected ingrowing toenail, whereas enlargements of all the lymph glands, including those in the armpits, groin and neck, point to a generalized disorder.

❷ Is the pain worse if you draw up your knee?
Few muscle strains are more likely to put a professional sportsman out of action than a groin strain. The muscles and tendons affected run underneath the inguinal ligament and allow you to bring your thigh up against the abdomen.

❷ Is the pain made worse by coughing or bending forward?
A slipped disc that is putting pressure on one of the nerves coming out of the spinal cord may cause pain to be referred along the nerve and into the groin. This may be the only manifestation of a slipped disc, with no pain being felt in the lower back at all. The pain is usually of a sharp, burning nature, is not made worse by manipulation or prodding in the groin area, but is certainly made worse by particular movements of the lower back, such as bending, twisting, stooping and coughing.

❷ Is your urine bloodstained?
The passage of a kidney stone, however small, from the kidney down the draining tube (the ureter) to the bladder can produce pain anywhere in the loin and the front of the abdomen, right down into the groin and the testicle on the affected side. The pain is usually excruciatingly sharp and often associated with bloodstained urine.

123

SUMMARY
PAIN IN THE GROIN

POSSIBLE CAUSE	ACTION
Hernia	Surgical support or surgery.
Lymph-gland enlargement	Identify cause and treat appropriately.
Muscle strain	Physiotherapy, anti-inflammatory medication.
Slipped disc	Rest, physiotherapy, medical and/or surgical treatment.
Kidney stone	Allow stone to pass spontaneously, lithotripsy (high-frequency ultrasound waves) to shatter stone, or surgery.

PAIN IN THE TESTICLES

When someone talks of 'kicking a man where it hurts most', most people are quite aware of the anatomical location being alluded to. The testicles, the delicate production factories of spermatozoa, are situated externally so that an optimum temperature for sperm production of 2°F lower than the rest of the body can prevail, but this of course also makes them more vulnerable to injury. All the structures within the scrotum (the 'ball bag' or sack of skin surrounding the testicles) are richly supplied with sensitive nerve endings, which can transmit discomfort and pain. Pain can sometimes be accompanied by swelling and/or other associated symptoms such as blood in the urine, pain passing water, or a high temperature. In some ways, the presence of pain is a reassuring sign in that a swollen testicle with no pain whatsoever suggests a cancer of the testicle, which is one of the commonest of all cancers in men between the ages of 20 and 40. Contrary to popular belief, cancer here rarely produces pain in the early stages, so any painless lump on one testicle alone should be reported to the doctor urgently. The good news is that thanks to the advances of modern medicine the cure rate is extremely high even in the later stages, with something like a 90 per cent success rate with surgery and radiotherapy, and possibly chemotherapy if the cancer has spread. However, there are a number of different causes of pain in the testicles, and the various symptoms that occur can help to put them in perspective.

❷ Has there been an injury?

Anybody who has ever suffered a knock in this area will remember for ever the pain experienced. Because the sensitive testicles are so vulnerable to injury, all contact sports should be played wearing supportive underwear or a jockstrap. Usually bruising and swelling are the worst consequences of injury here, which however alarming looking tends to settle within a few days with the help of supportive underwear and warm baths. The bruising and swelling secondary to a normal vasectomy operation will repair itself in the same way and in a similar amount of time.

❷ Is there blue discoloration above the testicle?

Just like the veins in the leg, the veins that drain blood away from the testicles in the scrotum can become varicose, in which case a 'varicocele' is formed. A varicocele feels like a bag of worms at the top of the testicle on the affected side, and the veins themselves can be tender to the touch. The doctor is usually able to ascertain that the veins are swollen without there being any testicular swelling.

❷ Is the pain located at the top or the bottom of the testicle?

At the back of each testicle, connected by a number of small ducts, is the epididymis. Sperm leaving the testicle travel along these ducts to the epididymis, leaving via the vas deferens, the tube that carries the sperm to the prostate gland and thereafter to the urethra within the penis. The epididymis can become inflamed or infected (epididymitis), in which case the top or bottom of the testicle will be extremely sensitive to the touch. The testicle itself is usually unaffected and antibiotic therapy generally solves the problem within a week or two.

❷ Is there a lump present in the groin as well as in the scrotum?

When a weakness in the muscular wall of the abdomen allows a loop of intestine to push through it, a lump appears on the outside. This is a hernia. In the groin area, a large hernia can

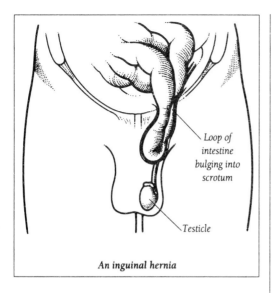

Loop of
intestine
bulging into
scrotum

Testicle

An inguinal hernia

extend downwards into the scrotum,
sometimes making it appear quite bulky. The
pain, which can be abdominal and/or scrotal,
is usually made worse by movement, coughing
or sneezing.

❷ Is there swelling on either side of the face as well?

Although mumps tends to occur mostly in
childhood, adult infections are occasionally
seen. Children are now vaccinated against
mumps, as well as measles and rubella, at an
early age, but any adult who has missed both
the vaccination and the illness won't have any
immunity and will therefore be vulnerable to
contracting the illness if exposed to it.
Although mumps normally causes swelling
of one or both of the salivary glands on either
side of the face, it can also produce swelling of
other glands, including the pancreas and the
testicles. In fact, significant pain and swelling
in one or both testicles is experienced in 10
per cent of cases of adult mumps, and in 10
per cent of these cases, some degree of
infertility also arises as a result of the condition
being left untreated.

If you think you might not be immune to
mumps and develop pain in the testicles after
being in contact with somebody who is
infected *you should inform your doctor urgently*
as steroids can prevent or reduce swelling and
preserve fertility.

❸ Have the pain and swelling arisen out of the blue?

Although the testicles are fairly mobile, there
is usually enough tissue holding them in place
to prevent them from twisting too far in one
direction. In the condition known as testicular
torsion, however, the testicle twists around
inside the scrotum, cutting off the blood
supply from above. As with any part of the
body when the blood supply is shut off, the
testicle will then swell and become painful.
Occasionally, as the swelling occurs, the
torsion will correct itself, in which case the
symptoms will disappear spontaneously.
However, some young men who experience
the recurrent but short-lived discomfort of
'temporary' torsion remain at risk of
'permanent' or persistent torsion. The real
problem arises when the blood supply is cut
off for more than six hours or so, after which
the testicle itself will not be able to recover
and will die. In these cases, *urgent* surgical
intervention to correct the torsion and a minor
procedure that permanently fixes the testicle
into the scrotum in a proper position can solve
the problem for good.

From time to time, neglected cases do result
in gangrene of the testicle on one side, which
then has to be removed. The good news is that
when this happens, people can still function
quite adequately firing on one cylinder, as it
were, and their future ability to perform
sexually and to father children is unaffected.

❷ Does the discomfort develop after sexual arousal?

Younger men in particular may experience physical discomfort in this area of the body as the result of unrequited love or 'blue balls', as the condition is more popularly known. Sexual excitement and stimulation not relieved by ejaculation can cause congestion in the epididymis and vas deferens, leading to a dull, aching sensation in the testicle area. Men who suffer from this discover for themselves that masturbation can relieve the pain, or that merely sleeping on the problem will result in relief of the discomfort by morning.

❷ Is your urine bloodstained?

The passage of even small kidney stones from the kidney downwards through the ureter into the bladder can often cause excruciatingly sharp referred pain in the testicle.

SUMMARY
PAIN IN THE TESTICLES

POSSIBLE CAUSE	ACTION
Trauma	Supportive underwear, hot baths, painkillers.
Varicose veins (varicocele)	Supportive underwear, surgery if necessary.
Epididymitis	Antibiotics.
Hernia	Truss or surgery.
Mumps	Steroids when swelling of the testicles occurs, to prevent infertility.
Permanent torsion	Urgent surgery required.
Unrequited love	Will resolve spontaneously.
Kidney stone	Lithotripsy or surgery if stone doesn't pass spontaneously.

PAIN IN THE PENIS

A number of different conditions may cause penile pain, any of which can produce ill-disguised hysteria in even the most stoical of men. The commonest cause might be described as injury due to overuse in the sexual sense, but there are one or two other problems that should always be considered.

❷ *Have you been overdoing it, romantically speaking?*

There are a number of structures on the penis that can become uncomfortable during sex, notably an over-tight foreskin that does not fully retract or a particularly short frenulum (the band of tissue on the underside of the penis, underneath the foreskin, which tethers the foreskin to the base of the penile head). In these cases, unlubricated intercourse or frequent intercourse with adequate lubrication can cause the foreskin to become sore or the frenulum to be stretched and torn. Usually, refraining from sexual marathons and the liberal use of lubricating jelly for him or Replens for her (both available from chemists) will be enough to avoid the problem.

❷ *Is there a rash?*

Genital herpes is a virus that can be passed from one person to another through unprotected sexual intercourse (practising safe sex by use of a condom protects against its transmission). It is thought that the virus reaches the tissues below the surface of the skin through a small breach, lying dormant for a short while before the characteristic tingling and itching occur, followed soon afterwards by a crop of small blisters with shiny, domed heads that later burst and become scabbed on top. At this stage the rash is tender and painful, especially if intercourse is attempted. Ideally this should be avoided when the virus is active since at this time the affected person is contagious, and also because secondary bacterial infection of the blisters is more likely to occur. Symptoms tend to last between seven and ten days in all, but attacks can recur from time to time, especially when the person is feeling run-down, tired or has some other infection such as a cold or flu. As well as the rash and the discomfort, there is often swelling of the glands in either side of the groin. Treatment involves warm salt baths and the administration of acyclovir by mouth or locally as a cream.

❷ *Is there any discharge from the penis?*

Nonspecific urethritis and gonorrhoea are the commonest of the sexually transmitted diseases causing pain when passing water and urethral discharge. There has usually been a history of unprotected sexual intercourse and there may also be swelling of the glands in the groin on both sides.

❷ *Has the pain been preceded by discharge some time in the past?*

Inflammation or infection of the prostate (prostatitis) can cause penile pain. The infection may be acute, i.e. of very recent origin, or long-standing, having been there for months.

It is usually due to a urethral infection caused by nonspecific urethritis or gonorrhoea, but may be the result of normally harmless bacteria living on the skin's surface being introduced through catheterization.

❷ *Is the foreskin red and tender?*

Balanitis, or inflammation or infection of the head of the penis, can be the result of a bacterial infection or thrush. Diabetics are particularly vulnerable to this because of their tendency to high blood sugars and skin infections, but anyone with a lowered immune response may be susceptible.

❷ *Does the penis bend when erect?*

In the condition known as Peyronie's disease, a painful area of scar tissue develops within the shaft of the penis toward one side, causing a painful angulation of the penis during erection. The cause of the condition is unknown and although megavitamin treatment has been used in the past it is not dramatically effective and in severe cases surgery is preferred.

❷ *Is the pain caused by permanent erection?*

Priapism describes a painful state of permanent erection, usually caused by a blood cloth (thrombosis) in one of the major veins that drain blood from the penis. It is secondary to injury or inflammation, or may be a result of generalized blood-clotting problems, when it tends to be seen in association with more significant illnesses such as leukaemia. Treatment may be medical or surgical.

❷ *Are your eyes red and joints swollen?*

Reiter's syndrome causes penile discharge and pain on passing water, together with inflammation of the eyes and joints. The condition usually responds to initial treatment with antibiotics within a few weeks.

❷ *Are there any swellings on the penis?*

Very occasionally there may be a penile tumour. Treatment may take the form of radiotherapy or surgery, or both.

SUMMARY
PAIN IN THE PENIS

POSSIBLE CAUSE	ACTION
Sexual overuse	Lubrication, hot salt water baths, antibiotics if necessary.
Genital herpes	Acyclovir cream or tablets.
Sexually transmitted diseases	Antibiotics.
Prostatitis	Antibiotics.
Balanitis	Treat with antibiotics. Test for diabetes.
Peyronie's disease	Megavitamin therapy is worth trying; otherwise surgery.
Priapism	Evacuation of blood clot, medical treatment of underlying conditio.
Reiter's syndrome	Antibiotic therapy.
Tumours	Surgery and/or radiotherapy.

PAIN PASSING URINE

Urine is produced as the kidneys filter the blood. It runs down the ureters into the bladder, where it is stored until a sufficient quantity stimulates the stretchy and elastic walls of the bladder, making the nervous system conscious of the need to empty the bladder. The bladder then contracts at the same time as the muscular valve or sphincter at the bottom end of the bladder relaxes. Urine is then released from the bladder to the urethra to the outside. Pain passing urine is known as dysuria, and often has a burning or scalding quality. Pain may occur before the urine stream begins, during it, or immediately after.

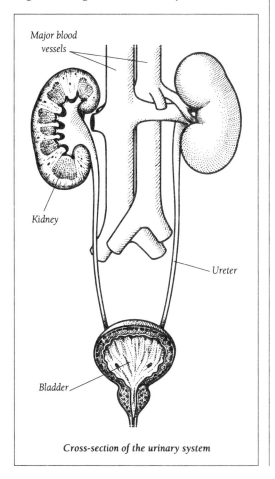

Cross-section of the urinary system

Major blood vessels

Kidney

Ureter

Bladder

Although the commonest cause is cystitis due to infection or inflammation of the bladder, there are a number of other causes that must be considered.

❷ *Is there discomfort and a burning sensation when urinating?*

These are the characteristic symptoms of cystitis, one of the commonest problems brought to doctors' surgeries. It is often of a recurrent nature or triggered by sexual activity, and is seen particularly in women. Women have a much shorter urethra (the tube from the bladder to the outside) than men, and consequently it is much easier for infection to find its way in. There is also less protection against ascending infections following sexual intercourse, but in 50 per cent of cases there is no proven infection anyway. Nevertheless a midstream specimen of urine should be sent off to the laboratory for testing to establish whether any true infection exists and consequently which antibiotics are required. One of the problems with cystitis is that inappropriate antibiotics are often used, with the result that although symptoms are improved, not all the bugs will be completely eradicated. This also reduces the effectiveness of such antibiotics in the future and encourages the development of particularly resistant organisms. Occasionally cystitis can allow ascending infection to the kidney, in which case kidney infection (pyelonephritis) ensues, with high temperatures, shaking fits (rigors) and back pain. Cystitis without infection may be due to inflammation of the urethra itself (urethral syndrome), a narrowed urethra or a small-volume bladder. Often a vicious circle is established in which the frequent desire to spend a penny is obeyed, resulting in a bladder of very restricted volume that feels full as soon as a small quantity of liquid is secreted from the kidneys.

Sexual cystitis is also common and is caused by traumatic irritation of the urethra as the result of sexual contact, often of an unaccustomed or unlubricated nature.

❷ Does the pain occur after sex?

Rough sexual foreplay or intercourse can irritate the urethra or bruise the base of the bladder, causing discomfort in the woman. Gentler sex with adequate lubrication and relaxation are important if these problems are to be avoided. Establishing a routine of emptying the bladder after sex in order to flush away any germs is also useful.

❷ Is there any vaginal discharge?

Infection with the fungus Candida produces thrush. Thrush is encouraged by taking any kind of female sex hormone, whether in the contraceptive pill or in hormone replacement therapy because the oestrogen contained in such preparations changes the nature of the vaginal secretions, allowing the infection to flourish. Diabetics are also vulnerable because of the high sugar levels of their bloodstream, and anyone who has taken a recent course of powerful antibiotics will also be more prone to it because these kill off many of the harmless bacteria that normally live in the vagina, thereby allowing an overgrowth of fungal elements to take over. Thrush generally causes soreness at the entrance to the vagina with cystitis symptoms (see above) and usually there is also a telltale, whitish, cheesy discharge from the vagina itself.

❷ Is there any discharge? Did it develop within days or weeks of unprotected sexual intercourse?

Nonspecific urethritis, a chlamydical infection can cause inflammation and discharge from the urethra. These inflammations may or may not cause discomfort when passing water, although infection with gonorrhoea certainly will.

❷ Is there any discomfort in the scrotum or back passage?

Any sexually transmitted disease that ascends to the prostate gland can produce infections of the gland (prostatitis) and discomfort when urinating or in the back passage.

Occasionally, bacteria not passed on by sexual intercourse may be responsible, especially following catheterization for surgical procedures.

❷ Is there any blood in the urine?

Kidney stones may move of their own accord in the flow of urine from the kidneys, down the ureter to the bladder and then beyond the bladder through the urethra to the outside. As the stone moves through the urethra it may scratch the sensitive lining, producing acute discomfort when urinating. Other symptoms include loin pain and the presence of blood in the urine.

❷ Are there any obvious trigger factors?

Some women find that certain elements in their diet can precipitate cystitis. Spicy foods, alcohol and coffee, for example, are often cited. Similarly, chemical irritants contained in scented soaps, bubble bath and talc can irritate the sensitive urethra, causing symptoms of frequency and burning very similar to those of cystitis.

It is important to wear all-cotton or natural-fibre underwear to minimise irritation. It is also wise to drink a large quantity of water – at least eight glasses a day – in order to flush out germs. Washing with plain water is also recommended.

SUMMARY
PAIN PASSING URINE

POSSIBLE CAUSE	ACTION
Cystitis	If infective: antibiotics; if non-infective: urodynamic investigations and urethral dilatation and bladder stretch if necessary.
Trauma	Avoid rough sex, ensure there is adequate foreplay, relaxation and lubrication. Empty bladder after sex.
Thrush	Antifungal cream, pessaries, or tablets.
Sexually transmitted disease	Appropriate antibiotics.
Prostatitis	Appropriate antibiotics.
Kidney stone	Allow stone to pass spontaneously or surgical removal.
Allergy	Avoid spicy foods, alcohol and coffee. Avoid scented soaps, bath oils, bubble baths and talc.

PAINFUL PERIODS

Normally between the onset of puberty and the end of the menopause a woman experiences regular and cyclical vaginal bleeding as a result of a series of hormonal fluctuations within her body. The changes are designed to prepare the uterus for implantation of a fertilized egg at the beginning of pregnancy, but when this does not occur, shedding of the lining of the womb takes place. However, although menstruation can be seen as an indicator of potential fertility, this cyclical occurrence is not always regarded in a positive light. Periods are not called the curse for nothing. They generally occur every 26–35 days and the amount of discomfort and lower abdominal cramping caused is variable, although most women will experience some discomfort during their lives. Some women complain of very little, but others come to terms from an early age with the fact that for two or three days every month of their reproductive lives they have to put up with moderate to severe pain. The cramp-like pain experienced during periods is caused by the release of chemicals called prostaglandins, which produce uncomfortable spasms in various structures contained in the pelvis. Happily there are now perfectly acceptable drugs known as antiprostaglandins that can inhibit the effect of these chemicals and reduce pain effectively without unnecessary side effects. Furthermore, the oral contraceptive pill, which is the commonest form of contraception in Britain today, significantly reduces not only the quantity of blood loss during a period but any pain as well. Nevertheless, whilst the bottom line is that period pain no longer has to be stoically endured, there are a number of potential causes, some more serious than others, and if you consistently suffer painful periods you should have a thorough gynaecological examination to identify the underlying problem. In the meantime, ask yourself the following questions:

❷ Have you always suffered lower abdominal cramps at the start of your period?
The hormone changes that occur throughout the menstrual cycle together with the cyclical changes that occur within the lining of the uterus lead to the build-up of certain chemicals known as prostaglandins, and these produce painful spasms in the pelvic structure. Although normal and not attributable to any underlying disease process, this physiological pain can certainly affect your quality of life, including your ability to work, for 2–3 days or more each month. Treatment can be given if this is the case, and anyway, it is quite unnecessary to endure discomfort purely because it is 'nature's way'.

❷ Did the painful periods begin after stopping the pill?
Women who have used the contraceptive pill for a number of years may have forgotten that when they started taking it, it not only reduced the quantity of bleeding during each monthly cycle, but also the pain. Thus when they stop the pill and return to heavier, more uncomfortable periods, the normal level of uterine discomfort comes as an unpleasant surprise.

❷ Have you had the coil (intra-uterine contraceptive device) fitted?
When a woman has a coil fitted by her doctor she will be warned that she may experience cramp-like pains for a day or two and that her periods may become heavier and more uncomfortable for 2–3 months. In some cases, the period pains remain bad and the coil has to be removed. This is basically because the coil is a foreign body lying within the cavity of the

womb and for some reason, in certain women, this can cause increased uterine contraction, particularly during a period. In this situation alternative methods of contraception should be sought.

❷ Is there abdominal and back pain together with pain on intercourse and interference with bladder and bowel function?

In this relatively common disorder, known as endometriosis, cells lining the inside of the uterus escape to other areas of the pelvis, particularly around the ovary, fallopian tubes and outside of the uterus, where they may bleed and cause irritation and pain coinciding with normal monthly bleeding. If any combination of these symptoms occurs, a gynaecologist should be consulted.

❷ Is your lower stomach always distended and is there a feeling of heaviness in your pelvis?

Fibroids are benign tumours of the muscular wall of the uterus, and extremely common. They may lie on the inside of the cavity of the uterus or lie within the wall itself, or develop on the outside of the uterus in the pelvis. They are by no means always painful, but when they bulge into the cavity of the uterus they can interfere with normal uterine functions and cause painful periods.

Nobody really knows why they occur, but they are always benign and are more common in women who have not had babies than in women who have. Small fibroids may well be asymptomatic and cause no problems at all, but larger ones cause pelvic congestion and a feeling of heaviness as well as the cramping spasms of painful periods. They are particularly likely to do this in the years leading up to the menopause, but if the symptoms are not too bad and the menopause not too far away,

gynaecologists often recommend no treatment as fibroids diminish in size after the change of life. In other cases, when the fibroids are very large and troublesome, and when the woman's family has been completed but her menopause is still some way off, surgical treatment of some kind may be necessary, perhaps in the form of a hysterectomy.

The presence of ovarian cysts should also be considered if these symptoms are experienced. They come in all shapes and sizes and even small ones can alter the delicate hormonal balance required for smooth cyclical activity, causing heavy, painful periods at times. They may be benign or malignant, but should always be investigated.

❷ Is the pain intermittent and unpredictable?

Polyps are fleshy, pear-shaped outgrowths from the lining of the womb that although benign do cause painful periods. Usually the solution lies in the simple removal of the polyp by means of a D & C or 'scrape' operation.

❷ Has there been any infection of, or injury to, the cervix in the past?

The blood lost during a period passes to the outside through the neck of the womb, or the cervix. If for any reason the cervical canal is narrow, the flow of blood from the uterus may be blocked, causing pain and discomfort. Dilatation (stretching) of the cervical canal may be required.

❷ Has there been any pelvic infection or discharge?

Pelvic infection involving the cervix, uterus or fallopian tubes produces swelling, congestion and discomfort. Normal period function may in turn be disrupted, leading to increased monthly pain.

SUMMARY
PAINFUL PERIODS

POSSIBLE CAUSE	ACTION
Physiological	Hot-water bottles; antiprostaglandin medication; painkillers; oral contraceptive pill.
Stopping the pill	Reassurance. Return to pill, or if pregnancy is planned, look forward to 9 months with no periods at all.
The coil	Remove within 3 months if pain remains troublesome.
Endometriosis	Hormone therapy or surgery.
Fibroids	Removal of fibroid alone or complete hysterectomy.
Ovarian cysts	If large, surgical removal.
Polyps	Surgical removal by D & C (dilation and curettage).
Narrowed cervix	Surgical dilatation.
Pelvic infection	Antibiotics.

LEG PAIN

As with pain in other sites of the body, pain in the leg may be caused by a single structure somewhere within the leg itself, or be referred from a distant area. When the origin of the pain is not obvious and where there has been no memorable recent injury, the source of the pain may at times be elusive.

In such cases it is worth looking at what the symptoms can tell us.

❷ Has the muscle suddenly become bunched up and painful?

Cramp is the protracted contraction of a muscle, usually the calf muscle, and can be intensely painful. It is caused by an imbalance of the minerals and salts in the body, particularly potassium and calcium, which is why cramp is also common in those suffering from a hangover. Occasionally cramp can follow unaccustomed, intense exercise, often occurring afterwards when the muscles are relaxed, for example when the sufferer is lying comfortably in bed. Immediate treatment consists of stretching the affected muscle – in the case of the calf muscle by pulling the toes up and towards the front of the shinbone – and rigorous massage. Sufferers should avoid excessive unaccustomed exercise, and pay attention to the type of footwear they are donning during the day (high heels may make things worse). Dietary modification is also worthwhile. Extra calcium from dairy products, especially low-fat milk, is important and so is plenty of potassium, found particularly in bananas, oranges and tomato juice. For recurrent cases, quinine tablets can be prescribed by the doctor.

❷ Is the pain in the back of the leg and is it made worse by bending forward?

This is caused by irritation of the large sciatic nerve (sciatica) that runs from the lower part of the spine down the back of the leg, sending out branches to various parts of the leg as far as the sole of the foot. Sciatica normally arises from a slipped disc in the lower part of the back and occasionally can be the only manifestation of this, there being no back pain whatsoever. There may be associated tingling and pins and needles in the leg on the same side, as well as possible muscle wasting and weakness.

❷ Are the joints stiff, with limited movement?

'Wear-and-tear' arthritis (osteoarthritis) in the weight-bearing joints of the hip and knees is particularly common, accounting for the majority of orthopaedic operations carried out in this country at the present time. It's worth pointing out that pain in the knee may actually arise from arthritis in the hip, but there will usually be the telltale signs of stiffness and limitation of movement in the hip joints if they are affected. Knee cartilage can also be torn through injury and the muscles and tendons surrounding joints in the leg may give rise to discomfort of one type or another.

❷ Do you suffer from varicose veins?

In this case, the source of the pain is obvious, as the dark-blue dilated, tortuous, cord-like structures are particularly visible, and when severe can certainly be most uncomfortable. The pain is caused by the distension of the vein wall as the result of increased pressure of the blood within it. Wearing elastic hosiery and support tights may reduce the discomfort, but if the pain increases injection therapy with a sclerosing agent or surgery will be necessary.

❷ Do you smoke and/or are you on the pill?

Anyone can develop a thrombosis or clotting of the blood, but the presence of any of the following risk factors will make the possibility more likely: having varicose veins, smoking, taking the pill, and not taking enough exercise. Thrombosis is particularly common in varicose veins, where the blood flow has become sluggish and the tendency to clot has become greater. In superficial veins the symptoms include soreness and redness over the affected vein, which is hard and solid to the touch. In deeper veins, however, the consequences can be much more serious as a blood clot may travel along it and lodge in a vital structure such as the heart or lung.

A travelling blood clot is called an embolus, and lung emboli are particularly common in women who have varicose veins or who have been laid up for rest after an injury or a surgical operation in hospital, particularly if the operation has been of a gynaecological nature, such as an hysterectomy. Other factors that increase the tendency of the blood to clot include taking the contraceptive pill and smoking. It is for this reason that a blood clot in the lung is not at all an uncommon reason for emergency admission to hospital in women between the ages of 20 and 50.

Deep-vein thrombosis usually begins in the lower leg, and other signs to watch for include swelling and redness of the foot, with pain in the calf muscle of the affected side. *Anybody experiencing such symptoms should call the doctor immediately as treatment and surgery are urgently required.*

❷ Does the pain come on during exercise?

Hardening of the arteries, most commonly associated with high blood cholesterol and smoking, can seriously interfere with the blood supply to the tissues of the leg. As the arteries become narrowed so the tissues are deprived of oxygen, causing pain. This tends to be made worse by exercise, which increases the demand for oxygen, and pain in the calf muscles

brought on by exertion or walking uphill is therefore a characteristic sign of arterial disease. There may also be changes in the skin, including loss of hair on the lower leg, pallor and a tendency to coldness and infection in the toes and feet.

Such symptoms should of course be reported to your doctor.

❸ Do you have any back pain?

Because pain is transmitted through the nerves, it is logical that any disorder of the nerves in the lower leg may give rise to problems. Pressure on the sciatic nerve from a slipped disc in the back can irritate the nerve, leading to sciatica and a sharp pain running into the buttock and down the back of the leg as far as the sole of the foot.

❹ Do you eat an adequate diet?

A diet lacking in the B group of vitamins can affect the nourishment of the nerves. This can in turn significantly alter the usual function of the nerves, leading to pins and needles, muscular weakness and pain in the leg. Vitamin supplements and/or an improved diet including lots of leafy green vegetables are required; your doctor will advise you.

❺ Did the pain come on very gradually?

Nerves need an adequate blood supply and a toxin-free environment. Disorders such as diabetes and alcoholism can both cause leg pain as the result of physiological damage to nerve tissue. In this situation, pins-and-needles-type pain followed by numbness and weakness in the extremities is often the first sign that something is wrong, and you should always consult your doctor about this combination of symptoms.

SUMMARY
LEG PAIN

POSSIBLE CAUSE	ACTION
Cramp	Initially, stretching and massage of affected muscle; later, correction of mineral imbalance with potassium and calcium salts. Quinine prescribed as necessary.
Sciatica	Identification of slipped disc, medical or surgical treatment.
Osteoarthritis	Physiotherapy, rest or exercise depending on activity of the arthritis, anti-inflammatory medication.
Varicose veins	Compression, sclerosant, injection or surgery.
Thrombosis	Stop smoking, avoid contraceptive pill, treat varicose veins, anticoagulant therapy.
Poor blood supply	Stop smoking, keep active and warm, surgery as required.
Nerve problems	Correct dietary deficiency. Adequate blood-sugar control in diabetes. Stop smoking and drinking.

FOOT PAIN

When people come to my surgery complaining of painful feet, the reason usually turns out to be badly chosen, ill-fitting shoes. This may seem obvious, but it's amazing how many people are surprised when I point out how narrow and pointed their shoes are. Bunching together of the bones of the foot with pressure on the overlying skin commonly leads to inflammation of the joints and nerves, which is how bunions and hammertoes begin, and to infections of the skin, all of which can be extremely painful at times. Fortunately these days, with our much better understanding of the role of good chiropody, the ulcers and bony deformities we used to see so much of in the past are becoming less common.

Nevertheless, the feet take the body's full weight, and bearing in mind that we usually walk several hundred thousand miles during the course of a lifetime, that most of us are overweight, don't wear tailor-made shoes and pay little attention to foot-care generally, then it isn't surprising that foot pain is still a very common problem. Also, there are a large number of joints in the feet that can be affected by all the conditions commonly causing problems in any joint. These include osteo- and rheumatoid arthritis. Localized problems such as gout and neuromas are frequently seen too.

❷ *Are you wearing the wrong shoes?*

Shoes bought off the shelf in high-street shops rarely fit perfectly. In an ideal world, shoes would be made on a personalized basis to suit every foot whatever the shape and size. As this is not the case, it is important to make sure with children's shoes that there is plenty of room for the foot to grow in, and with adults' shoes that there is adequate room for movement, even if the end result may not be particularly attractive. If everybody in the world wore boring, 'sensible' shoes, as my mother used to call them, far fewer people would be suffering and hobbling about than is currently the case.

❷ *Are you overweight?*

Over the years, excess weight will stretch the supportive ligaments in the sole of the feet, leading to fallen arches. Shoes without arch supports underneath do not help. Regular exercise to strengthen the feet and weight control are therefore recommended.

❷ *Is the big toe alone affected?*

With gout, the joint at the base of the big toe becomes acutely tender to the touch, bright red and swollen. It is a throbbing type of pain, severe enough for the sufferer to remove his or her shoe and sock and sit with the foot elevated and a pack of frozen peas placed upon it. The cause is the build-up of uric acid in the body. We all make a certain amount of this as it is derived from the breakdown of protein-like substances in the body and in the diet, but some people seem more vulnerable to attacks of gout. Gout may occur in other small joints of the body, but is most common in the big toe.

❷ *Do you have long-standing pain in your heel?*

When muscles and tendons attach themselves to bones, they can, over a period of many years, form a bony outgrowth from the main part of the bone, called a 'spur', with a sharp point that digs into surrounding structures, causing pain. A common site is underneath the heel, and this is a common explanation for long-standing discomfort in this area, and may be accompanied by inflammation of the tendon called 'policeman's heel'. The discomfort classically eases off as the day goes on but comes back with a vengeance after resting with the feet up or first thing in the morning.

139

Cortisone injections, along with good chiropody and appropriate footwear, are usually effective, although occasionally surgery is required.

❷ *Are other joints playing up?*
The many little joints in the foot can be affected by osteo- and rheumatoid arthritis. Examination of the foot by a doctor is essential.

❷ *Do you experience a sharp, stabbing pain when walking?*
Little swellings of the nerves (neuroma) running between the toes can cause intense and very sharp pain when walking. A cortisone injection can sometimes be remedial, but occasionally surgery is required.

❷ *Are there circulation problems?*
Poor blood supply affecting the nutrition of the tissues in the feet can lead to pain. Raynaud's disease is characterized by an increased sensitivity to cold and is common amongst women. The fingers and toes will become pale, white and then blue in even moderately cold weather, and pain is then likely to occur. The other cause of poor blood supply to the feet is hardening of the arteries higher up in the leg or in the small vessels of the foot itself, as in diabetes. A doctor should always be consulted.

❷ *Do you suffer from back problems?*
Foot pain may be experienced as the result of abnormalities of the nerves much higher up the leg or even in the small of the back. Often nerve pain in the foot is associated with pins and needles and tingling. There may also be weakness of the muscles.

SUMMARY
FOOT PAIN

POSSIBLE CAUSE	ACTION
Poor-fitting shoes	Change shoes. See a chiropodist. Avoid pressure on deformed joints.
Being overweight	Weight loss, regular exercise, proper supporting footwear.
Gout	Anti-inflammatory or preventive medication. Dietary adjustment.
Spur	Cortisone injections and/or surgery.
Arthritis	Identify type and treat appropriately.
Inflamed nerve (neuroma)	Cortisone injections or surgery.
Poor blood supply	Raynaud's disease: use vasodilator drugs, stop smoking and keep warm. Hardening of the arteries: stop smoking, with surgery if necessary.

5

ABNORMAL
BLEEDING

The symptom of bleeding, or haemorrhage, is usually an alarming one. It isn't so bad if the source of the bleeding can be explained. Any kind of cut or laceration to the skin, for example, is bound to result in some blood loss, whilst women of reproductive age would worry if they did not see a monthly period. But abnormal and unexpected bleeding can be terrifying, and the sight of this dramatic, bright-red internal fluid is enough to make some of the strongest amongst us pass out. Even a small amount of blood when diluted in other body fluids such as urine looks a great deal worse than it really is.

IN POINT of fact, in most one-off episodes of bleeding from any of these sources there is a simple and harmless explanation. And scary though visible bleeding may be, it can also be a very useful symptom because it draws our attention to any problems going on within us. Intestinal bleeding, for example, will show up in the motions, staining them a dark, tar-like colour. Even small quantities can be detected using chemical reagents, and this is one of the most useful tests for the relatively common cancer of the bowel, which would otherwise exist silently and often without the patient knowing about it. Haemorrhage when it occurs at the back of the eye can be seen by a doctor or optician with the help of a special torch called an ophthalmoscope. High blood pressure can force blood through tiny breaks in the vessels over the delicate retina, the light-sensitive membrane at the back of the eye, producing a flame-shaped bleeding that helps confirm the diagnosis. Bloodstaining in various body fluids can point to the presence of kidney, bladder or lung infections, nasal

problems, or disorders relating to the female reproductive system. Underlying abnormalities within the bone marrow itself, where the blood components are made, may give rise to abnormal bleeding from almost any site, as may the presence of liver disease or coagulation defects.

For this reason, no recurrent bleeding from any source in the body should be ignored. There may indeed be a harmless explanation, but you should never assume that a streak of blood coughed up is merely due to the rupture of a small blood vessel lining the lung passages, or that a small amount of blood in the toilet bowl is necessarily caused by piles. Recurrent bleeding should always be investigated so that the source can be found.

The following section explains what happens when we bleed, and the possible consequences of any abnormalities in the blood-clotting process.

HOW CLOTTING OCCURS

Most people are aware that blood circulates around the body through veins and arteries. Arteries are blood vessels with relatively thick, elastic walls. They carry blood at pressure from the heart to the various tissues around the body, which take their oxygen from the red blood cells as they pass through. The blood is then re-collected into the veins, which are less elastic and more fragile blood vessels with thinner walls, and they then carry the blood back to the heart and lungs for recirculation. On the whole, arterial blood is brighter red than venous blood as it carries more oxygen. Injuries to arteries produce heavier bleeding, often with spurting, because the blood is under pressure. Blood loss from a vein tends to ooze but will clot fairly quickly.

When most people experience bruising or bleeding it is usually restricted to a particular site, and is the result of a local problem such as an injury, an infection, an ulcer or a tumour. In these circumstances, the clotting process will then be activated. First of all, when a blood vessel is damaged, its wall will contract, enabling it to reduce both its own size and the size of the laceration. Small fragments in the blood called platelets then appear, covering the breach, which then has special clotting proteins or factors deposited on it, which coagulate and form the platelet 'plug'. Any one of these processes may be affected by certain circumstances, for example where there is a weakness of blood vessels (hereditary haemorrhagic telangiectasia), or of platelets (bone-marrow abnormalities such as leukaemia), or of clotting factors (liver disease, haemophilia). In these cases, bleeding may appear in multiple sites. On the whole, platelet-plug problems cause superficial bleeding, usually in the skin (bruising) in the way of nosebleeds, or otherwise as vaginal bleeding.

This tends to happen in people taking anticoagulant drugs, and in those with vitamin K deficiency or liver disease. Problems with the clotting factors themselves cause bleeding in deeper tissues such as the muscles and joints, and are the result of a deficiency of individual clotting factors, as is seen in haemophilia, Von Willebrand's disease and Christmas disease.

Any doctor talking to a patient with generalized bleeding should therefore ask if he or she has ever bled excessively in the past, or had any relatives with bleeding problems. More specifically, they need to ask if the patient has ever had a tonsillectomy, any major abdominal or orthopaedic surgery, or dental extractions, and if so, if there was any abnormal bleeding. Investigations should then be carried out to exclude underlying problems within the clotting mechanism itself.

The rest of this chapter looks at bleeding from the various sites of the body in turn and examines the possible causes.

BRUISING

Most people noticing a bruise on their arm or leg raise an eyebrow and wonder how it got there. Usually they will be able to attribute it to a trivial knock or scrape they received during the course of the last few days, but if spontaneous bruising, or bruising with increasing regularity and severity occurs, they quite correctly begin to worry about it. For people with any of the hereditary blood-clotting disorders such as haemophilia, Von Willebrand's disease or Christmas disease (named after the first patient), such symptoms will be expected. In these conditions, congenital abnormalities of the blood's clotting mechanisms mean that one of the many different proteins involved in the clotting process is missing. The result is deep-seated bleeding in the internal organs or in the tissues of the muscles or joints, but bruising under the skin is also likely. These disorders run in families and regular and excessive bleeding occurs from birth. A congenital weakness of the walls of certain blood vessels known as telangiectasis also causes sufferers to experience bleeding in the same site on numerous occasions.

Generally speaking, however, there is usually a simple explanation for bruises appearing, but because they can sometimes signify a more serious underlying condition, it is worth examining the nature of your symptoms by asking yourself the following questions:

❷ Has there been any injury?

Direct or indirect blows to the skin will damage the underlying blood vessels, causing them to ooze blood and show up as a dark blue patch within a few minutes. The clotting mechanism takes over to reduce any further bleeding, but an immediate application of cold pressure can make the blood vessel contract, thereby reducing the bruising.

❷ Is your skin becoming more lined and wrinkly?

As the years go by, our skin becomes drier, thinner and less elastic. As a consequence, the blood vessels beneath the surface are more exposed and spontaneous bleeding from them is much more likely to occur, which is why elderly people often find numerous small purple-coloured haemorrhages on the backs of their hands. The condition is known as senile purpura, and is normal and harmless.

❷ Is your skin irritated or sore anywhere?

Any kind of allergic irritation of the skin, for example following an insect bite or a bee sting, can cause itching, swelling, and bleeding.

❷ Are you tired and anaemic with swollen joints?

Some of the auto-immune diseases, such as rheumatoid arthritis or polyarteritis, where the body produces antibodies against its own tissues, can reduce the number of platelets in the blood, and these are not then able to produce efficient clotting of the blood. Sufferers will therefore bruise more easily.

❷ Are you taking any medication?

People taking anticoagulant drugs, for example to treat deep-vein thrombosis of the leg, a blood clot on the lung, or a heart attack, will need to monitor the dosage of their medication very carefully as too much can cause excessive bleeding and bruising. Certain other drugs are also known to have a similar effect, including quinine, used in the treatment of leg cramps at night, and quinidine, used in the treatment of disordered rhythms of the heartbeat. Even some antibiotics and water tablets (diuretics) can produce spontaneous bruising.

❷ Have you a yellowish tinge to your skin and/or the whites of your eyes?

If you are bruising easily and also develop jaundice, the chances are that you have liver disease. The liver produces vitamin K, an essential ingredient in the blood-clotting process. People with cirrhosis, chronic hepatitis or other liver diseases are all likely to develop this combination of symptoms.

❷ Has your body shape changed? Are your limbs thin but your body heavy?

Cushing's syndrome is caused when over-activity of the adrenal glands situated just above the kidneys leads to the production of too much natural cortisone. The fault may lie with the adrenal glands themselves or there may be an abnormality in the pituitary gland at the base of the brain. Cortisone tends to break down protein in the body, including in blood-vessel walls, which as a result are rendered more fragile and breakable. Bruising is a common sign in Cushing's syndrome.

❷ *Are you taking steroids of any kind?*
Steroids administered in large and protracted dosages for severe asthma, or for auto-immune diseases, can produce bruising under the skin as a side effect. Close monitoring is necessary.

❷ *Have you had a cold or flu-like illness?*
Even fairly trivial viral infections can sometimes result in damage to the number and quality of blood platelets (blood cells that play an important role in the coagulation of blood). People especially sensitive to the effects of these viruses may need to be treated with cortisone,

and if the spleen, the organ mainly responsible for the reprocessing of blood cells, is affected, it may have to be removed. The viruses stimulate the production of antibodies in susceptible people, which damage platelets at the same time as eradicating the viruses themselves. Steroids prevent the antibodies from doing this. Steroids taken in small dosages for short periods will not cause problems.

❷ *Do you suffer from frequent infections and anaemia?*
The various forms of leukaemia, and other related conditions that affect the bone marrow, can cause bruising. Indeed, spontaneous and generalized bruising along with weakness and anaemia are important symptoms of leukaemia. But this is relatively rare.

SUMMARY
BRUISING

POSSIBLE CAUSE	ACTION
Trauma	Apply cold pressure to stop the bleeding.
Ageing skin	None.
Allergic reaction	Antihistamines or steroids.
Autoimmune disorders	Steroids and/or transfusion.
Medication	With your doctor, identify and discontinue drug responsible.
Liver disease	Dietary adjustment and medication.
Cushing's syndrome	Medication and/or surgery.
Steroids	Reduce dosage.
Viral illness	Steroid treatment. Removal of spleen if condition very serious and unresponsive to other treatment.
Leukaemia, bone-marrow disorders	Chemotherapy, platelet transfusions.

BLOODSHOT EYES

Whenever we meet someone, the focus of our attention is usually the eyes, so any degree of redness there appears very obvious indeed. In the most dramatic cases, the white of the eye can be transformed into a livid red colour, either in a small patch or extending right across the whole of the white of the eye. Usually, however, the eye just looks pink and 'angry', and generally speaking it usually looks worse than it actually is.

There are many causes of 'red eye' and sometimes the distribution of the redness can help in identifying the particular problem. For example, swollen blood vessels under the eyelids themselves together with discharge signify infection and inflammation in this area (conjunctivitis), whilst swollen blood vessels predominantly around the iris, the coloured part of the eye, especially when there is additional pain and visual disturbance, can often signify the presence of a more serious inflammation of the cornea, the clear part of the eye, or inflammation within the main structures of the eye inside.

To determine the cause of your symptom, ask yourself the following questions:

❷ Is the redness mainly under the lids?

If this is the case, the problem is conjunctivitis, which can be either allergic or infective in origin. If there is any pus or discharge coming from the eye, the cause is probably an infection, but if there is irritation and itching without any discharge, it is probably an allergic reaction.

❷ Has the white of the eye suddenly turned bright red?

With subconjunctival haemorrhage, a large part of the white of the eye is transformed into a bright red splash of colour. In this case, minor trauma to the tiny blood vessels on the eye's surface causes the vessels to rupture and then spread out. It can be the result of something as simple as rubbing your eyes over-vigorously, and the good news is that it is usually quite trivial. However, the patch tends to stay bright red because the released blood cells are near enough to the air to stay relatively well oxygenated, unlike a bruise under the skin, which will turn a blue-yellow colour. It usually takes 2–3 weeks for the colour to fade completely.

❷ Is the redness mainly around the iris (the coloured part of the eye)?

In this case, the redness may be associated with inflammation within the eye itself (iritis), with increased pressure of the fluid within the eye (acute glaucoma), or with inflammation of the cornea (keratitis), the clear part of the eye at the front.

❷ Is there a gritty sensation in the eye?

There may be a foreign body such as a fleck of dust or grit embedded on the very sensitive surface of the eye.

❷ Is the red eye painful?

Pain suggests something more than just conjunctivitis. Pain can be caused by a foreign body, by inflammation of the cornea (keratitis), by inflammation within the eye itself (iritis), by acute glaucoma, or by a number of generalized diseases, including diabetes and autoimmune diseases such as rheumatoid arthritis and systemic lupus erythematosus.

❷ Is there any visual disturbance?

Whilst conjunctivitis can produce a temporary blurring of the vision, usually cleared by blinking, more important inflammations of the cornea (keratitis) or within the eye itself, as the result of shingles, for example, will affect vision more significantly.

❷ Is there any change to the size and shape of the pupils?

Pupil size is not affected by conjunctivitis, but if the problem is inflammation of the cornea, a foreign body, or inflammation within the eye itself, differences between the two pupils can be seen.

❷ Is the eye very tender to touch?

Anything affecting the front of the eye such as conjunctivitis will make the eye sensitive to the touch. Glaucoma can make the entire eyeball tender. It occurs when the pressure of the fluid within the eyeball builds up. When this happens slowly, over many years, there is little pain or redness, but the vision will gradually deteriorate. However, when it happens suddenly, in acute glaucoma, there will be intense pain and redness. *Urgent treatment is required* to save the sight.

SUMMARY
BLOODSHOT EYES

POSSIBLE CAUSE	ACTION
Infective conjunctivitis	Antibiotic drops or ointment.
Allergic conjunctivitis	Decongestant, steroid or allergy-preventer drops.
Subconjunctival haemorrhage	Clears spontaneously.
Iritis (inflammation in the eye)	Medical treatment (usually steroids) for underlying cause.
Acute glaucoma	Drops or iridectomy (operation to allow fluid drainage).
Keratitis (inflammation of the cornea)	If infective, antibiotics. If inflammatory, steroids.
Foreign body	Removal under local or general anaesthetic.
Diabetes	Regulate blood sugar with tablets or insulin.
Autoimmune disease (rheumatoid arthritis, systemic lupus erythematosus)	Steroids. Supportive treatment.

BLEEDING FROM THE EAR

Small quantities of blood from the ear are usually the result of superficial irritation of the skin lining the ear canal. Profuse bleeding is almost always caused by serious injury.

❓ Is the ear painful to the touch, especially if you gently pull it?

This is suggestive of a boil or infected spot on the skin lining the ear canal. The skin is stretched very tightly over the bone here, with little room to expand, so acute pain may result.

❓ Is the ear itchy inside?

Infected eczema that has been scratched with a fingernail or cotton bud could be responsible.

❓ Did you have terrible earache deep inside the ear before the blood appeared?

Occasionally acute infections produce bleeding from the eardrum itself. This is particularly common in children with recurrent ear infections.

❓ Have you been exposed to a very loud noise or sudden air-pressure changes?

Occasionally the eardrum can bleed when it is ruptured following a very loud noise or sudden pressure changes, as can happen in situations such as deep-sea diving or flying in an aircraft.

❓ Has there been any head injury?

A larger amount of blood literally pouring from the ear is a more sinister sign, and is more usually seen when there has been a fracture of the skull as the result of a serious head injury, generally one bad enough to cause loss of consciousness. Should this be the case, *urgent transportation of the patient to hospital is essential* for further investigation and treatment.

SUMMARY
BLEEDING FROM THE EAR

POSSIBLE CAUSE	ACTION
Boil	Antibiotics by mouth, surgical drainage in severe cases.
Infected eczema	Antibiotic and anti-inflammatory drops or cream.
Acute infection	Antibiotics.
Ruptured eardrum	May heal spontaneously. Otherwise, surgical repair.
Head injury	Urgent hospitalization.

NOSEBLEEDS

There are many forms of nosebleeds, and generally speaking they are fairly harmless. Problems can range from a simple episode affecting one nostril to recurrent nosebleeds on one or other side, or even the occasional torrential haemorrhage from both nostrils with bleeding occurring not only down the front of the nose, but also down the back of the throat. Common causes include direct injuries to the face, picking and other interference to scabs just inside the nasal cavity, and spontaneous rupture of the little blood vessels lining the sensitive membrane inside the nose.

Most people are familiar with the first-aid measures required for a simple nosebleed. The patient pinches the nose between forefinger and thumb just below the bony bridge in the middle section. The pressure should be kept up for at least ten minutes, with the head pushed forward between the knees. Ten minutes is how long it normally takes for blood to coagulate, so trivial nosebleeds will settle within this time scale. Generally, however, the patients who visit their doctor with nosebleeds have troublesome, recurrent and sometimes heavy bleeding that has encouraged them to believe there may be some other underlying problem that requires attention.

❷ Do you have regular nosebleeds?

These are more common in children, but can be seen in adults. They usually occur on one side of the nose only, and can happen any time, without warning. They are precipitated by cold weather, physical exercise, sneezing and having a cold.

The problem is usually due to a weakness within the walls of a blood vessel within a patch of the lining membrane called Little's area, and treatment of this with cautery (burning), under local anaesthetic in hospital is generally recommended.

❷ Has there been any injury?

Obviously any trauma to the nose is likely to cause immediate bleeding, and any uncorrected damage to the sensitive mucous membranes lining the nasal passages, or to the bony structure itself, can cause recurrent nosebleeds. Nasal fractures where there has been displacement are best straightened surgically, and any long-standing inflammation of the lining passageways should receive attention.

❷ Have you always tended to bruise easily?

A number of inherited disorders including hereditary haemorrhagic telangiectasia, are characterized by fragility of blood vessel walls, and these can often come to a person's attention through nosebleeds. There is often a family history of abnormal bruising or nose bleeds, and any tendency to readily bleed with or without trauma may have been present for some time. Treatment involves cauterizing the weak blood vessels individually.

❷ Have you only recently tended to bruise easily?

Excessive bleeding from any site can be the first sign that the blood is not clotting as efficiently as it should. This can happen when the components of the blood itself are faulty, a problem that occurs in conditions ranging from simple virus infections through to very rare conditions such as leukaemia.

❷ Have you had your blood pressure checked recently?

It is always worth checking the blood pressure of anyone over 50 who complains of nosebleeds because occasionally it can be found to be significantly raised. When this happens, the elevated blood pressure damages the walls of the blood vessels, causing them to rupture and bleed profusely. Occasionally blood can haemorrhage not only from the front of the nose, but also at the back, leading to swallowing of the blood and subsequent vomiting. In these cases pressure on the front of the nose is insufficient, and *admission to hospital is urgently required* to prevent further blood loss and clinical shock. Treatment involves packing the nasal cavity from back to front to put pressure on all areas of the bleeding blood vessel. In due course, when the bleeding is under control, the blood pressure itself should be brought within normal limits.

SUMMARY
NOSEBLEEDS

POSSIBLE CAUSE	ACTION
Weak blood vessel	Cautery.
Nasal trauma	Nasal packing. Surgical correction of crooked nose (deviated septum) if necessary.
Congenital disorders	Cautery for nosebleeds. Transfusion if necessary.
Clotting disorders	Prevent platelet destruction from whatever cause, platelet transfusion. Transfuse with blood-clotting proteins.
Raised blood pressure	Medical treatment to stabilize blood pressure. Urgent hospital admission if severe haemorrhage from front and back of nose occurs.

BLEEDING GUMS

The gums are pink and fleshy as a result of their excellent blood supply. They are vulnerable to infection and inflammation. Being well supplied with nerve endings, they quickly tell us when something is wrong.

❷ Do your gums bleed when brushed?

It's really quite common for people to notice that their gums bleed a little if they brush their teeth overvigorously. Provided it happens only occasionally this is not sign of an underlying problem. However, when the teeth are not brushed often or adequately, tartar can build up around the base of the teeth and this can make the gums bleed in their own right.

❷ Are your gums swollen and sore?

Chronic inflammation of the gums (gingivitis) can erode the gums and the underlying bone, eventually leading not only to bleeding but to the loss of your teeth.

❷ Do you wear dentures or are you prone to mouth ulcers?

Ill-fitting dentures can cause bleeding, as can mouth ulcers and cold sores.

❷ Do you visit the dentist regularly?

Without regular brushing and dental treatment, dental caries and gum disease can occur. Abscess formation around the teeth also often causes bleeding.

❷ Are you diabetic?

Infections are more common in diabetics generally, and their gums do not escape.

❷ Is your diet satisfactory?

Scurvy used to be commonplace amongst sailors whose gums bled and teeth fell out due to the complete lack of vitamins C and K in their diet. Deficiencies of these vitamins still occasionally occur, but these days scurvy is rare.

SUMMARY
BLEEDING GUMS

POSSIBLE CAUSE	ACTION
Vigorous teeth brushing	Gentler brushing. Flossing. Visits to hygienist.
Gingivitis	Dental treatment.
Dentures	Check correct fitting.
Mouth ulcers	Steroid pellets to hold against ulcer, antiseptic paint, lozenges.
Dental caries and abscesses	Dental treatment.
Diabetes	Stringent dental hygiene and control of blood sugar.
Dietary deficiency	Plenty of fresh fruit and vegetables and milk. Vitamin C supplements.

VOMITING BLOOD

When blood is vomited it is almost always the result of bleeding disorders of the gullet, the stomach or the first part of the small intestine. The blood may then act as an irritant in the stomach and promote sickness. Depending on the site of the problem and its severity, blood may appear as a mere streaking in what is vomited or what is brought up may appear to consist entirely of blood. The colour of the blood can vary. Blood that is fresh and has not yet been acted upon by stomach acid will be bright red in colour, whereas blood from lower down the digestive system will be darker red or black and typically resemble coffee grounds.

There are a number of possible reasons for blood in the vomit (haematemesis). When trying to discover the exact cause, doctors investigate either by passing a fine, hollow tube down the gullet into the stomach and intestine (endoscopy), or with barium X-rays. Many cases of this type of bleeding will stop spontaneously, but if continuous bleeding results in low blood pressure and circulatory failure, blood transfusion and surgery to stop the source of the bleeding may be required.

❷ Did you vomit blood after a heavy nosebleed?
Bleeding from the back of the nose that is subsequently swallowed can irritate the lining of the stomach and be brought back up.

❷ Has any repetitive vomiting preceded the bleeding?
A tear in the lining of the gullet caused by persistent and violent vomiting can lead to the vomiting of bright red or dark-coloured blood. This is commonly seen after a night of alcoholic binging, and the blood lost through a tear in the gullet in this situation can lead to sometimes quite profuse bleeding. Usually, the bleeding will settle spontaneously.

❷ Have you been suffering from persistent indigestion?
Constant irritation of the lining of the stomach (gastritis) for whatever reason can cause bleeding. This may occur spontaneously or in response to dietary factors such as spicy or fatty foods coupled with a high alcohol intake. Smoking and caffeine are also important factors. Certain medications can also cause inflammation of the stomach lining, which may lead to bleeding. Examples are aspirin and aspirin-related products. Steroid drugs are also guilty of producing this effect.

❷ Do you suffer from recurrent sharp pain in the stomach area?
This suggests the possibility of a peptic ulcer. An ulcer is a breach in the lining membrane of any organ, in this case the stomach. Many of us have superficial ulcers for much of the time but they heal spontaneously within a few days, just like ulcers that can develop in the mouth. When an ulcer becomes deeper, however, it may penetrate the underlying structures of the stomach wall itself and can occasionally erode a blood vessel sitting at the base of the ulcer. In the case of an artery, this can result in sudden and dramatic haemorrhage leading to pain and copious vomiting of blood. Symptoms are pain in the pit of the stomach, usually worse between meals or in the middle of the night. The pain is usually well localized enough for the sufferer to be able to put a finger on the site of the pain. The pain is often alleviated by antacids, including milk, and exacerbated by alcohol, smoking and fatty or spicy foods.

❷ Are you or have you been a very heavy drinker? Have you recently been jaundiced?
Cirrhosis is an inflammation of the liver. There are a number of potential causes, the commonest being chronic alcohol consumption

and hepatitis. The liver becomes shrunken and scarred, leading to congestion of blood in the veins. This in turn leads to congestion in other veins, including those running up under the lining of the oesophagus which become varicose: swollen, congested, tortuous and liable to break. When they do, torrential bleeding can occur. *Vomiting blood from this source is a medical emergency.*

❷ Have you lost a lot of weight?
Cancer can also cause stomach bleeding,. Erosion of a blood vessel in the stomach wall occurs, leading to blood loss within the stomach followed by vomiting. Additional symptoms usually include sudden and dramatic weight loss, indigestion and loss of appetite. There may also be anaemia, and a palpable lump in the abdomen.

❸ *Do you tend to bruise easily?*
Anyone with an increased tendency to bruise or bleed easily because of problems with the clotting mechanism or because of anticoagulant therapy is obviously more likely to develop bleeding from within the stomach. Easy bleeding syndrome, as it is known, has no underlying cause and is not serious in itself.

SUMMARY
VOMITING BLOOD

POSSIBLE CAUSE	ACTION
Heavy nosebleed	*If bleeding persists, admission to hospital for packing of nose. Otherwise, no treatment needed.*
Persistent vomiting	*Anti-emetic treatment, antacids.*
Gastritis	*Avoid aspirin, steroids, alcohol, caffeine, tobacco. Antacid therapy.*
Medication	*Avoid aspirin. With your doctor, identify and then discontinue or reduce dosage of drug responsible.*
Peptic ulcer	*Dietary modification, antacids, H2 blocking drugs. Proton pump inhibitors for resistant ulcers. If there is severe blood loss with collapse, immediate emergency care to arrest haemorrhage, blood transfusion.*
Varicose veins in the oesophagus due to cirrhosis of the liver	*Emergency medical and surgical treatment.*
Stomach cancer	*Surgery.*
Easy bleeding syndrome	*Medical correction if appropriate.*

BLEEDING FROM THE NIPPLE

Any blood emanating from the nipple should be checked by a doctor. It might well turn out to be something as simple as a cracked nipple or even trauma as the result of breast-feeding, but it is essential to exclude the possibility of an underlying cancer of the breast, whether or not a lump can also be felt. The following questions should help you to identify the possible cause of any bleeding in this area:

❷ Is the nipple dry, sore and cracked?

A cracked nipple, inflamed eczema or trauma caused by breast-feeding can all produce these common symptoms.

❸ Is the bloodstained discharge coming from one nipple only, and is there any lump below the nipple area?

Sometimes very tiny growths in the breast ducts themselves can produce bleeding, so these should always be checked out carefully. One-side bleeding from the nipple, with or without underlying lumps in the breast, should always be investigated urgently. X-rays of the breasts (mammography) can be offered to most women over the age of 35, and a nationwide breast screening policy for all women between the ages of 50 and 65 is currently in operation.

SUMMARY
BLEEDING FROM THE NIPPLE

POSSIBLE CAUSE	ACTION
Cracked nipple, inflamed eczema, breast-feeding	*Protective, antiseptic barrier creams, breast pumps if necessary.*
Breast lump below nipple	*Urgent investigation. Surgery if necessary.*

153

EXCESSIVE VAGINAL BLEEDING

At the beginning of the cycle, oestrogen stimulates the thickening of the lining of the uterus to prepare it for a possible pregnancy. Halfway through the cycle, or, more precisely, 14 days before the next expected period, an egg is released from one ovary, an event that coincides with a surge in the production of progestogen, another female sex hormone. This one causes the cells lining the uterus to swell even further, preparing them for the implantation of any fertilized egg. If this fails to happen, production of both female sex hormones diminishes, resulting in the shedding of the cells lining the womb, which are expelled from the uterus to the outside by way of muscular uterine contractions. The average blood loss is about 30 ml in each period, although there is enormous individual variation. Heavier periods, although normal and not attributable to any underlying disease process, can nevertheless produce a level of discomfort that can alter a woman's quality of life and affect her ability to work for 2–3 days or more each month. Treatment is required if this is the case, and anyway, it is quite unnecessary to endure discomfort purely on the basis that it is nature's way.

Sometimes, however, excessive vaginal bleeding can be the result of an underlying disorder. If this is a possibility, your doctor will carry out a vaginal examination to detect any obvious changes in the pelvic organs. A speculum is usually inserted into the vagina so that inspection of the cervix can be carried out and a cervical smear taken. Blood tests can also help to determine the underlying cause. Often it will turn out to be something easily curable such as a reaction to the contraceptive coil, but when it isn't, referral to a gynaecologist will be necessary so that additional tests and possibly treatment can be started. As a general rule,

however, all women should have a smear test every three years as a matter of routine. It is also important to remember that good general health, nutrition, exercise and hygiene are all necessary for 'normal' menstrual function.

However, if you do have problems with excessive vaginal bleeding, consult the following check list of questions to help you identify the possible underlying cause of the conditon:

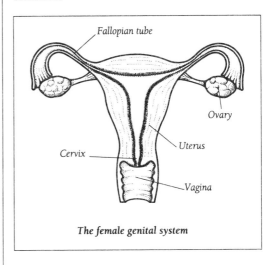

The female genital system

❷ *Have you been under a lot of stress recently?*

Often the onset of heavier or irregular periods coincides with stressful life events such as bereavement, leaving home, relationship difficulties or a change in jobs. These psychological tensions can have a profound influence on the hypothalamus and pituitary glands at the base of the brain, which have an overriding controlling function in the production of the female sex hormones responsible for a normal menstrual cycle. If you are experiencing such lifestyle factors, keep an accurate diary for at least three months to assess the pattern. If the excessive bleeding is still unresolved after this time, other causes should be considered.

❷ Are you in your late 40s or early 50s and have you had any hot flushes lately?

During the menopause there is a gradual diminution in the production of oestrogen as eggs are no longer produced, or produced less often by the ovaries. Such hormonal fluctuations lead to hot flushes, insomnia, irritability, weigh gain, skin changes, and, most commonly, to excessive and irregular bleeding. Keep a diary of your periods, including duration, quantity of blood loss and pain, because these can be helpful when consulting your doctor as to the best available treatment. These include hormone replacement therapy, a D&C (dilatation and curettage), hysterectomy or a new technique called an endometrial resection where only the blood-shedding lining of the womb is removed.

❷ Have you noticed swelling of the lower abdomen and the need to empty your bladder more often?

Large fibroids, which are muscular swellings in the wall of the uterus, may enlarge to the extent that swelling of the abdomen and pressure on the bladder occurs. Smaller fibroids, however, may only cause excessive bleeding, especially if the fibroids grow towards the internal cavity of the womb as opposed to the outside. As in the case of ovarian cysts, sometimes only an internal examination by a doctor will detect the presence of the fibroid. They are amongst the commonest causes of excessive bleeding.

❷ Have you had a coil fitted in the last 3 months?

Although the intrauterine contraceptive device or coil suits most women, a minority experience heavier or irregular bleeding after it has been fitted. Generally speaking, minor symptoms will settle down within 3 months, but if this is not the case or if the symptoms are severe, the coil should be removed and an alternative method of contraception chosen.

❷ Do you take the mini-pill?

The mini-pill, or progestogen-only pill, needs to be taken every day at the same time for 28 days in a row. There is no oestrogen component and menstrual irregularities, including excessive bleeding, are more common with this type of pill. If the periods do not settle down within 3 months, or if the symptoms are severe, an alternative method of contraception should be chosen.

❷ Have you lost or gained weight for no apparent reason?

Thyroid-gland disorders are not uncommon causes of excessive bleeding. The gland is the body's natural thermostat and controls the general speed at which the body works. An over- or underactive gland can upset the menstrual cycle, but often such changes are noticed in the context of weight gain (underactive gland) or weight loss (overactive gland) when no attempt at dieting has been made.

❷ Are you or could you be pregnant and miscarrying?

Pregnancy normally causes absent periods. However, where pregnancy has been established, excessive bleeding may be a sign of miscarriage or of a ruptured ectopic pregnancy. Miscarriage occurs in about one in five of all pregnancies, often for no explained reason, and produces lower abdominal, cramp-like pain and bleeding, sometimes profuse. An ectopic pregnancy is one that has established itself in the fallopian tube rather than in the lining of the womb. As the growing foetus stretches the narrow wall of the fallopian tube, it may rupture causing brisk haemorrhage and pain. In either case it would be unlikely for excessive pain to occur until at least four weeks after the missed period. *If there is a possibility that you are pregnant and you experience these symptoms, see your doctor urgently.*

❷ Do you suffer from backache and pain on intercourse?

These symptoms together with an increasing desire to pass urine and infertility indicate endometriosis. Here the tissue that normally lines the womb and bleeds at monthly intervals has escaped along the fallopian tubes to the ovary and the outside walls of the uterus, bladder, fallopian tubes and, occasionally, the intestines. Bleeding may occur from these sites at monthly intervals, producing inflammation and long-term adhesions within the pelvis.

❷ Have you noticed slight bleeding after intercourse?

This is most likely to be experienced in the presence of a cervical erosion (roughening of the neck of the womb), or in the presence of a cervical polyp (see above).

❷ Is the bleeding only slight but present most of the time?

This is suggestive of a polyp or an erosion of the cervix, the neck of the womb. A polyp is a pear-shaped, fleshy outgrowth from the lining of the womb or cervix that can become irritated and bleed from its surface. It is benign.

❷ Did the bleeding start up again several months after the menopause?

Postmenopausal bleeding occurs by definition a year after the last menstrual period. However, any bleeding occurring several months after what is thought to be the menopause should be regarded with a high degree of suspicion since this when cervical and endometrial cancer are commonest. *Urgent investigation by your doctor or gynaecologist is essential.*

❷ Have you had any vaginal discharge, pain and a high temperature?

This suggests an infection either of the womb itself (endometriosis) or of the fallopian tubes (salpingitis). If long-standing, the inflammation is referred to as pelvic inflammatory disease, the most important complication of which is possible infertility. *These symptoms should be reported to a doctor as soon as possible.*

❷ Have you noticed swelling in your lower abdomen or deep-seated pain or discomfort during intercourse?

These symptoms are suggestive of a large ovarian cyst, although small ovarian cysts can cause excessive bleeding without there being any other symptoms. Only a doctor's internal examination can detect such a silent cyst, and therefore excessive bleeding requires full examination if symptoms are prolonged.

❷ Have you any clotting disorders in your blood or do you take anticoagulants?

Whilst anyone who knows she has a clotting disorder or is taking anticoagulants would be aware of an increased tendency for unexplained bleeding, it is easy to forget these underlying complaints and regard vaginal bleeding as due to a gynaecological cause. However, if the anticoagulant dosage is not appropriate or the clotting disorder inadequately controlled, excessive bleeding may occur.

❷ Have you any vaginal discharge?

Most forms of sexually transmitted disease can produce some vaginal discharge and irritation, but will rarely cause menstrual abnormalities unless the infection ascends to the lining of the uterus and to the fallopian tubes. If this occurs, abdominal pain and fever generally ensue, and at that point excessive vaginal bleeding may occur. *Prompt treatment is required.*

SUMMARY
EXCESSIVE VAGINAL BLEEDING

POSSIBLE CAUSE	ACTION
Stress	Share problems with friends or family. Professional counselling, stress management, psychotherapy.
The menopause	Hormone replacement therapy, D&C (dilatation and curettage), hysterectomy or endometrial resection.
Fibroids	Myomectomy (removal of fibroid alone), or hysterectomy if fibroid large and family has been completed.
Coil	Choose alternative method of contraception.
Mini-pill	Choose alternative method of contraception.
Thyroid-gland disorder	Restore thyroid function through drugs or surgery.
Miscarriage	May settle spontaneously, although D&C (dilatation and curettage) may be required.
Ectopic pregnancy	Urgent surgery to stem bleeding and remove affected fallopian tube and ovary.
Endometriosis	Hormone treatment and/or surgery.
Cervical erosion	Cautery using silver nitrate.
Polyp	Surgical removal.
Endometrial cancer	Hysterectomy or anti-cancer therapy.
Cervical cancer	Cone biopsy or hysterectomy and anti-cancer therapy.
Pelvic inflammatory disease	Antibiotics and pain relief. Hospitalization.
Ovarian cyst	May settle spontaneously, otherwise surgery with anti-cancer therapy if malignant.
Clotting disorder or anticoagulants	Check blood-clotting status and use blood-clotting factors by transfusion or adjust dose of anticoagulants.

IRREGULAR AND UNEXPECTED PERIODS

On average periods last from two to seven days and can be light, moderate or heavy. Although most women experience a period every 28 days, the actual interval between cycles can be as short as 21 days or as long as 35. The cycle is governed by a complex chain of events that begin in the brain and affect the ovary and uterus in turn, leading to the monthly flow of blood from the lining of the womb.

Any departure from the regular monthly cycle can cause a great deal of inconvenience and worry. Such problems include bleeding between periods, bleeding after sexual intercourse, bleeding despite taking the oral contraceptive pill, periods missed for a month or two at a time, and periods occurring every two to three weeks. The underlying cause could be a problem anywhere in the complex sequence of events that lead to the monthly cycle, and working out the exact cause may require patient evaluation of the person's lifestyle, a full physical examination and a series of investigations.

❷ Are you suffering from stress of any kind?

There is no doubt that emotional worries can create temporary psychological disturbances that affect the first step of the menstrual cycle in the higher functions of the brain itself. This is why, for example, teenage girls who have already begun their periods may notice significant irregularities or stop having them when they move away from home for the first time, or experience emotional problems.

❷ Are you taking the contraceptive pill?

Missing one pill rarely causes difficulties, but forgetting to take more than two often does. Taking the daily contraceptive pill keeps the lining of the womb in a pregnancy-like state in which shedding of the lining does not take place. If more than two pills are missed, the lining of the womb will break down and a small amount of 'spotting' or breakthrough bleeding will occur. The reliability of the pill as a contraceptive will also be lost.

❷ Are you taking any medication?

A number of drugs and medications can interfere with the normal level of sex hormones in the female body, resulting in irregular periods. It is always worth asking your doctor about the medications you have been prescribed.

❷ Are you breast-feeding?

The hormones released during breast-feeding can inhibit the normal menstrual cycle. For this reason, periods may not return to normal in breast-feeding mothers for several months after childbirth.

❷ Do you feel constantly hot and are you losing weight?

These symptoms suggest an overactive thyroid gland, which can cause menstrual irregularities. With an overactive thyroid gland, the presence of too much thyroxine hormone stimulates the body's metabolism to work faster than normal, so that other common symptoms include diarrhoea, excessive sweating, a fast pulse, palpitations, increased appetite and intolerance of hot weather.

❷ Do you feel constantly cold and have you gained weight?

An underactive thyroid gland causing the metabolism to slow down can lead to menstrual irregularities. Associated symptoms include constipation, coarse, thinning hair, intolerance of cold and thickening of the skin on the lower leg.

❷ Is the bleeding fairly light but continuous?

Polyps are benign, fleshy growths that emerge from the lining of the womb or from the lining of the cervix. They can alter the frequency and amount of menstrual blood flow.

❷ Is there a bloodstained discharge?

The cervix may develop an 'erosion' or roughening of its surface, and may develop polyps or indeed cancer. An internal examination and smear test are necessary.

❷ Has there been any fever, vaginal discharge and abdominal pain?

Pelvic infection caused by a sexually transmitted disease can not only lead to infertility but may also result in menstrual irregularities. Usually there is a history of vaginal discharge and abdominal pain, with or without a high temperature, and *these symptoms should be urgently investigated and treated.*

❷ Did the 'period' begin more than a year after your last period?

Post-menopausal bleeding *should be urgently investigated* by a gynaecologist. It should be considered the result of a malignancy until proved otherwise. It is far better to be safe than sorry.

SUMMARY
IRREGULAR AND
UNEXPECTED PERIODS

POSSIBLE CAUSE	ACTION
Stress	Adjustment of lifestyle, stress management.
Oral contraceptive pill	Explanation. No action required.
Medication	Discuss discontinuing or reducing dosage of drug responsible with your doctor.
Breast-feeding	No action required.
Thyroid disorders	Medical or surgical treatment.
Polyps	Surgical removal.
Cervical 'erosion' (erythroplakia)	If smear normal, cauterization.
Cervical cancer	Laser treatment, cone biopsy, surgery, radiotherapy.
Pelvic infection	Antibiotics and/or surgery.
Post-menopausal bleeding	Urgent investigation and treatment in hospital.

ABSENT PERIODS

The absence of normal monthly bleeding can be as alarming as excessive vaginal bleeding to the woman concerned, who may worry that it is a sign of an underlying disease. Fortunately, this is hardly ever the case and most of the causes of absent periods are reversible. However, a big mistake that some people make is to assume that because they are not having their periods there is no chance of their becoming pregnant. This is certainly not the case. Ovulation can still take place even when periods are absent and contraceptive precautions are therefore recommended to anyone enjoying an active sex life.

❷ Have your previously regular periods suddenly stopped?

If this is the situation, there is an underlying hormonal imbalance that is creating the problem. The commonest cause of absent periods is pregnancy and the first question you should ask yourself is whether there is any possibility at all of your having conceived.

❷ Are you taking the pill?

The oral contraceptive pill tends to lessen the flow of menstrual blood in all women, but occasionally may lead to periods being absent altogether, on either a one-off or a regular basis.

❷ Are you breast-feeding?

Hormones released during breast-feeding can inhibit the normal menstrual cycle. For this reason, periods may not return in breast-feeding mothers for several months after childbirth, which is why in the past breast-feeding was relied upon as a form of contraception. However, even though periods may be absent during this time, this should not be regarded as a reliable method of contraception.

❷ Have your periods not yet started?

Nowadays girls tend to start their periods from the age of 11 or 12, and it is unusual not have started by the age of 15 or 16. It's worth asking whether your mother was late starting because this often runs in families. Emotional factors such as changing school, losing a parent or relationship difficulties can often delay the start of menstruation, but the possibility of an underlying illness such as anaemia or depression should be excluded. Often the hormones have not yet been kick-started into action and this may be the result of some eating disorder such as anorexia nervosa. Investigations need to look at the entire chain of events that lead to a normal menstrual cycle, which in the first instance will involve blood tests and X-rays.

❷ Are you particularly worried about anything?

Emotional worries can cause temporary psychological disturbances that affect the first step of the menstrual cycle in the brain's higher functions, causing the sufferer to stop having periods or to experience irregularities.

❷ Are you underweight for your height, exercising vigorously or crash dieting?

Any of these factors can temporarily put the body in starvation mode and cut off the pituitary hormones, which in turn govern menstrual function. When weight is regained, the periods will usually resume spontaneously. In the eating disorders bulimia and anorexia, absent periods are very common indeed.

❷ Are you in your late 40s or early 50s or have you had your ovaries removed surgically?

During the menopause the levels of circulating oestrogen fall dramatically so that periods no longer occur.

❷ *Has your weight changed recently and unwanted hair begun to be noticeable?*
Glandular irregularities affecting the ovaries and adrenal glands may lead to absent periods. Tumours in these glands produce excessive amounts of female hormone. Greasy skin, acne, body and facial hair may be among the first symptoms noticed. Thankfully, these disorders are relatively rare.

SUMMARY
ABSENT PERIODS

POSSIBLE CAUSE	ACTION
Pregnancy	Counselling and support.
The pill	Reassurance.
Breast-feeding	No action required.
Emotional or psychological	Reassurance counselling, social support.
Weight problems and eating disorders	Psychotherapy, dietary supervision, antidepressants.
The menopause	Hormone replacement therapy if symptoms troublesome.
Ovarian or adrenal tumour	Surgical excision. Radio- or chemotherapy.

BLOOD IN THE URINE

Blood in the urine is always a worrying sign, particularly as a little bit of blood goes an awfully long way once it is diluted in a large volume of urine. Because of this, patients often report the loss of a large quantity of blood when in reality they have probably lost a couple of teaspoonfuls. Nevertheless, they are quite right to be concerned as one of the oldest maxims in medicine is never ignore blood in the urine. In most instances it will simply be coming from the bladder, where an infection has irritated the lining (cystitis).

When infection is not the cause, however, the entire urinary system has to be considered as bleeding can come from any part of it, from high up in the kidneys to further down in the urethra. The colour of the blood itself will be a good clue to the source of the bleeding. Blood coming from the kidney area will often produce a browny tinge to the urine, whereas blood coming from just inside the urethra (the tube connecting the bladder to the outside) will appear brighter red in colour. If there is any doubt about the nature of the problem, your doctor will carry out a number of tests to identify the source of the bleeding. These include an MSU (a midstream urine specimen) to test for the presence of infection, and a 'culture and sensitivity' test, when the laboratory cultures any bacteria that may be growing in the urine over 48 hours. This also helps to determine to which antibiotics that particular bug would be sensitive.

In order to exclude the possibility of cervical cancer being the source of the bleeding, a cervical smear will be taken at the same time, and a cystoscopy, where the lining of the bladder is viewed through a special telescope passed through the urethra under general anaesthetic, is often the next step. Ultrasound scans of the kidney and bladder may also identify various problems and if the cause still remains in question two further options are an IVP, in which the patient is injected with a special dye that is excreted through the kidneys to allow X-ray viewing of the urinary system, and a CAT scan.

❸ Do you need to empty your bladder more often than usual?

The very common symptom of frequently needing to empty your bladder, even for small amounts, is most usually associated with cystitis, although it can also happen after radiotherapy treatment given for almost any pelvic tumour. Drink plenty of water to flush away germs.

❸ Is the pain continuous?

Unlike colic which comes and goes, the presence of continuous pain suggests an infection or inflammation of the kidney itself. The pain is usually of a dull, aching nature and is usually felt in the back.

Ascending infection from cystitis may lead to infection in the kidney, but auto-immune diseases such as polyarteritis nodosa and lupus erythematosus may damage the cells within the kidney, leading to bleeding and loss of normal function. In this case, there may also be high blood pressure, a decrease or increase in the amount of urine passed, swelling of the eyes, hands and feet; and the patient may also experience general malaise and anaemia.

❸ Does it hurt when you urinate?

Pain passing water when there is blood in the urine is usually associated with an infection in either the bladder or the urethra. It may, however, be the first sign of a sexually transmitted disease such as nonspecific urethritis or gonorrhoea. In the latter, urethral discharge is usually an accompanying feature.

❷ Do you also have an excruciating, knife-like pain that comes and goes?

The intense spasmodic pain of kidney colic is quite unique, and is usually described as knife-like. When associated with blood in the urine, it is almost always due to kidney stones on the move. Kidney stones tend to move down from the kidney through the ureter, which is richly supplied with sensitive nerves.

❷ Do you see the blood as you start to empty your bladder or towards the end?

Normal clear urine that becomes bloodstained towards the end of the stream suggests that the blood is coming from the bladder. Possible causes include cystitis, benign polyps and malignancies. Simple mechanical irritation can also sometimes be responsible. Many long-distance runners experience blood in the urine as a result of the continuous pounding the bladder takes against the pubic bone as the abdominal organs jolt up and down. Blood seen at the start of the stream suggests a much more superficial source of the bleeding, perhaps just inside the urethra itself, caused by a sexually transmitted disease, trauma from unlubricated sexual intercourse, hospital catheterization or the insertion of a foreign body, or in the prostate as the result of prostate enlargement, either benign or malignant, or prostatitis, infection within the prostate gland. Blood mixed evenly throughout the stream suggests haemorrhage from higher up in the kidney area.

❷ Is there persistent blood in the urine without any discomfort?

These symptoms make the more common and benign conditions such as infection and stones less likely. The possibility of a benign or cancerous tumour in the bladder or kidney arises, as does the possibility of an autoimmune disorder. *Urgent investigation is required.*

❷ Are you passing thick clots of blood?

Bleeding heavy enough to produce clots is usually caused by tumours in the bladder or kidney, either benign or malignant. *Urgent consultation with your doctor is necessary.*

❷ Have you suffered any kind of blow directly to your back in the last few days?

Occasionally, a significant blow to the back can bruise or even rupture a kidney. As well as pain and bruising over the site of the trauma, there may often be blood in the urine the next time the victim goes to the loo or, if unconscious, is catheterized. For this reason, patients attending Accident and Emergency departments with back injuries are asked to wait until they have passed a sample of urine, even after they have been clinically examined and given the all clear.

❷ Are you taking any medication?

There are a number of substances, such as beetroot, that can be excreted through the kidneys that will give the urine a reddy-orange tinge resembling blood without any blood being present. Laxatives containing the dye phenolphthalein can also have this effect, as can Pyridium, used as a locally reacting anaesthetic for any sort of discomfort in the urinary system, and Rifadin, used in the treatment of tuberculosis.

However, people who take anticoagulants should be warned that bloodstaining of the urine can occur if the dosage taken is excessive. In this case, checks should be made to determine the appropriate.

❷ Is there any irregularity of the heart rhythm? Do you have a heart murmur? Have you recently suffered a stroke?

Any of these factors would make the possibility of an embolism more likely. Emboli are blood clots that form on the walls of damaged arteries and then break off and travel around in the blood stream. When one reaches a sufficiently narrow artery, it will lodge there, blocking off the supply of oxygen to any structures nourished by that blood vessel. If the clot is not dissolved within a few hours by the body's natural anticoagulant system, the cells in those structures will die. In the kidney, cell death leads to blood in the urine.

SUMMARY
BLOOD IN THE URINE

POSSIBLE CAUSE	ACTION
Infection of bladder (cystitis), kidney, urethra or ureter	Identify organism responsible. Antibiotics. Follow-up to ensure resolution and exclude recurrence.
Kidney stone	Small stones treated by highly focused ultra-sound waves (lithotripsy), large ones surgery.
Mechanical irritation of the bladder	High fluid intake and rest.
Prostate enlargement	If benign (90 per cent), medical treatment or surgical excision or laser ablation if severe. If malignant, surgical excision and radiotherapy.
Prostatitis	Antibiotics.
Tumours, benign or malignant, in kidney, bladder and ureter	Surgery and/or radiotherapy.
Sexually transmitted disease	Accurate diagnosis and antibiotics.
Direct injury	Possible surgery.
Trauma to urethra	Hot salt-water bathing. If caused by catheterization, no treatment necessary. If caused by foreign body, removal of foreign body, patient education. If caused by unlubricated sex, abstinence for a few days.
Medication	Reassurance for staining of urine from medicinal dyes (Rifadin, Pyridium, laxatives). Reduce dosage of anticoagulants, depending on blood-clotting tests.
Embolism	Anticoagulants.
Autoimmune disorder of the kidney	Steroids or immunosuppressants.

BLOOD IN THE SEMEN

Few symptoms are more guaranteed to have anxious men rushing to the surgery than ejaculated blood. As a symptom, it seems to be associated with the irrational but firmly held fear that their 'bits' are about to fall off. In fact, the truth of the matter is that the blood is almost always harmless.

❷ Did the symptom appear out of the blue?

Temporary congestion of the veins in the prostatic area may be at fault. However, gradual, benign enlargement of the prostate, which occurs in the majority of men as they grow older, although it only leads to symptoms in one in three men over the age of 50, could also be responsible. Associated symptoms in this case would be emptying the bladder more often, a poor urinary stream with little pressure, dribbling, difficulty starting, and blood in the urine. A small percentage of prostatic enlargements are due to cancer within the gland and the associated symptoms are almost identical. The older the man, the greater the risk, so these kind of urinary problems should never be ignored.

❷ Do you have, or have you recently had, any penile discharge or discomfort?

Any low-grade infection of the prostate gland as a result of sexually transmitted disease or catheterization can occasionally cause bloodstaining of the semen. Antibiotic treatment will clear this up.

SUMMARY
BLOOD IN THE SEMEN

POSSIBLE CAUSE	ACTION
Congested veins	A 'one-off' episode may be ignored. Otherwise, consider surgery.
Enlarged prostate (benign)	Repeated symptoms may require medical treatment with the drug finasteride, or surgical excision.
Infection	Antibiotics.
Enlarged prostate (cancer)	Surgery, hormone therapy, chemotherapy, radiotherapy.

BLOOD IN THE MOTIONS

This is a very important symptom indeed. Bleeding can be the result of a variety of causes anywhere along the considerable length of the gastrointestinal system, which runs between the food pipe and the anus. Whilst blood emanating from above the stomach, from the mouth, throat or oesophagus, is usually vomited, blood coming from a source below the stomach will generally make the motions a darker colour. Bleeding from within the stomach itself can go either way.

The colour of the blood reported is therefore an important clue to the source. Fresh red blood suggests the blood is coming from a fairly superficial site, for example the bright red streaks seen with piles. Blood that has come from higher up, however, and which has been altered by the actions of digestive enzymes, acids and juices, and which has lost the oxygen it once contained, may produce jet-black stools with a tar-like consistency. Quantities of blood loss are difficult to estimate, but just two teaspoons of blood will be enough to colour the motions black. Daily blood loss of this nature is quite sufficient to produce anaemia, with its symptoms of pale skin, shortness of breath and fatigue, if it occurs over a period of time.

The causes of blood in the motions are manifold, and most of them are benign and eminently easy to treat without drastic intervention. However, because serious disorders of the gastrointestinal system can remain relatively 'silent' until bleeding becomes obvious through discoloration of the motions, doctors obey a cardinal rule that any sign of blood from the bowel should be regarded as a possible sign of underlying cancer until proved otherwise. Investigations will involve a full blood count to determine the degree of any anaemia resulting from chronic blood loss, plus various endoscopic tests to look down the gullet and into the stomach, or up through the rectum and bowel towards the stomach. Any abnormal tissue can then be viewed directly or biopsied for an accurate diagnosis. Barium X-ray examinations, either barium meals or barium enemas, still have a place in diagnosis too.

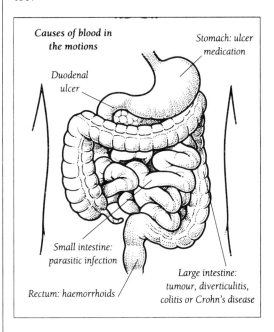

Causes of blood in the motions

Stomach: ulcer medication

Duodenal ulcer

Small intestine: parasitic infection

Rectum: haemorrhoids

Large intestine: tumour, diverticulitis, colitis or Crohn's disease

❷ Is the blood only on the outside of the motion or on the toilet paper?
This would indicate that the blood is coming from a more superficial site, as is the case with haemorrhoids (piles), for example, perhaps the commonest cause of blood in the motions. Accompanying symptoms can also include pain and the swollen lumpiness of the varicose veins, which can be felt as they push out through the anus. A simple examination carried out by the doctor will confirm the diagnosis, but if this proves not to be the case, further investigations are essential.

❷ Is there any accompanying pain?
Pain felt when actually going to the lavatory

suggests a problem located within the rectum itself. Haemorrhoids or a fissure (a split in the sensitive lining here) may be the cause. On the other hand, a well-localized, dull, aching pain in the abdomen occurring when the sufferer is not going to the loo is more suggestive of an inflammation of the bowel (colitis), an infection or a bowel tumour.

❷ Is there any anal itching?

Local irritation due to eczema or fungal infection leading to itching and scratching at the back passage may cause bleeding.

❷ Is indigestion a problem? Do you have a burning pain in the centre of your stomach that is worse between meals?

Two of the commonest causes of blood in the stools are inflammation of the lining of the stomach (gastritis) and peptic ulcers.

❷ Are you taking any medication?

Prescribed medications can cause problems, as is the case with certain antibiotics, including gentamicin, erythromycin, lincomycin and clindamycin, but so can steroids and aspirin and aspirin-related products used in the treatment of arthritis. Potassium supplements for people who are on certain diuretics (water tablets), especially if they are also taking digitalis, a drug to control disordered rhythms of the heart that can cause blood in the motions by itself, can also be responsible. The potassium has an irritant effect on the lining of the gut and there have been a few cases of bleeding as a result. Dark motions can also be produced by iron supplements, taken for anaemia and during pregnancy, and perhaps the commonest of such causes, by charcoal biscuits to control flatulence, by liquorice-based products used in the treatment of stomach ulcers, stomach settlers, bismuth-containing preparations to treat diarrhoea, and

even by blueberries. In this case, the motions will be black, but won't have the tar-like consistency they have when blood is present.

❷ Is there fainting and weakness?

These symptoms combined with blood in the motions suggests a heavy bleed from, for example, a severe peptic ulcer, which can then be a *potentially life-threatening situation*. Investigation of the cause here takes second place to correcting the blood loss through hospitalization and blood transfusion.

❷ Do you pass mucus as well as blood?

Generalized inflammatory diseases of the bowel such as ulcerative colitis and Crohn's disease may also produce abdominal discomfort, weight loss and anaemia. These conditions usually start in young adulthood and produce ulceration and thickening of the bowel wall. Although some kinds of colitis are infective in origin and temporary, neither of these two disorders has been adequately explained in terms of cause. The passage of blood with mucus rectally is suggestive of their presence. The bleeding may be so high up in the bowel that the motions are black, or so low down in the bowel that the bleeding is red. Somewhere between these two extremes is more likely, so that maroon-coloured blood is perhaps more suggestive of these conditions.

❷ Is the blood mixed uniformly with the motions, or is it on the outside of the motion?

Blood mixed with the motion itself suggests that the bleeding is occurring higher up in the gastrointestinal system, for example as the result of peptic ulcers in the duodenum or stomach, or of tumours of the stomach wall. Ulceration in the oesophagus (oesophagitic) or ruptured blood vessels in the oesophagus from excess vomiting are also possibilities.

❷ Have your bowel habits altered recently?

Are you opening your bowel more or less often than has been usual during your life? If there have been recent changes, perhaps accompanied by loss of appetite and/or weight loss, and particularly if the motions have taken on a ribbon-like consistency, the presence of blood, especially when dark, is suggestive of a tumour of the stomach or bowel. Occasionally bowel tumours can make people feel they want to open their bowels again, even after they have just been emptied, but irritable bowel syndrome can do this too.

❷ Is there diarrhoea?

Diarrhoea and constipation can both be caused by underlying cancers of the bowel, but infection and inflammation of the bowel (colitis) can also produce diarrhoea with bleeding.

❷ Have you travelled abroad to any exotic locations recently?

Occasionally people report after a trip abroad, especially to tropical countries, that they have bloody diarrhoea. Parasitic or bacterial infections may well be responsible, in which case a laboratory examination of a stool sample can identify the causative organism and determine the appropriate treatment.

❷ Are you or have you been a chronic heavy drinker?

When the liver is damaged by excessive alcohol intake it scars. This is called cirrhosis. Like any scar tissue it is solid and hard and the blood flow within it becomes sluggish and congested. This in turn leads to congestion in other blood vessels, including the veins lining the gullet. These become varicose and likely to rupture and bleed, sometimes quite profusely. *Urgent medical and surgical treatment is required.*

❷ Do you suffer from angina? Have you ever had a stroke? Do you have high blood pressure?

Most of us are familiar with the common consequences of hardening of the arteries, namely heart attacks and strokes. However, the blood vessels that supply the intestine can also become narrowed as we grow older, and when the blood flow is sufficiently constricted a section of the gut may perish, leading to pain and bleeding into the intestine.

❷ Do you bruise easily?

Just as there can be congenital abnormalities and weaknesses in the walls of the blood vessels in the nose, skin and elsewhere in the body, vascular malformations can also occur in the gut, causing sudden, unexplained bleeding.

❷ Has any accidental damage to the back passage occurred?

Casualty officers are fully aware that blood in the motions may be caused by trauma to the back passage, which can occur as a result of anal intercourse or the introduction of foreign bodies, although patients often won't admit to such activities.

❷ Are you over the age of 50, suffering from occasional low abdominal pain?

A common condition in anyone over the age of about 50 is diverticulosis, in which the muscular wall of the large bowel becomes weakened, largely through failing to eat enough roughage over the years, with the result that little pouches from the lining of the bowel push through the muscle coating in finger-like projections. These can trap the contents of the bowel and become inflamed, in which case diverticulosis becomes diverticulitis. This can produce abdominal pain, temperature and occasionally bleeding.

SUMMARY
BLOOD IN THE MOTIONS

POSSIBLE CAUSE	ACTION
Haemorrhoids	If mild: ointment, creams and suppositories; if moderate: suppositories, injection with sclerosing agents or surgical 'banding' to cut off the blood supply; if severe: surgical excision.
Local irritation	Creams and ointments. Surgical correction for fissure.
Gastritis, peptic ulcer	Avoid alcohol, caffeine, smoking and fatty or spicy foods. Antacids. For peptic ulcer, the above plus H2 antagonist drugs and proton pump inhibitor.
Medication	With your doctor, identify and discontinue drug responsible.
Colitis (ulcerative colitis, Crohn's disease)	Medical treatment at first, surgical treatment if necessary.
Oesophagitis, excessive vomiting	Antinausea drugs and antacids.
Cancer of the bowel	Surgical treatment and/or anti-cancer therapy.
Cancer of the stomach	Surgery and/r anti-cancer therapy.
Parasitic or bacterial infection	Antibiotic treatment if appropriate.
Cirrhosis of the liver with bleeding varicose veins	Urgent medical and surgical treatment.
Hardening of the arteries	Surgery for thrombosed parts of intestine.
Blood-vessel abnormality	Surgery to cauterize weak blood vessels.
Trauma	Surgical repair if appropriate.

169

7

LUMPS AND SWELLINGS

Lumps and swellings, particularly in the neck, breasts, head, armpit and wrist, are extremely common reasons for attendance at doctors' surgeries and often cause a great deal of worry and concern. The greatest fear of all is that the bump – which often has been noticed for the very first time – may represent some form of cancer, so let me just say here and now that very, very few of these lumps and swellings ever turn out to be any form of malignancy. Most have a simple explanation of a benign nature, and usually represent the result of some trauma or mild inflammation. A helpful rule to remember is that any lump which is painful and has developed suddenly is most likely to be due to infection or to recent injury, whilst a lump that has appeared gradually over a period of time and is quite painless should be regarded as a malignancy until proved otherwise. It may well turn out to be something quite trivial such as a sebaceous cyst, but some cancers can present themselves in this way, so such symptoms should never be ignored.

Given the understandable concern such symptoms engender, what should we do about them? It is just as wrong and foolish to ignore a new finding such as a bump as it is to worry about it unduly. In order to understand the true nature of a lump – or tumour, as the medical profession calls all such swellings – whether benign or malignant, consider the following points:

POSITION

Describing the location of any lump or swelling is important, although it won't in itself necessarily pinpoint the source of the problem. For example, whilst the source of a breast or thyroid lump will be fairly easy to identify, a lump in the abdomen can arise from any one of a number of internal structures. Nevertheless, it is always worth knowing as near as possible where the swelling is.

SIZE

Generally speaking, large tumours are more significant than small tumours, although this is not necessarily the case. For example, in the kidney and liver, a very large tumour can sometimes represent a cyst that may not interfere with the normal function of the organ in which it is growing, and which may be easily removed. Conversely, a malignant melanoma on the skin may remain quite small, hardly bigger than the blunt end of a pencil, and yet be capable of spreading to distant sites in the body such as the lungs and the liver. So, when describing a mole to the doctor, its actual size is of some importance, those larger than the end of a pencil in diameter being suspicious, and smaller ones less so. Doctors generally measure tumours in square centimetres, and then keep an eye on their progress.

SHAPE

The shape and contour of the lump may indicate the source. A lump in the parotid salivary gland for example, will produce an L-shaped swelling in front of and underneath the ear, whilst a thyroid swelling may take the shape of the thyroid gland as it sits in front of the windpipe. An enlarged spleen has a characteristic shape, and an obstructed bladder will produce a balloon-shaped swelling, with the fully rounded part situated somewhere around the naval and the tapering part disappearing behind the pubic bone.

COLOUR

Different types of swellings are different colours. The characteristic boils of infections, for example, are red and inflamed, lumpy bruises are bluey-yellow in colour, and melanomas are generally dark brown to black, although this is not universally so. Xanthomata are yellowy, waxy-looking lumps on the skin that represent collections of fat and cholesterol in those people who have inherited an increased tendency towards heart disease. Strawberry birthmarks are swellings so-called precisely because of their bright red appearance, which is due to a collection of dilated blood vessels lying very near the skin's surface.

TEMPERATURE

Most tumours will be of the same temperature as the rest of the body, but any degree of excessive heat generation suggests infection or inflammation. Thus an actively inflamed joint in someone with rheumatoid arthritis or gout, for example, will feel particularly hot, and a deep-seated abscess will also feel a different temperature to the surrounding tissues.

TENDERNESS

It is a common misconception that cancer is always painful. In fact, in the early stages it is very rare for cancers to produce pain unless there is pressure on sensitive surrounding structures. It is for this reason that malignant breast tumours are often not discovered until later on, as they cause very little discomfort. The presence of pain is much more likely to signify inflammation or acute infection. One example of an acutely tender lump is a neuroma, a small swelling on a nerve. The neuroma itself won't hurt if squeezed, but because it is attached to healthy nerve tissue, there will be a sharp, knife-like pain every time it is touched.

MOBILITY

A tumour firmly fixed to an underlying structure is more worrying than a lump that moves about freely. For example, a mobile breast lump suggests the tumour is benign, whereas a lump that is fixed is highly suspicious. A lump in the groin that suddenly bulges on coughing or sneezing is diagnostic of a hernia. However, a tumour that pulsates when you feel it suggests a swelling on or around a blood vessel, and a large swelling in the lower abdomen that pulsates could signify the present of an aortic aneurysm, a dangerous swelling on a major artery, that is a surgical emergency, requiring urgent hospitalization.

CHARACTER

Consider what the tumour feels like. Lipomas, which are harmless, consist of a collection of fat cells bound tightly together by a surrounding shell or capsule. They are rubbery in consistency and feel like firm marshmallows under the skin surface. A ganglion, on the other hand, is a cystic swelling near a tendon. It is firmer and more tense, and feels as if it is filled with fluid under pressure. A collection of fluid around the testicles (a hydrocele) is a not uncommon occurrence in men, and a swelling here will be characteristically soft, mobile and obviously full of fluid. It feels just like squeezing a small balloon filled with water.

SURFACE TEXTURE

Is the lump smooth or irregular on the surface? A smoothly enlarged thyroid gland is common in a goitre where the whole gland is either under- or overfunctioning, but an irregular outline to an enlarged thyroid is more likely to indicate one or more nodules, which will require more urgent investigation. In the same way, a smooth surface to an enlarged liver suggests a general enlargement and is commonly seen in chronic alcoholism with cirrhosis.

An irregular liver, however, suggests the secondary spread of cancer from another abdominal organ and is therefore more worrying.

NUMBER OF SWELLINGS

In neurofibromatosis, there will be multiple small lumps on the nerves, and these can occur at any site of the body. People who suddenly notice one lipoma, or fatty lump, often have several more over the trunk of their body or thighs. People with generalized infections or blood disorders may have enlarged lymph nodes at various sites of the body, including the neck, armpits and groin. Women with chronic mastitis may have general lumpiness of both breasts with associated tenderness, which although inconvenient perhaps, is nevertheless reassuring in that it is unlikely to be linked to

an underlying cancer. However, certain cancers may spread to distant sites and cause various lumps and bumps elsewhere. Breast cancer, for example, may extend to the lymph glands and liver, and occasionally these secondary tumours can be detected by a doctor before the primary one.

These are the sort of characteristics that can be described to the doctor over the phone prior to a consultation. They will give the physician a good idea of the nature of the tumour and how urgent the consultation should be. Once the doctor has taken a look and made a diagnosis, he or she will want to confirm the diagnosis in a number of ways. For example, it is possible to ascertain whether a large lump is connected to an abnormality of the underlying blood vessels by listening to it with a stethoscope. A family history of similar lumps or bumps can be particularly relevant in conditions such as thyroid disease, breast disease or neurofibromatosis. With a lump in the groin suspected of being a hernia, the doctor can use the stethoscope to listen for the presence of bowel sounds, which are fairly unmistakable and will certainly point to this diagnosis. If fluid is suspected of filling the lump, say around the testicle or in a pocket just below the kneecap, then he or she might shine a torch through the skin. The light is easily transmitted through fluid, showing up the full size of the lump nicely. This is called 'transillumination'. Finally, X-rays or internal scans may be used to highlight the exact location and nature of the tumour, although a biopsy, which is a surgical procedure in which a piece of the tissue itself is examined under the microscope, is really the only definitive way of deciding the exact nature of the beast. Once this is determined, appropriate therapy can be decided upon.

THE TOP TEN LUMPS AND SWELLINGS

LIPOMAS

Anyone who is overweight is particularly susceptible to developing tightly encapsulated areas of fat cells that feel firmer than the surrounding fatty cells. These lumps are called lipomas and they can range from the size of a pea to that of an apple. They are mainly situated on the trunk, but in obese people are also noticed on the arms and legs. They are totally benign and are only surgically excised for cosmetic reasons or if they rub against overlying clothing and cause pain.

FIBROMAS

A fibroma is a lump arising from fibrous tissue in or underneath the skin. The lump is quite firm and hard but reasonably mobile and is always benign. Surgical removal is only required if cosmetic or other symptoms dictate.

BRUISES

Bruises can be swollen in the early stages of injury as the result of blood and serum leaking into damaged tissues, but older bruises can also become swollen for a second time. What happens is that the blood collected in the bruise attracts fluid from the circulation, so that a little pocket of liquid results. This is known as a hygroma, which usually requires no treatment as it resolves spontaneously, although in some instances withdrawal of the fluid through a needle is attempted.

ABSCESSES

An abscess is simply a collection of infected fluid at any site of the body. As the infection develops, so the lump tends to get larger, and in the case of skin abscesses it will often 'point' towards the skin's surface. There may be a fluctuant spongy dome overlying the abscess through which the underlying pus will naturally drain in time, but often surgical drainage under local anaesthetic is required.

SWOLLEN LYMPH GLANDS

Lymph glands in the body swell as the result of infection or inflammation. For example, if you have a sore throat, the glands draining that part of your body will swell, causing painful lumps in the side of your neck. Just as an infected blister or cut on your foot or leg will lead to painful swellings in the groin. Generalized infections such as glandular fever and brucellosis, however, produce swelling of all the glands of the body, a phenomenon also seen in various forms of blood cancer such as Hodgkin's disease and the chronic leukaemias. The lymphatic-gland swelling associated with acute infections usually needs no other treatment than antibiotics but long-standing swelling of several lymph glands requires further investigation and treatment.

BLOCKED DUCTS

If the drainage ducts and channels of various glands become blocked, the gland itself will swell. When this happens to the sebaceous glands, which make oil to lubricate the surface of the skin, blackheads, whiteheads and ultimately acne and boils can occur, whilst blockage of the salivary-gland ducts, perhaps as the result of infection or a stone, can lead to swelling of the salivary glands. Sebaceous cysts are often very slow-growing, are the normal colour of your skin as they lie beneath its surface, and to touch often show evidence of trapped fluid below. Occasionally they can become infected from bacteria on the surface of the skin, in which case redness, further swelling, pain and a cheesy discharge from the duct itself can occur. Large infected sebaceous cysts should be excised. Small infected sebaceous cysts may respond to antibiotics.

SCROTAL SWELLINGS

Swellings in the scrotum are relatively common. They may represent a swelling of the testicle itself, but more commonly varicose veins draining the testicle – in which case they are called varicoceles – or a collection of fluid in the envelope around the testicle itself (a hydrocele) are responsible. Each of these has particular characteristics that allow the diagnosis to be made. The congested veins of varicoceles lie above the testicle, feel like a bag of worms to the touch, and are bluish in colour, whereas a hydrocele, feels like a small balloon full of fluid. When a pocket torch is shone through the fluid, the light passes right through, confirming that the fluid is clear. Swellings of the testicle itself are firmer, with a much more defined margin and will not transilluminate in this way. Both varicoceles and hydroceles may require surgery.

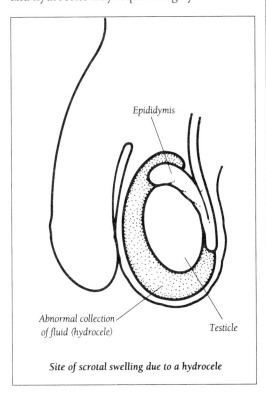

Epididymis

Abnormal collection of fluid (hydrocele)

Testicle

Site of scrotal swelling due to a hydrocele

DISTENSION OF THE BLADDER

When the outflow of urine from the bladder is obstructed, usually due to an enlarged prostate, the bladder can go into retention, which can be extremely uncomfortable. The bladder swells and forms a balloon-shaped bulge, acutely tender to the touch, rising up as far as the navel in extreme cases. Treatment involves passing a tube through the penis and into the bladder (catheterization) to relieve the obstruction and drain the urine, and is *urgently* required. Obstruction of the bladder rarely happens in women, but may happen as the result of nerve damage, multiple sclerosis or a slipped disc.

BONY SPURS

Bony outgrowths, or exostoses as they are called, commonly occur on various sites on the skeleton, but especially where there is the pull of strong tendons, the undersurface of the heel being a prime example. In this case, there will be inflammation and bruising of the surrounding tissues, making you feel as though you are constantly walking on a sharp stone. Occasionally, if it cannot be relieved by the attention of a chiropodist or by an injection of cortisone, surgery may be necessary.

CANCERS

Cancers can manifest themselves on the skin in various forms. A rodent ulcer is one of the commonest forms of cancer. It appears on the face, usually between the corner of the eye and the corner of the mouth, and looks like a small spot that refuses to heal. It scabs over from time to time, on each occasion the surface crust flaking off, only to be replaced by another as the ulcer gradually becomes larger and starts to eat deeper into the skin surface. Although technically speaking a rodent ulcer is a type of cancer, it never spreads to other parts of the body and is easily dealt with by surgery or radiotherapy. It is particularly common in people over the age of 60. A more serious form of cancer is the malignant melanoma, which can arise from both old and new moles. A mole that has increased in size, has changed colour, bled or irritated should always be regarded as suspicious. Malignant melanoma is on the increase in Britain, particularly in fair-haired, pale-skinned individuals taking frequent trips to sunny climes, and is a major cause of death from cancer in people aged 20-45. Any suspicious mole should therefore be seen by the doctor urgently. Finally, there are other types of skin cancer that can produce lumps, and these usually irritate and bleed. Again, most of them occur in areas of skin usually exposed to sunlight, such as the scalp, face, arms, legs and neck. It should never be assumed that these are minor infections or trivial blemishes and they should always be checked over by a doctor.

SWOLLEN JOINTS

Swollen joints can arise for a number of reasons, many of which are mechanical and related to injury, but some of which are the result of infection, problems with the internal metabolism or more generalized disorders such as rheumatoid arthritis. Generally, with injury or a metabolic disorder such as gout, only one joint will be affected whereas with generalized disorders such as rheumatoid arthritis many joints may be. A very hot, red joint would suggest active rheumatoid arthritis or an infection, whilst a cold swelling is associated with mechanical disorders such as cartilage tears.

❷ *Has there been any mechanical injury?*
Sometimes following an injury a flake of cartilage or bone can escape into the joint fluid, and when the sufferer moves, it is caught by the moving bone ends, causing recurrent

inflammation and swelling of the joint. X-rays can often identify the foreign body, but sometimes arthroscopy, the passing of a special tiny telescope into the knee joint, has to be done.

❷ *Does the knee click and give way?*
A cartilage tear is a common and disabling injury amongst sportsmen and women in particular, and is usually sustained as the result of twisting the knee with the full body weight planted firmly on the leg. The joint puffs up quickly after the tear and 'clicking' sensations are common. It can cause disruption to the function the joint and produce significant swelling. There is usually a history of injury.

❷ *Has fluid appeared around the joint?*
The internal lining of the joint, or synovial membrane, produces a fluid that allows movement of the bone ends. If the membrane becomes inflamed (synovitis) for any reason, for example due to injury, viral infection or generalized arthritic conditions such as rheumatoid arthritis, the result is a puffy joint that feels very unstable.

❷ *Is there very localized tenderness?*
Ligaments are strong bands of tissue that hold the joint components together. When a joint is strained the ligaments can become inflamed, puffy and extremely painful. They have a poor blood supply and are therefore slow to heal, but the underlying cause can usually be identified because there is well-localized pain on pressure.

❷ *Do you bruise and bleed easily?*
Bleeding into a joint as the result of trauma or a clotting disorder such as haemophilia can produce swelling and discomfort in that joint. The body will naturally reabsorb a small amount of blood, but large amounts will need

to be aspirated through a needle as otherwise secondary arthritis can follow.

❷ Have you lost weight? Are you pale?

This suggests an inflammation condition. These include disorders such as psoriasis, which, although predominantly a skin condition, can also produce arthritis. Rheumatoid arthritis and ankylosing spondylitis can have far-reaching effects.

❷ Does the swelling develop when you overuse the joint?

Often referred to as wear-and-tear arthritis, osteoarthritis is the commonest type of rheumatism. There is stiffness and pain in the joints, particularly weight-bearing joints such as the hip and knee, and there may also be deformity and a 'grating' feeling. Osteoarthritis is particularly common in the elderly and in younger people who have had previous trauma

to the joint, and is therefore always worth bearing in mind when swelling occurs.

❷ Is the big toe alone affected?

Gout is caused by uric acid building up in the bloodstream and crystallizing in the synovial fluid that lubricates the joint, producing severe pain and inflammation. Classically it occurs in the joint at the base of the big toe, but in some people it may affect other small joints. Other features of gout include fleshy nobbles on the backs of the fingers or the earlobes (tophi).

❷ Has there been a recent infection?

Joints may become infected by viruses such as German measles (rubella) or by bacteria, as is the case with septic arthritis and gonorrhoea. Other infections can produce a secondary response in which the antibodies produced damage the lining of the joint, and this occurs in rheumatic fever and Reiter's syndrome.

SUMMARY
SWOLLEN JOINTS

POSSIBLE CAUSE	ACTION
Foreign body	Identify and remove.
Cartilage	Meniscectomy (cartilage removal).
Synovitis	Identify cause. Medical or surgical treatment.
Ligament damage	Physiotherapy or surgical repair.
Bleeding into the joint	Aspiration of large amounts of blood by needle. Treat underlying cause.
Inflammatory conditions	Identify cause. Medical or surgical treatment.
Osteoarthritis	Rest, gentle exercise, physiotherapy, medication, surgery.
Gout	Medication.
Infection	Identify underlying cause. Medical treatment

BULGING EYES

There are only two conditions likely to cause the symptom of bulging eyes, which when it happens is certainly very obvious to all concerned. One is an overactive thyroid gland, known as hyperthyroidism, in which case one eye tends to bulge more than the other. When the underlying problem is an ocular tumour, however, only one eye will be affected.

❷ Have you lost weight and do you feel constantly hot?

Over the course of time, and whether or not it is treated, an overactive thyroid may cause fatty material to accumulate behind the eye in the bony eye socket. Eventually this produces the appearance of bulging, staring eyes, with white visible all around the cornea and iris when the person looks straight ahead (normally some of the iris, the coloured part of the eye, is covered by one or other of the eyelids). This condition is known as proptosis and is accompanied by the other symptoms of an overactive thyroid, namely a fast pulse, flushed skin, sweating, diarrhoea, weight loss and heat intolerance.

❷ Is just one of your eyes apparently enlarged?

Very occasionally one eye can bulge as the result of lumps or bumps developing behind the eyeball. These may be of a benign or malignant nature and may or may not involve visual disturbance. Haemorrhage occurring within or behind the eye for any reason can have a similar effect. However, these conditions are extremely rare.

SUMMARY
BULGING EYES

POSSIBLE CAUSE	ACTION
Hyperthyroidism	Medication with tablets. Radiation treatment or surgery.
Tumour or haemorrhage	Identify cause. Medical or surgical treatment.

SWOLLEN GUMS

The problem of swollen gums usually finds its way to the dentist because it is so often related to poor dental hygiene, but there are a potential number of medical causes.

❷ Are the gums red and hot as well as swollen?

Gums can become infected by viruses, bacteria or fungal organisms, which can end up producing an abscess, resulting in swelling.

❷ Do you take medication for epilepsy?

A number of drugs can produce gradual and irreversible swelling of the gums, especially those used to control epileptic seizures, for example phenytoin and phenobarbitone. If significant swelling occurs it may be possible to change to an alternative medication.

❷ Do your dentures fit correctly?

If dentures have rough edges or pinch the gums, the result can be inflammation.

❷ Could it be a sensitivity to mouthwashes and toothpastes?

These products contain various compounds that can produce irritation and allergy in the gums. Simple saltwater gargles and special toothpaste for sensitive teeth are recommended.

❷ Is the diet adequate?

Deficiencies in the diet, especially of vitamin C, can cause bleeding gums, and although rare in Britain, may be seen in people on severe diets or in elderly people living alone.

❷ Are you pale and tired and do you suffer from frequent infections?

Very occasionally, bleeding from, and inflammation of the gums are seen in various forms of leukaemia. However, by the time this happens the leukaemia is fairly far advanced and there have usually been other signs and symptoms.

SUMMARY
SWOLLEN GUMS

Possible Cause	Action
Infection	Antiviral agents, antibacterials, or antifungals. Abscess drainage if necessary.
Medication	With your doctor, identify and then discontinue or reduce dosage of drug.
Ill-fitting dentures	Return to dentist for attention.
Sensitivity to mouthwashes and/or toothpastes	Use a different brand.
Malnutrition	Correct deficiency.
Leukaemia	Medical treatment.

A SWOLLEN TONGUE

A swollen tongue soon makes itself felt by making talking and eating difficult. In some situations, the swelling may be accompanied by colour changes in the tongue, for example as the result of an infection. Examining the nature of such accompanying symptoms will help to pinpoint the possible cause of the problem.

❷ Is your tongue red and shiny?

This is a typical result of iron-deficiency anaemia, along with pallor of the skin and shortness of breath.

❷ Are there white patches on a red tongue?

A red tongue liberally splashed with tenacious white material suggests a thrush infection.

❷ Is your tongue black and hairy?

Whilst this certainly looks alarming, it is generally seen when fungal overgrowth occurs after taking powerful antibiotics or as the result of heavy smoking.

❷ Did the swelling begin after eating or drinking anything?

Just as our skin becomes red, hot and swollen in response to a wasp or bee sting, so various allergies can cause the tongue and lips to swell. In susceptible individuals this commonly occurs after eating such allergenic foods as strawberries and shellfish, in which case it is a significant warning sign because occasionally it can be associated with swelling at the back of the throat and respiratory obstruction. It is therefore a potential medical emergency and should be referred to a doctor immediately for treatment. Antihistamine preparations are usually used, but occasionally much more potent adrenaline has to be administered.

❷ Do you feel cold all the time? Have you gained weight?

Underactivity of the thyroid gland (myxoedema) can produce, amongst other things, macroglossia or a swollen tongue. Other more common symptoms include abnormal sensitivity to the cold, weight gain, constipation, coarsening and loss of body hair, loss of the outer third of the eyebrows and reduced sweating.

❷ Have you been experiencing double vision lately?

The pituitary gland is a tiny gland sitting at the base of the brain that governs the overall function of the glands. A tumour in the pituitary area may lead to an increased secretion of growth hormone, resulting in renewed growth of various parts of the body after the normal growth that occurs at puberty. A swollen tongue may therefore be seen in association with enlargement of the lower jaw, hands and feet. Double vision and headaches may accompany pituitary tumours, which are almost always benign.

❷ Has there been any injury to the tongue?

Infection of the deeper layers of the tongue usually occurs as the result of physical damage. However, because the enzymes in saliva provide the tongue with a natural resistance to infection, this is not all that commonly seen.

❷ Are you a heavy smoker?

I have deliberately put this at the bottom of the list because any malignancy involving the tongue is rare. However, smokers, and particularly pipe smokers, where the smoke stream is usually directed to a localized area of the tongue, can develop leucoplakia, a condition characterized by white patches on the tongue, which if neglected may develop into cancer. Certain forms of leukaemia can also involve the tongue as a secondary feature by making it swell, although I have to say that when I worked for some time on a leukaemia ward in a hospital, I never saw a single case.

However, any smoker who develops a long-standing painless white patch on the tongue should certainly have it looked at, biopsied and treated. Needless to say, he or she should also stop smoking.

SUMMARY
A SWOLLEN TONGUE

POSSIBLE CAUSE	ACTION
Anaemia	Iron tablets or injections.
Thrush	Antifungal medicine.
Fungal overgrowth	Antifungal medicine. Stop smoking.
Allergy	Antihistamines, adrenaline if necessary.
Underactive thyroid gland	Thyroid-replacement medication.
Pituitary gland dysfunction	Surgery or radiotherapy.
Deep infection	Antibiotics.
Malignancy	Biopsy followed by surgery or radiotherapy.

SWELLINGS IN THE NECK

Most lumps and swellings in the neck are trivial and simply due to sebaceous cysts or fat-cell collections (lipomata), which are also frequently seen in other parts of the body. Other types of neck swellings tend to be restricted to either the side or the front of the neck. If the lump is to the side, this suggests an enlargement of the lymph or salivary glands, whilst a lump in the middle of the neck over the trachea (windpipe) indicates a swelling of the thyroid gland. Most swellings in the neck are short-lived and trivial and will settle down on their own. Lumps that last longer than two weeks, however, should be taken seriously as they could represent a more serious disorder such as a malignancy, in which case they require urgent investigation and treatment. Many specialist ENT centres such as the one at the Queen Elizabeth Hospital in Edgebaston recognize this and offer walk-in 'lump in the neck' clinics where patients can be seen as soon as a swelling is noticed so that an early diagnosis can be reached. The earlier the diagnosis, the greater the chance of a cure should the problem turn out to be serious. Generally speaking, though, any lump you have only just noticed should not give great cause for concern.

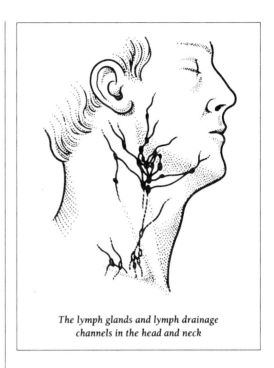

The lymph glands and lymph drainage channels in the head and neck

❷ Are the lumps at the side of the windpipe, just below the jaw?

The lymph glands are responsible for combating and draining infection or inflammation at various sites of the body, and in the neck this means the whole of the face, head and skull. The glands concentrate the action of antibodies and antibody-producing cells against the invading germs, thereby allowing the body to fight the disease process. In tonsillitis, therefore, not only do the tonsils themselves swell, but so do the glands lying adjacent to the carotid artery and jugular vein at the side of the windpipe as they are the next line of defence. Short-lived, lumpy and painful swelling of these glands occurs in acute infections, for example as the result of throat infections, dental infections, sinusitis, ear trouble and injuries affecting the scalp. The glands themselves will settle down within a matter of days once the original source of the infection has settled.

❷ Have the lumps been there for more than two weeks? Are there any elsewhere in the body?

Long-standing (chronic) swelling of the lymph glands in the neck where there is no obvious local source of infection suggests a generalized disorder such as glandular fever, tuberculosis or brucellosis. In these conditions there may well be swelling of the lymph glands in other parts of the body, particularly the armpits and groin. Occasionally, glandular enlargement may represent a response to malignancy elsewhere in the body or even a malignancy of the glands themselves, as is the case in Hodgkin's disease and other types of lymph-gland cancer (lymphoma).

❷ Is the swelling just in front of the neck, under the ear?

This is likely to be due to enlargement of the parotid salivary gland and is most often the result of mumps infection. Mumps generally causes swelling on one side at a time, and is most commonly seen in children. With the advent of the MMR (mumps, measles and rubella) vaccine, however, it is becoming increasingly rare.

Mumps can affect other glands in the body, notably the other salivary glands just below the jawline at the side of the neck and under the chin, but also the pancreas, ovaries and testicles. The incubation period is between two and three weeks and the patient is infectious from one week before the swelling of the gland and up to two weeks afterwards. The salivary gland usually remains swollen for 7–10 days.

❷ Does the swelling come and go? Is it provoked by eating?

Any blockage of the tubes from which saliva is produced can cause intermittent enlargement of the salivary glands. As eating results in increased amounts of saliva, the swelling is generally most noticeable at mealtimes. Blockages are usually the result of stones in the salivary ducts or of infection.

❷ Is there a smooth, puffy-looking swelling over the front of the windpipe?

This generalized, smooth enlargement of the thyroid gland is called a goitre and may be associated with altered activity of the gland itself. Usually goitres are soft, but they can also be hard and lumpy, and at times they can be quite large, causing compression of the windpipe behind and a dramatic increase in collar size. Accompanying symptoms include any signs of altered activity of the gland. With an overactive gland, therefore, weight loss, heat intolerance, palpitations and diarrhoea would be likely to occur.

Underactivity, on the other hand, would cause weight gain, intolerance of cold weather, constipation and coarse thinning hair.

❷ Is there a lopsided enlargement or a single firm lump in front of the windpipe?

In this situation, most of the thyroid gland is normal except for one tiny area that forms a nodule. A thyroid nodule is a symptom to be taken somewhat more seriously than a goitre because it is more often associated with an underlying malignancy. One of the tests the doctor will perform is a radioactive scanning test to see whether or not the nodule is producing thyroxine hormone like the rest of the gland. If it is, it is called a 'hot' nodule, but if it isn't, it is called a 'cold' nodule. Cold nodules require further urgent investigation to exclude the possibility of a malignancy. The good news is that thyroid cancers tend to be slow-growing and are very likely, therefore, to be curable.

❷ Is the swelling below and in front of the ear, and has it been present for more than two weeks?

In anyone over the age of 30 this raises the possibility of a tumour in the parotid salivary gland. These are generally benign, slow-growing and well localized to the substance of the gland itself. Surgical treatment is effective and the earlier the diagnosis the better the results. *Therefore it is imperative that you see your doctor about this combination of symptoms as soon as possible.*

SUMMARY
SWELLINGS IN THE NECK

POSSIBLE CAUSE	ACTION
Acute or chronic infection of the lymph glands	Symptomatic relief for viral infections, antibiotics for bacterial infections.
Viral infection of salivary glands (mumps)	Pain relief.
Thyroid goitre	Surgery if large (thyroidectomy).
Salivary-gland stone	Surgery to remove stone.
Bacterial infection of salivary glands	Antibiotics.
Malignancy of lymph glands	Chemotherapy and/or radiotherapy, surgery, bone-marrow transplantation.
Thyroid nodule	Surgery followed by radioactive iodine treatment if malignant.
Parotid tumour	Surgery. Radiotherapy if malignant.

SWELLINGS IN
THE ARMPIT

Every couple of weeks in general practice I will see a patient who complains of a lump under the arm. Almost without looking I know that the lump will be either a blocked sebaceous (oil-producing) gland or an enlarged lymph node just beneath the surface of the skin. But I always take a look anyway. Firstly, because the treatment for each of these is different, and secondly because just occasionally the swelling will turn out to be something unexpected and perhaps more urgently in need of treatment.

❷ Is the lump very near the surface, tender and reddened?

Sebaceous cysts are particularly common in hairy areas of the body, armpits included, because of the large number of oil-producing glands there. In these hot, moist areas, there is an increased tendency for the gland ducts to be blocked by the build-up of oily material called sebum in the underlying gland itself. A cyst then develops, which may become infected, in which case the lump will become red and tender as well. Such cysts are close to the skin surface and if you look closely, preferably with a small magnifying glass, you can identify a small central punctum, or opening, which represents the blocked opening of the blocked duct.

It is sometimes possible to express the white cheesy material from the cyst between finger and thumb when the pressure within the gland or the pressure of the infection is making the pain much worse.

Generally, however, when infection has occurred, incision with a scalpel under local anaesthetic is sometimes necessary to drain the infected matter.

❷ Is the lump quite difficult to locate, firm and very mobile?

Lymph glands in the armpit are responsible for draining any infection or inflammation that occurs in the arm or breast on that side. When there is an infection, perhaps around the fingernails (paronychia), or a laceration or wound that has become infected, these glands will swell, producing a tender lump. If the other lymph glands in the body, for example in the neck and groin, are also enlarged, this suggests a more generalized disorder such as glandular fever, or a blood disorder, including cancer of the lymph glands themselves, as in Hodgkin's disease.

If no local infection is uncovered by the doctor's initial search, he or she will then look for possible causes of generalized lymph-gland inflammation, using blood tests and lymph-gland biopsy.

❷ Is there any sign of a breast lump on the same side?

As well as draining infection and inflammation, lymph glands also enlarge in response to a nearby or distant malignancy. Swollen glands in the armpit, or axilla, to give it its technical name, can therefore be due to cancer of the breast, of which there are something like 25,000 new cases every year in this country. It is for this reason that doctors will also examine the armpits when any lump in the breast is noticed. Unfortunately, breast cancer also involving the lymph glands in this area suggests that the tumour is spreading, which means that *urgent consultation with your doctor is essential.*

❷ Did you notice the swelling when you started taking the pill or when you became pregnant?

Just occasionally the top outer corner of the breast extends way up towards the armpit itself, where it may be felt as a tender swelling, particularly at the times when the rest of the breast tissue would normally be sensitive, for example when taking the oral contraceptive pill for the first time, or during pregnancy. The characteristic consistency and behaviour of such a lump, identical as it is to the rest of the breast, usually helps confirm this diagnosis.

SUMMARY
SWELLINGS IN THE ARMPIT

POSSIBLE CAUSE	ACTION
Sebaceous cyst	Leave to resolve spontaneously or surgical drainage.
Enlarged lymph gland	If due to local infection, identify source and treat, if combined with generalized swelling of glands, identify underlying cause and treat appropriately.
Malignancy	Treat underlying condition. Chemotherapy and/or radiotherapy.
Aberrant breast tissue	No treatment required.
Lipoma	Surgical treatment for cosmetic reasons only.

BREAST LUMPS

The discovery of a breast lump in any shape or form is quite justifiably a cause for concern. Breast cancer is far too common in this country compared to other parts of the world, and despite advances in medical technology generally over the last two decades, there has not been the tremendous improvement in breast-cancer treatment to match. Having said that, 90 per cent of women noticing a small lump in their breast or armpit will prove to have a benign tumour rather than cancer. But for the remaining 10 per cent who do have a malignancy, the sooner that lump is detected the easier it will be to diagnose and treat. For early operable breast cancers, the survival rate is good. Ninety per cent of women are alive and well ten years after their operation. For more advanced cancers the outlook is not so healthy. It is for this reason that doctors still advise women to be 'breast aware' by gently examining their breasts every three months or so to check whether any changes have occurred. Ninety per cent of all lumps are discovered by women themselves rather than a doctor, so I for one certainly believe that this checking routine is important. Special breast X-rays performed after the age of 35 can also be useful, but in this country there is no national breast-screening programme that examines women under the age of 50 in this way. Mammography is, therefore, largely restricted to women with a palpable lump suspected of being malignant.

When examining your breasts, you should check for the following: any change in shape or size, any enlarged veins, any areas where the skin appears thicker than usual, and any dimpling of the skin or resemblance to the pitting seen in orange peel. Also, any ulceration of the overlying skin, any new inturning of the nipple, any discharge from the nipple, any swelling under the armpit, any swelling of the

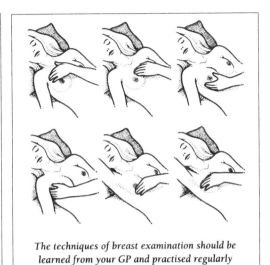

The techniques of breast examination should be learned from your GP and practised regularly

arm itself. If a lump is found, important characteristics to note are its size, whether or not it is tender and painful, whether it feels hard or soft, and whether it is mobile or fixed to underlying tissues. On the whole, small, tender, soft lumps that are freely mobile are benign, whilst painless, solid lumps that are fixed to the underlying wall of the chest are much more serious. However, these are only guidelines and any lump of this nature should be referred to the doctor and if necessary, mammography, biopsy and/or surgical removal of the lump can be performed.

❷ *Are your breasts often tender before your periods?*

Some women develop naturally lumpy breast tissue that becomes more noticeable at a certain stage of the menstrual cycle. Such mastitis, as it is called, does not have to be put up with indefinitely, and it may be worth consulting your doctor for help.

❸ *Have your breasts become generally more lumpy?*

If these changes are new and different to

normal, they could be due to numerous small breast cysts, otherwise known as benign mammary dysplasia. The underlying reason is rapid fluctuation in sex-hormone levels. It is usually worst in the upper, outer quarter of the breast area and is more common in women in their twenties and thirties, women who have had irregular periods, and women who have never had children.

General lumpiness of the breast in itself is not unusual, so no treatment is necessary. However, frequent self-examination and regular checks by your doctor or practice nurse are advisable, and will go a long way towards reassuring you.

❷ Is the lump tender and soft, and does it move freely under the fingers?

If so, it is most likely to be a cyst caused by fluid retention in one of the breast ducts. These are more common in women in their twenties and thirties who have not had children. They are benign and can usually be drained by aspiration through a needle.

❷ Is the lump fixed and painless?

Lumps that are relatively solid and fixed to the skin are more often due to malignant changes than soft, mobile lumps are, and therefore require *urgent examination and investigation by a doctor.*

They can sometimes be quite large, and are more significant the older you are. Tests will include a mammogram, a special X-ray of the breast, and/or a needle biopsy. If microscopic examination reveals cancer, a decision then has to be made about treatment. Options include removal of the lump by itself (lumpectomy), removal of the breast (mastectomy), or mastectomy with other therapy, which may include radiotherapy, chemotherapy and/or hormone therapy as extra 'insurance' against tumour cells coming back.

❷ Is there bruising of the breast, with a hard lump beneath?

This suggests a recent knock, which has resulted in a harmless bruise below the surface. It is not cancerous.

❷ Is the lump accompanied by redness and pain?

This combination of symptoms is often due to infection or abscess formation within the breast tissue and is usually associated with breast-feeding or the postnatal period, when infection can creep into the breast ducts from outside and set up the inflammation. Antibiotics and poultices are very effective.

❷ Does the lump have puckered or dimpled skin?

This could be caused by a recent injury to the breast tissue, to inflammation of an underlying breast duct, or to a breast cancer. Have it checked out.

❷ Has there been any change in the size of a breast?

This could be due to a large cyst, to pregnancy or to the changes that occur in the week before your period. Inform your doctor if the changes don't settle quickly.

❷ Are your nipples inverted?

If you have always had inverted nipples there is no need to worry, as this is harmless. If the inversion happens suddenly, however, it could be due to trouble with the underlying breast ducts, in which case you should have the problem checked by a doctor, although these changes are very seldom cancerous.

❷ Is there any discharge from the nipple?

Fluid from the nipple may be milk-like and creamy, yellowy-green, or bloodstained.

Discharge occurs during pregnancy, at certain times in the menstrual cycle, after an abortion or miscarriage, or sometimes through frequent stimulation during love play. *Bloodstained discharge should always be reported to the doctor urgently as it may represent the first sign of a tumour.* Many types of growths in the milk ducts could be responsible for this, most of which will be benign. Even cracked nipples and minor infection can produce some bloodstaining. Just occasionally, however, bleeding signals an underlying cancer, so urgent investigation and treatment is required.

❸ *Are you taking any medication?*
Very occasionally, breast lumps or enlargement can be the result of taking certain medications. Common offenders include the diuretic spironactolone, which can cause breast enlargement in men as well as in women. Drugs to reduce blood pressure such as beta-blockers and Aldomet should also be considered, along with chlorpromazine, a long-acting tranquillizer often used in the treatment of mental illness.

SUMMARY
BREAST LUMPS

POSSIBLE CAUSE	ACTION
Mastitis (fluid retention)	*Explanation and reassurance, plus supportive bra, pain relief if necessary, diuretics before each period. Consider oral contraceptive pill.*
Benign mammary dysplasia	*As above. Aspiration of fluid from large cysts through a fine needle if necessary.*
Cyst	*If small, observe until the next period is finished. If large, aspirate through a fine needle.*
Injury	*No treatment necessary as it will resolve itself.*
Cancer	*Mammography and/or biopsy. Medical or surgical treatment, with or without radiotherapy.*
Medication	*With your doctor, isolate culprit and discontinue medication.*

A SWOLLEN ABDOMEN

A swollen abdomen is not at all uncommon, and more often than not is actually stomach distension produced by a slap-up meal! Other common causes of generalized abdominal swelling include trapped air building up and irritable bowel syndrome, the main features of which are bloating, dull, aching, cramp-like pains, wind and alternating diarrhoea and constipation. During the early stages of pregnancy there may also be generalized swelling due to hormonal changes, and I have often seen kidney infections and premenstrual changes in the week or so before a period have similar effects. Swellings can also be localized to a particular area of the abdomen, possible causes being an enlarged spleen due to a chronic infection or glandular fever, an obstructed bladder, or tumours of the colon or large bowel.

When a doctor examines a swollen abdomen, he or she will look to see if the distension is spread generally across the whole abdomen. If it is, this suggests the presence of wind, as the trapped gas is distributed fairly evenly throughout the intestine. If, on the other hand, it is mainly in the sides, this indicates an accumulation of fluid, which may have an abnormal underlying cause such as cirrhosis or a tumour. In this situation any accompanying weight loss is another warning sign.

❷ Have you just had a large meal?

Overeating is the most obvious cause of abdominal swelling. There will be a clear time relationship to the previous meal, with a gradual diminution in the size of the belly as the food is digested.

❷ Do you regularly suffer from bloating, abdominal cramps and wind?

These are the characteristic symptoms of irritable bowel syndrome. There will also be episodic and alternating diarrhoea and constipation, plus the frequent urge to empty the bowel, which is seldom relieved by doing so. It is important to exclude other causes of these symptoms through sometimes exhaustive investigations, especially because the symptoms may be mimicked by problems as serious as cancer of the bowel.

❷ Do you worry a lot and tend to gulp your food?

Anyone suffering from the nervous habit of air swallowing, or aerophagia, unintentionally gulps down large quantities of air, which can lead to stomach distension and is normally accompanied by belching and flatulence. The good news is that the condition is benign, and simple re-education and counselling for anxiety are usually all that is required.

❷ Could you be pregnant?

You would be surprised how many women complain to the doctor about their growing abdominal girth, not thinking that they could be pregnant. Any woman of reproductive age should therefore always be asked about the timing of her last period and whether she is using any form of contraception. A pregnancy test can be carried out, but an internal examination will reveal an enlarged uterus and give a rough idea as to the dates of the baby's gestation. Sometimes in very early pregnancy there can be marked abdominal swelling, but this is fluid retention due to hormonal changes, which soon settles down again.

❷ Does your bladder feel as if it's about to burst?

Obstruction of the bladder is acutely painful and causes distension in the form of a balloon-shaped swelling with its rounded top somewhere up near the navel. *It requires urgent relief by catheterization.*

❷ Is the lump causing protrusion of the belly-button?

Hernias around the navel, known as 'paraumbilical' hernias, are fairly obvious because the enclosed intestine can be pushed back through the weakness in the muscle wall with the forefinger. An 'incisional' hernia resulting from weakness in the muscle due to previous surgery will also have similar characteristics.

❷ Are the whites of your eyes or your urine a browny colour?

Both infections of the gall bladder (cholecystitis) and gallstones can seriously interfere with the normal process of digestion and cause swelling of the abdomen. Usually there also is a dull, aching pain in the right upper part of the abdomen that comes and goes (colic), possibly with jaundice, indigestion, wind, dark urine and pale stools. The swelling is not necessarily restricted to that part of the abdomen, but the presence of the symptoms described above generally allows the doctor to make the diagnosis.

❷ Are you a heavy drinker?

Cirrhosis of the liver can occur in a number of conditions, but is most commonly caused by excess and long-term intake of alcohol. In this condition, the liver can no longer perform the various functions it was designed for, and serious consequences occur. The liver may be enlarged and tender, but in the later stages it becomes shrunken and scarred. Other telltale signs are a red nose and 'spider naevi', little red spots on the skin of the chest and face with spidery blood vessels running away from the central spot. There may also be loss of facial hair, reduction in the size of the testicles, and a reduction in sex drive, all of which are the result of a build-up of oestrogen, which the failing liver is no longer able to break down

and get rid of in the normal way. For the same reason, men with cirrhosis may also experience an increase in breast size. As the condition becomes more advanced, there is a build-up of pressure further along the blood vessels leading to the liver, causing fluid to be forced out of the circulation and into the abdominal spaces. The resulting abdominal swelling is known as ascites.

❷ Are your ankles swollen too?

A weak heart fails to pump blood adequately around the body. As a result, there is a build-up of pressure in the veins, congestion of fluid within the lungs, with resulting shortness of breath, particularly when lying flat, and accumulation of fluid within the abdomen. Eventually the build-up pressure causes fluid to leak into other tissues, including the ankles and feet, a very common symptom in both heart failure and constrictive pericarditis, a condition where the surrounding envelope of the heart becomes rigid and tight, also leading to a build-up of pressure in the veins.

❷ Are your periods heavy and/or irregular?

Fibroids are benign muscular lumps in the wall of the uterus. They are not at all uncommon and should always be thought of when a woman complains of lower abdominal distension. Usually they are quite small, but some women can develop more sizable ones, larger than a grapefruit in some instances, in which case they become very obvious. They usually develop before the menopause and they tend to shrink afterwards, when the uterus diminishes in size as the result of lowered oestrogen levels.

❷ Do you feel a pressing heaviness in your lower abdomen or pelvis?

Ovarian tumours, whether they are benign

cysts or more solid malignant growths, can cause abdominal swelling simply because of their size, although with the latter, the formation of very large quantities of fluid may be the first sign of the disorder. Occasionally, ovarian cancer is picked up during routine internal examinations, particularly in women over the age of 50, but because it causes so few early symptoms, it is one of those cancers that tends to come to the doctor's attention late on in its development, when it may be causing abdominal swelling, discomfort, irregular bleeding and pain on intercourse, often when treatment is less effective. For this reason, *any woman with progressive abdominal distension that is not associated with weight gain, particularly if she is over 50, should urgently seek the attention of her doctor.*

❸ Have you passed any blood with your motions?

Cancer of the colon can produce a lump that you can feel in the abdomen, usually, but not always, on the left-hand side. Other symptoms include alternating constipation and diarrhoea, weight loss and general tiredness and malaise. There may also be bleeding into the gut, producing blood mixed with the motions or blood lost on its own into the toilet, but this is by no means invariably the case.

❹ Do you feel generally exhausted? Has your belly grown but your arms and legs become thinner?

A number of other organs in the abdomen can become altered by benign or malignant conditions. Most of these organs consist of many layers so that in the stomach, for example, growths can arise from the stomach wall, from its lining, or from the blood vessels that supply it. Malignant conditions can also spread to the abdomen from elsewhere, for example from the breast. In the late stages of these disorders, the abdomen can be distended by fluid, which when aspirated and looked at under the microscope reveals cells identical to those from the source of the original problem.

191

SUMMARY
A SWOLLEN ABDOMEN

POSSIBLE CAUSE	ACTION
Over-eating	Alter quality or quantity of food eaten.
Irritable bowel syndrome	High-fibre diet, stress management and counselling, antispasmodics.
Air swallowing	Reassurance, treatment of underlying anxiety.
Pregnancy	Confirmation.
Bladder obstruction	Urgent catheterization.
Hernia	Surgical repair.
Gall-bladder problems	Medical or surgical treatment.
Cirrhosis of the liver	Medical treatment if reversible; surgical treatment for vein congestion if not.
Heart failure	Restrict fluid and salt. Diuretics, digitalis, other drugs to stimulate the heart. Surgery for constrictive paricarditis.
Fibroids	Remove fibroid or hysterectomy if fibroid large and family completed.
Ovarian cancer	Surgery, chemotherapy or radiotherapy.
Colonic cancer	Surgery and radiotherapy.
Other tumours	Identify cause. Medical and/or surgical treatment.

SWELLINGS IN THE GROIN

It is usually fairly easy to pinpoint the cause of swellings in the groin because apart from the common lumps and swellings that can affect the skin and underlying tissues in any area of the body, there are only a limited number of possibilities to consider here.

❷ Are several small, firm lumps present?

Just as the lymph glands in the neck become enlarged as a response to infection or inflammation anywhere in the head or neck, so the lymph glands in the groin become enlarged when problems occur anywhere in the legs or lower abdomen. A badly infected ingrowing toenail or an infected sports wound often produce the characteristic red lines of ascending infection that can be seen running up the leg from the source of the trouble towards the groin. This is evidence of infection being carried away by the lymphatic drainage system to the glands to be dealt with by the white blood cells and antibodies that they help to manufacture.

Some more generalized disorders such as Hodgkin's disease or a malignancy of the lymph glands themselves can also produce swelling in the groin, in which case glands in other parts of the body such as the armpits and neck will be swollen as well. In these conditions there are usually other constitutional symptoms such as anaemia, lethargy, tiredness and loss of appetite and weight. Certain virus infections such as glandular fever can also be responsible, as can chronic infections such as brucellosis and tuberculosis, in which case glands in the neck and armpit areas will also be enlarged.

Finally, it is always worth considering an allergic reaction to certain medications since occasionally these turn out to be the culprits.

❸ Is there a single soft swelling?

The groin is perhaps the commonest area of all for a hernia, which is caused when a loop of intestine pushes through between weak muscle layers. For this reason, when the doctor listens over the hernia with a stethoscope, he or she can sometimes hear the sounds produced by normal bowel function. There is usually a soft bulge that becomes more obvious on straining or standing upright, and which can usually be pushed back in place with the fingers. When the person coughs or sneezes, a little shock wave can be felt over the hernia, a symptom known as a cough impulse. Hernias can be small, the size of a fingertip, or at times very large, moving right down into the scrotum in a man and filling it completely. They are always a little uncomfortable, generally because the underlying muscle layers are forcibly pushed apart. Occasionally the edges of the muscle will squeeze the part of the bowel pushing through it, with the result that the blood supply to that part of the intestine can be completely cut off. When this happens the hernia cannot be pushed back into its proper place, and if neglected gangrene of the underlying intestine with intense pain and generalized infection of the lining of the abdomen (peritonitis) can follow. This is known as a strangulated hernia and is a surgical emergency requiring hospitalization and treatment.

❹ Does the lump feel full of fluid?

Sebaceous cysts are formed when the duct of a sebaceous gland is blocked, and they are therefore often found in the hairy areas of the body, where oil-producing glands are more common. They lie very near the surface, are usually dome-shaped and slightly paler than the surrounding skin, and there may be an identifiable tiny hole at the surface of the skin where the blocked duct is situated. Sometimes the sebaceous cyst will ooze thick, cheesy material of its own accord but generally the chronically thickened wall of the cyst means that a spontaneous cure is unlikely and surgical removal will be required. If infection gets in from the outside, the cyst will become hot, tender and red in which case antibiotics followed by curative surgery, will be necessary.

SUMMARY
SWELLINGS IN THE GROIN

POSSIBLE CAUSE	ACTION
Swollen lymph glands	If localized, treat underlying infection; if generalized, antibiotics if caused by chronic infection. Surgery, radio- or chemotherapy if caused by malignancy.
Hernia	Surgery under general or local anaesthetic. Frail, elderly people may be happy with a surgical truss if necessary.
Sebaceous cyst	Small cysts may resolve spontaneously once infection treated. Surgically treat infected cysts more than 1 cm in size to prevent spread of infection.

SWELLINGS OF THE TESTICLES

Swellings of the testicle and scrotum are by no means uncommon and whilst highly alarming to most men, they generally have some eminently treatable and reversible cause. The alarm is all the more apparent when the swelling is painful, but in fact the presence of discomfort or pain is by no means always such a bad thing. Suffice it to say at this point that a totally painless swelling of one testicle is actually a much more sinister sign as testicular cancer in men aged between 20 and 40 is not all that uncommon and is likely to begin in this way, although there are other conditions that can produce painless swellings in this area.

❷ Is the swelling painful and has there been any injury?

Significant trauma to the testicle is incapacitating, which is why special self-defence courses for women concentrate on aiming for this sensitive area! The testicle and its surrounding tissues are richly endowed with nerve endings and there is really very little to protect the testicle from damage. Sumo wrestlers have learned the knack of massaging their testicles upwards, out of the scrotum and into the inguinal canal before combat to protect them from harm, but this is not practical for most adults who have not been taught the technique from a young age and so most men will always be vulnerable. Acute trauma produces swelling and heat, but unless there is a large amount of bruising the treatment is rest and support, followed a few days later by hot baths. Pain relief may also be necessary.

❷ Do you also have swelling in front of the ear or under the jaw?

Orchitis is a painful swelling of the testicle, usually on one side, where there has been no history of trauma. When it occurs together with swollen salivary glands, this is highly suggestive of mumps, which not uncommonly causes orchitis in about 10 per cent of sufferers, although bacterial infections can also be responsible. Treatment for the latter is with broad-spectrum antibiotics, probably for at least 2–3 weeks.

❷ Is the testicle swollen just at the top or bottom?

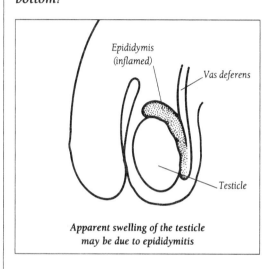

Apparent swelling of the testicle may be due to epididymitis

The epididymis is the tube along which sperm manufactured in the testicle is transported towards the prostate and from there to the outside. It can be infected by micro-organisms or congested by sperm, with acute tenderness as the result. Normally the doctor is able to distinguish between infection of this tube and infection of the testicle itself as they are anatomically separate, although occasionally both may be inflamed together.

❷ Did the swelling and pain begin suddenly?

Torsion, or twisting, of the testicle may result in interruption of the blood supply, causing acute pain and swelling in the testicle on one side. This is because the artery that feeds the testicle comes vertically downwards from above into the scrotum, so that when the testicle twists, the artery does too. Most men are endowed with special strands of fibrous tissue that tether the testicle in the scrotum and prevent this from happening. In a small proportion of young men, however, these physiological 'guy ropes' are inadequate, allowing the testicle, which is very mobile anyway, even in normal people, to rotate more than just a few degrees. The condition may correct itself, in which case the symptoms will disappear spontaneously. However, some young men who experience recurrent but short-lived discomfort from 'temporary' torsion remain at risk of 'permanent' or persistent torsion. The real problem arises when the blood supply to the testicle is cut off for more than six hours or so, after which time gangrene and testicular death will occur. This in itself is not life-threatening but obviously the testicle will become non-functional and if gangrenous will have to be removed surgically. This does not affect fertility as men can function perfectly adequately with a single testicle.

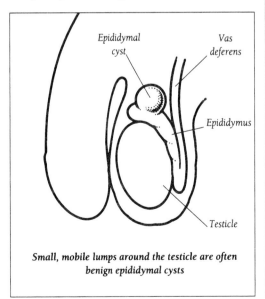

Small, mobile lumps around the testicle are often benign epididymal cysts

❷ *Is there a single small lump to be felt?*
It is not at all uncommon to find fluid-filled cysts around the epididymis. These may gradually enlarge and produce discomfort but are usually quite distinguishable from inflammations of the epididymis or of the testicle.

Aspiration under local anaesthetic with a needle is sometimes possible, but occasionally open surgery is performed.

❸ *Is the swelling painless, filling the scrotum and going up as far as the groin?*
Strictly speaking a hernia is not a swelling of the testicle at all, although it may appear so. What happens is that a hernia in the groin can push downwards into the scrotum and be noticed by the man concerned as a lump.

Generally speaking, hernias are not painful unless they 'strangulate', which means that the loop of intestine being pushed through the weak muscle of the abdominal wall becomes pinched at the base, cutting off the blood supply to the intestine. The intestine then becomes painful and potentially gangrenous.

This constitutes a surgical emergency and must not be ignored.

❹ *Is the swelling painless, and does it feel like a balloon full of water?*
A hydrocele is a collection of fluid around the testicle that can sometimes become quite large. It is possible to distinguish between swelling of the testicle itself and a hydrocele, and one simple test involves transilluminating the area with the light from a pocket torch. The fluid of a hydrocele will be illuminated, unlike a solid swelling of the testicle.

Temporary hydroceles are sometimes seen in newborn babies, or after minor trauma in adults, and are not serious, but occasionally they need to be surgically treated to prevent recurrences.

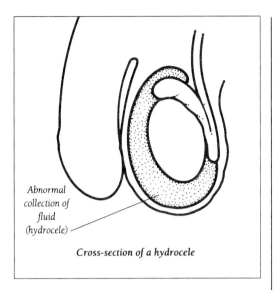

Abnormal collection of fluid (hydrocele)

Cross-section of a hydrocele

❷ Is the swelling painless and bluish in colour?

When the veins that drain the testicle become permanently congested, they become swollen, bluish and tortuous, just like varicose veins in the legs, and in the scrotum resemble a bag of worms. Treatment for varicoceles is not usually necessary unless they are severe, in which case surgery can be carried out.

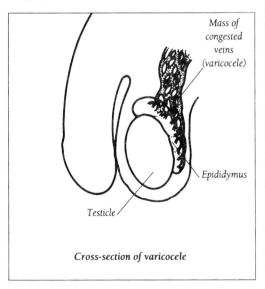

Mass of congested veins (varicocele)

Epididymus

Testicle

Cross-section of varicocele

❸ Is the swelling painless and only on one side?

Cancer of the testicle is the commonest cancer in men aged between 20 and 35. There are two main types, both of which start with a painless swelling of one testicle that may be noticed either by the man himself or by his sexual partner. One is a seminoma, which arises from the cells that produce sperm. The other is called a teratoma and consists of several different types of cells. The symptoms are generally very similar. The good news is that when detected early there is an excellent cure rate, reaching something like 90 per cent, even when the cancer has spread to other areas of the body. For this reason men are now being strongly encouraged to carry out self-examinations, just as women do with their breasts.

SUMMARY
SWELLINGS OF TESTICLES

POSSIBLE CAUSE	ACTION
Trauma	Pain relief, supportive underwear, hot baths later.
Orchitis	Antibiotics.
Epididymitis	Antibiotics.
Permanent torsion	Urgent surgical treatment.
Scrotal cyst	Surgery if causing symptoms.
Hernia	Surgical treatment, or surgical truss for the elderly and frail.
Hydrocele	Small ones may reabsorb spontaneously. If not, and if uncomfortable, surgery.
Varicocele	Treatment not usually required, surgery sometimes needed if uncomfortable or causing infertility.
Cancer	Surgical removal of testicle with radio- and/or chemotherapy.

LUMPS IN AND AROUND THE RECTUM

Lumps and swellings may appear with or without pain in this particularly private and personal area for a number of reasons. Although they can give great cause for concern, the majority of them are completely benign.

❷ Has there been any bright red bleeding?

Haemorrhoids (piles) are basically varicose veins in an awkward and uncomfortable place. They can be of varying degrees of severity, the mildest causing discomfort and anal irritation, the moderate sort causing bleeding as well, especially after passing a motion, and the most severe bleeding heavily at any time and sometimes prolapsing through the anus to the outside where a painful, palpable lump can be felt. Occasionally this will 'thrombose', which means that the blood within it becomes stagnant and clots, resulting in swelling and great discomfort, especially when sitting. Treatment for the mild to moderate symptoms involves creams, ointments or suppositories, but for the more severe kind a special technique known as 'banding' can cut off the blood supply to the varicose veins permanently, whilst sclerosing injections can be used to glue the walls of the veins together and permanently empty them of blood that way. Occasionally surgery is required to remove the veins altogether.

❷ Can you feel fleshy skin tags around the back passage?

It is quite common for people to notice that the skin surface around the back passage has become irregular and lumpy, and for these skin tags, as they are called, to become inflamed and sore. They may represent the long-term results of a pile that has thrombosed and shrunken away into scar tissue, but they may simply be naturally forming little skin pouches. Either way they can easily be surgically removed under local anaesthetic if necessary.

❷ Are many, quite firm lumps present?

Anal warts are multiple, fleshy lumps that gradually become larger. They are not uncommon and are very similar to warts seen on the hands and other parts of the body. They may be transmitted sexually or by contamination from warts on the fingers, and can be treated effectively with the application of special chemicals such as podophyllin paint, available on prescription from the doctor.

❷ Is the lump exquisitely tender?

Abscesses can occur around the back passage just as they can anywhere else. Obviously this is an area that is difficult to keep scrupulously clean and contamination with bacteria is therefore likely. Abscesses can be quite large and deep-seated and are clearly painful and uncomfortable, particularly when sitting. Small abscesses may respond to antibiotics if treated early enough, but generally speaking the larger ones need to be surgically drained and left open to heal from the deep part of the abscess upwards towards the surface.

❷ Are you a man over the age of 50 with difficulty passing urine?

Occasionally an enlarged prostate will make the sufferer feel as though he is sitting on a golf ball. There is nothing to feel on the outside but the swelling of the prostate gland pushes back against the rectum, giving this feeling of there being 'something there'.

The doctor may be able to detect this enlarged prostate through a rectal examination with a gloved finger. Treatment will involve surgery if the prostate is significantly enlarged and if there are also urinary obstructive symptoms.

● *Have you noticed any altered bowel habits? Have you passed any blood or mucus recently?*

A tumour in the rectum or in the last part of the large bowel might cause symptoms of discomfort or swelling around the back passage, although it would usually have to be quite large to do this. If in doubt, the doctor can examine the back passage and last part of the intestine with an instrument called a proctoscope or with a gloved finger. However, in most instances of swellings around the back passage, this diagnosis will be ruled out.

SUMMARY
LUMPS IN AND AROUND THE RECTUM

POSSIBLE CAUSE	ACTION
Haemorrhoids (piles)	Cream, ointment, suppositories, 'banding', sclerosing injections or surgery.
Skin tags	Local anaesthetic and removal if necessary.
Anal warts	Podophyllin paint.
Perianal abscess	Antibiotics if small; surgical drainage if large.
Enlarged prostate	Surgery.
Tumour	Surgery and/or radiotherapy.

SWOLLEN LEGS

There is no doubt that swelling of one or both legs is a common problem. Usually there is a physiological cause, in other words the swelling is a normal response to a particular circumstance. For example, the patient may have sprained an ankle recently, with resulting puffiness of the surrounding tissues, and if a woman is premenstrual, there may be fluid accumulation around the feet just as there is in the breast tissue. People who travel by aeroplane often notice that their feet swell during the flight as a result of the lowered cabin pressure, whilst in the summer many people notice that their ankles and feet swell simply because their veins are more dilated and tend to leak a little more lymphatic fluid. Occasionally, however, the cause will be more serious and require more vigorous investigation and treatment.

❷ Are the veins in your legs swollen, tender and tortuous?

Varicose veins are not only cosmetically unattractive and obvious but they can also be uncomfortable. They tend to affect the veins over the calf muscle first, but then the large vein on the inside of the ankle, running upwards past the knee and into the thigh, can become dilated and tortuous. Varicose veins are particularly common after childbirth or in people who are overweight, but any condition that increases abdominal pressure and compresses the veins higher up, for example cirrhosis of the liver and heart failure, can cause the problem. As a result of the increased pressure of blood within the veins, there is a tendency for fluid to leak through the vein walls and accumulate in the tissues of the feet and ankles, causing swelling. (Although fluid can accumulate anywhere in the body, the law of gravity means that it naturally moves downwards.) Swelling caused by varicose veins tends to affect both legs and can be vastly improved by the wearing of surgical-support stockings and by elevating the feet when resting. In long-standing varicose veins pigmentation around the ankles is also very common. Blood leaking from the veins either spontaneously or through rupture of the vein walls, leads to iron derivatives from the red blood cells being deposited, causing dark brown staining of the skin.

❷ Is the area red and hot as well as swollen?

Whether it is the result of an ingrowing toenail, chilblains, bunions, athlete's foot, injury or underlying diabetes, any type of infection of the foot can allow bacteria into the tissues underneath the skin, resulting in cellulitis. In cellulitis the skin is very red and hot to the touch and the extent of the infection is clearly marked. Usually the lymph glands in the groin are swollen as antibodies to the infection are produced, but there will also be considerable swelling in the affected leg.

❷ Is the calf tender and swollen?

Whilst varicose veins affect the surface or superficial veins of the legs, bang in the middle of the legs is a much more important system of veins where in certain circumstances clotting, or thrombosis, can occur. A clot in the deep veins is a serious condition. As well as causing swelling of the ankle and foot on that side, the clot can extend higher up the vein or break off and be carried in the circulation towards the heart and lungs, where it can have potentially very serious results. In deep-vein thrombosis, the calf is sometimes painful and sore to the touch, and there may be redness and a hot sensation in the foot and ankle as well as swelling. To prevent further extension of the thrombosis, *urgent medical treatment with anti-coagulants is required.*

❷ Is your abdomen distended?

Any disorder within the abdomen causing pressure on the veins will produce swelling of the legs as fluid leaks out of the thin vein walls. Pregnancy will do this, but so will other swellings in the abdomen such as ovarian cysts. Liver disease, particularly cirrhosis, will produce a build-up of pressure in the veins; kidney disorders will lead to a build-up of fluid in the body that may accumulate in the legs.

❷ Are both legs swollen and is there any shortness of breath?

This combination of symptoms is characteristic of a weak heart unable to pump blood efficiently around the circulation. This weakness leads to a build-up of pressure in the veins carrying deoxygenated blood to the heart, and as a result fluid leaks out of the veins and into the surrounding tissues. When fluid leaks into the lungs, it causes congestion and shortness of breath, whilst in the legs it produces accumulation of fluid around the feet. Sufferers may also find that swelling caused by a weak heart can be worse at night. The swelling itself, however, is easily treated with diuretic tablets, which get rid of excess fluid from the body. Pericarditis, or inflammation of the envelope covering the heart, can also interfere with the heart's pumping action, producing similar symptoms.

❷ Are you on regular medication?

A number of drugs used therapeutically by doctors can cause swollen legs, particularly steroids, including oestrogen, used in hormone replacement therapy, and the oral contraceptive pill, anti-inflammatory agents used in the treatment of arthritis, the male sex hormone testosterone, used controversially to treat the male menopause and to stimulate libido in women, and drugs used in the treatment of high blood pressure.

❷ Is there any swelling of the face?

This is unusual in most causes of swollen legs but may occur in allergic conditions, in conditions where there is inflammation of the covering layer around the heart (pericarditis), where the thyroid is under-active, or in trichinosis, a rare disorder in the UK, which is contracted through eating infected pork.

❷ Is there any yellowing of the whites of the eyes?

The characteristic symptoms of liver disease include enlargement of the breasts in men, together with loss of facial hair, shrunken testicles and a diminished libido. In either sex it may cause jaundice, 'spider' naevi (little red spots with spidery blood vessels running away from the central spot) on the face and chest and a flapping tremor of the hands.

❷ Do you always feel cold and have you put on weight?

You could have an underactive thyroid gland, one of whose characteristic features is a thickening and swelling of the lower legs known as pre-tibial myxoedema. In this case, it is impossible to indent the swelling by pressing with the fingertip. (In most other cases of swelling of the legs or feet, this indentation is usually present and is known as 'pitting' oedema.)

❷ Is there the possibility of severe malnutrition?

Malnutrition can lead to swelling of the legs and abdomen due to the lack of protein in the diet. Because there is not enough albumin, a form of protein, in the blood, fluid cannot be retained in the circulation, and instead seeps out of the blood vessels, accumulating in the tissues in the belly and around the feet. A very severe diet could have this effect, but it is not commonly seen in this country.

❷ *Has your urine output changed for no obvious reason?*
Abnormal kidney function producing too much or too little urine and anaemia may also lead to swelling of the feet and ankles.

SUMMARY
SWOLLEN LEGS

POSSIBLE CAUSE	ACTION
Physiological (heat, injury, premenstrual tension)	Support bandaging or stockings, diuretics if necessary.
Varicose veins	Surgical support stockings, sclerosant injections, surgical treatment.
Infection	Antibiotics.
Deep-vein thrombosis	Anti-coagulants, strapping, elevation and rest.
Pregnancy	Check blood pressure and urine to exclude pre-eclampsia.
Heart failure	Medical treatment, diuretics.
Medication	With your doctor, identify the offending drug and discontinue.
Allergy	Antihistamines.
Ovarian cysts	Surgery.
Liver failure	Antibiotics, lactulose, liver transplant.
Pericarditis	Anti-inflammatory drugs, diuretics, surgery for extreme 'constrictive' types.
Underactive thyroid	Thyroid-replacement treatment.
Malnutrition	Adequate protein intake.
Trichinosis	Anti-worm treatment.
Kidney failure	Dietary adjustment, blood-pressure control, blood transfusion, steroids, diuretics, dialysis, transplant.

8

PERSONAL SYMPTOMS

Personal symptoms are embarrassing symptoms. They are the antisocial and much-dreaded afflictions that most of us suffer from at some stage in our lives but which of course nobody wants to admit to.

In this situation a doctor can be very useful, not just because he or she may easily conjure up successful remedies, but because the medical profession can find appropriate scientific terminology to 'label' such unpleasant symptoms as part of a physical condition, offering sufferers an acceptable reason beyond their control for such problems, and thereby absolving them from all blame. It is the very perception or even accusation that lack of personal hygiene may be to blame that makes so many people self-conscious enough to avoid seeking help at all.

However, suffering in silence, as so many do, can lead not only to paranoia and self-criticism, but at times to more profound psychological problems.

The good news is that all of the 'personal' symptoms discussed here are treatable. The more interesting news is that with any one of them there may be a significant underlying medical disorder as the root cause – even more reason to summon up the courage to visit your doctor and have the problem properly sorted out.

Acne and body-hair changes, for example, may just be a normal physiological development during puberty, but can just as easily be the result of a glandular condition or even the side effect of certain medications. Halitosis is usually due to a person's diet but can also reflect digestive or sinus disorders. Incontinence may well be attributable to weak pelvic-floor muscles, but can also indicate cystitis, diabetes, multiple sclerosis or a slipped disc.

HAIR LOSS

There is no doubt that baldness causes a lot of grief to a lot of people. It is a problem that particularly affects men. Hair loss in women is much less common, but when it occurs the effects are that much more socially devastating. There is an hereditary element, and women's hair usually becomes thinner after the menopause, but earlier significant hair loss may well be due to easily reversible causes such as anaemia or an underactive thyroid gland.

Sufferers will go to enormous lengths to try to remedy the situation, encouraged by the large number of commercial organizations and products whose main purpose is to make them believe that there is a solution. Although in the vast majority of cases hair loss is not the result of an underlying medical condition and is therefore not treatable, some medical conditions do have this side effect, so it is worth asking yourself the following questions:

● *Have you inherited your receding hairline?*

Hereditary baldness, or male pattern baldness, tends to run in families, although it can certainly skip a generation. This means that the son of a bald father can retain a full head of hair, only to see his own son lose his. Patterns can also differ within a generation, so that brothers may be quite differently endowed with hair. This type of baldness tends to begin at the temple area or on top of the head at the crown. The problem is basically related to the male sex hormone testosterone, which for some reason in susceptible individuals causes loss of the hair roots. Previously the only remedies suggested were wigs or hair transplants which were both expensive and cosmetically not terribly effective. Hope has emerged in the form of minoxidil (Regaine), which when applied regularly may cause a reduction of hair loss and a slower regrowth of some hair.

● *Are you suffering from stress?*

New research has suggested that stress may be a factor in hair loss as it is well known to reduce the blood flow to the hair roots, resulting in their premature destruction. Quite why some individuals should react in this way to stress and not others is yet to be explained. Suggested treatment includes relaxation therapy, inversion therapy (hanging upside down by the feet) and the application of specially formulated potions.

● *Have you recently had a baby?*

The sudden hormonal fluctuations in the bloodstream caused by pregnancy can produce fairly sudden hair loss but hair growth will be restored within 3–6 months of childbirth.

● *Are you going through the menopause?*

Hair usually becomes thinner after the menopause. This can be prevented and partially reversed by HRT.

● *Do you feel cold all the time and have you gained weight?*

Coarse, thinning hair can be the result of an underactive thyroid gland producing too little thyroxine hormone. The resultant slowing down of the body's metabolism also leads to constipation, intolerance of cold weather and a thickening of the skin on the lower leg. The hair loss is reversible when the underlying condition is treated.

● *Do you feel hot all the time and have you lost weight?*

Hair loss can also be caused by an overactive thyroid gland where the over-production of the thyroxine hormone stimulates the metabolism to work faster than normal. Symptoms also include an increased appetite, diarrhoea, excessive sweating and a fast pulse. Again, the problem is reversible when the underlying condition is treated.

● *Do you also suffer from double vision?*

Sudden hair loss can be the result of benign tumours of the pituitary gland, which sits at the base of the brain and governs many of the hormone functions of the body. The good news is that the hair loss is reversible when the underlying condition is treated.

● *Do you feel constantly weak and tired?*

Anaemia caused by iron deficiency may result in thinning of the hair and this is particularly true in women. It is always worth asking your doctor to perform a simple blood test to rule out anaemia if you notice that there are more hairs than usual on your pillow in the morning or around the bath plug after washing.

● *Is your hair falling out in clumps or patches?*

Autoimmune disorders are caused when, for unknown reasons, antibodies produced by the body to attack foreign invaders act against the body's own tissues. Alopecia areata is one example of an autoimmune disease that produces patches of baldness over the scalp and in the beard area in men. In this case, the antibodies destroy the hair follicles. The hair loss can persist for several months. Usually after this time it settles spontaneously, although the hair when it regrows may be of a different colour. Hair loss of this kind can also occur in systemic lupus erythematosus. A family history of vitiligo (white patches on the skin) or thyroid disorders makes this more likely.

❷ Is there a skin disorder affecting the scalp, knees and elbows?

Psoriasis is a condition of the skin where there are red patches with excessive silvery scale overlying the surface. The appearance is similar to that of severe dandruff, but at the edge of the hairline there is often the telltale redness and soreness that characterizes the condition. Hair loss may occur spontaneously or as the result of itching and scratching. It is treated by using coal-tar shampoo and steroid lotions.

❸ Are you taking any medication?

Certain drugs may lead to hair loss particularly drugs used in chemotherapy, and this is a predictable but reversible side effect. Vitamin A toxicity may also produce hair loss (it is always unwise to take too much of any vitamin). Radiotherapy will kill off the hair roots just as chemotherapy does, but again this effect is usually reversible when treatment finishes.

❹ Have you had an infection recently?

After any high temperature or serious illness patients will often experience an increase in the fallout rate of the hair, producing marked thinning. The hair regrows when the underlying condition improves.

❺ Do you blow-dry and/or perm your hair?

There is no doubt that various manipulations of the hair, for example overtight rollers or too much high-temperature blow-drying, will damage the hair roots, causing the hair to fall out. Certain dyes and other chemicals used in perming may also be responsible.

SUMMARY
HAIR LOSS

Possible Cause	Action
Heredity	There is no proven medical treatment except for Minoxidil, available on private prescription. Otherwise, hair transplants, wigs, toupees.
Ageing	Untreatable as yet.
Stress	Relaxation therapy, inversion therapy.
Pregnancy	Hair regrows spontaneously within 3–6 months of childbirth.
The menopause	Consider hormone replacement therapy.
Thyroid disorders	Medical or surgical treatment to restore thyroxine hormone to normal levels.
Pituitary-gland tumours	Surgical excision or radiotherapy.
Iron-deficiency anaemia	Dietary adjustment, iron supplements.
Autoimmune disorders	Steroid injections into the scalp may be helpful.
Psoriasis	Coal-tar or steroid preparations.
Medication	If caused by radio- or chemotherapy, hair will regrow spontaneously when treatment stops. Stop or reduce dosage of vitamin A to allow hair to regrow spontaneously.
Fever	Recovery is spontaneous when fever goes.
Hairdressing techniques	Avoid perming, crimping, too much blow-drying, overtight rollers.

UNWANTED HAIR

Unwanted hair can produce just as much embarrassment and anxiety in women as baldness does in men. The medical name given to the condition where hair grows in areas where normally it does not is hirsutism, and there may or may not be some masculinization associated with it, for example, a deepening of the voice, increased muscular development, loss of hair on the head, clitoral enlargement, an increased sex drive, the development of facial hair, reduction in the size of the breasts and alteration in the normal menstrual cycle. Hirsutism generally represents some underlying medical disorder and therefore needs investigation and treatment. Hypertrichosis, on the other hand, simply describes thicker and more widespread hair without masculinization and this may have other explanations, including heredity.

❷ Does the rest of your family have a similar problem?

There is no doubt that the amount of body hair we have depends on our racial and geographical origins. Mediterranean women, for example Greeks, Italians, Arabs and Jews, tend to be more generously endowed with darker and thicker body hair than Chinese or Scandinavian women. This degree of hairiness is genetic in origin and therefore runs in families. There is no need here for medical treatment, but should there be a wish to reduce the amount of hair for cosmetic reasons, various beauty treatments including electrolysis are widely available.

❷ Have your periods become less frequent or stopped altogether?

During the change of life the reduction in the circulating levels of oestrogen marks the end of the reproductive era, after which time the unopposed effects of testosterone make their presence felt. The resulting increase in body hair is physiological and entirely normal, and any of the various beauty treatments such as electrolysis can be used if so desired.

❷ Are you taking any medication?

Testosterone used to treat decreased libido or chronic fatigue in women may produce unwanted body hair as a side effect, but the anabolic steroids used by body builders to gain extra muscle bulk are much more likely to do this. Other drugs, usually of a hormonal nature, such as danazol, used to treat very heavy periods and endometriosis, are also well known to have this side effect too when taken in significant doses.

❷ Do you experience pain or discomfort on intercourse?

Ovarian cysts and tumours, whether benign or malignant, can either increase the amount of testosterone made by a woman, or decrease the amount of oestrogen. In either situation, excess hair may result. Such cysts can sometimes produce pain during sexual intercourse, although usually they are found during a doctor's internal examination and confirmed by an ultrasound scan.

❷ Do you take body-building steroids?

Hair growth is governed largely by the sex hormones. The male sex hormone testosterone in particular promotes hair growth, which is why women taking anabolic steroids for body-building purposes commonly experience hair growth on the moustache and beard areas, around the nipples, down the middle of their abdomen below the navel, and in other areas.

❷ Did the hair growth appear gradually with changes in body weight?

Benign or malignant tumours affecting the adrenal gland, for example, alter the sex-hormone balance, causing too much testosterone to be produced, and this can result in hirsutism. A blood test and a CAT scan can make the diagnosis.

❷ Have your hands, feet and jaw grown larger over the last year or two?
Tumours of the pituitary gland can produce excess growth hormone, resulting in a condition known as acromegaly in which the hands, feet and lower jaw become larger, and acne and hirsutism also occur.

❸ Has the weight of your trunk increased at the expense of your arms and legs?
In Cushing's syndrome an over-active adrenal gland is associated with an accumulation of fat over the back of the neck – the so-called 'buffalo hump' – and the body generally resembles an orange on sticks as fat accumulates on the torso but the arms and legs remain thin. The patient often looks moon-faced as a result of the extra cortisone being produced, and flushed skin and increased hair growth are also experienced.

SUMMARY
UNWANTED HAIR

POSSIBLE CAUSE	ACTION
Heredity	Plucking, waxing, sugaring, depilatory creams, electrolysis.
The menopause	Consider hormone replacement therapy.
Medication	With your doctor, identify drug responsible and reduce dosage or discontinue.
Ovarian cysts	Medical or surgical treatment.
Adrenal-gland tumours	Surgery.
Acromegaly	Radiotherapy or surgery.
Cushing's syndrome	Reduce steroid dosage if responsible; surgery or radiotherapy if a tumour is responsible.

FLUSHING AND BLUSHING

Most people have experienced the uncontrollable sensation of blushing when they have been angry, embarrassed or made to feel guilty about something. This kind of blushing tends to affect only the head and neck. Here, small blood vessels or capillaries controlled only by the automatic part of the nervous system respond involuntarily to an emotional stimulus by dilating wide open, thereby dramatically increasing the blood flow and producing the characteristic redness and sweating. Some people are particularly susceptible to this trick of the nervous system because it stops them from being able to present a cool and collected persona, they can feel seriously handicapped by it. In the past little could be done about it, other than to help the individual deal with his or her response to certain situations through counselling and psychotherapy.

These days, however, drugs called beta-blockers can stop blushing by preventing the capillaries and other blood vessels in the skin from opening up. Beta-blockers are available on prescription and although they should not be taken long-term, are certainly worth taking prior to particular situations likely to precipitate the problem. However, blushing and flushing can also be symptomatic of a variety of underlying conditions.

❷ Could you be going through your menopause?

Hot flushes are a common symptom of 'the Change', although some women are affected a great deal more than others. Thus, whilst some women sail through the menopause with virtually no problems whatsoever, others can be plagued by frequent, distressing and embarrassing flushes that can even wake them at night. The flushes are caused by the sudden reduction in levels of the female sex hormone

oestrogen, and are associated with a number of other symptoms caused by the same problem, including vaginal dryness, thinning of hair, loss of elasticity of the skin, irritability, insomnia, fatigue, anxiety and depression. Fortunately, modern women no longer have to put up with this and modern doctors no longer advise them simply to grin and bear it. Hormone replacement therapy, which these days really has very few unwanted side effects, can dramatically decrease the frequency of the hot flushes, if not eradicate them.

❷ Do you have a high temperature?

When the body's temperature is elevated, the skin will automatically try to lose the excess heat by allowing the blood vessels to dilate. This in turn produces the flushed, reddened skin that is the normal response to any kind of infection.

❷ Are you drinking heavily?

Alcohol has a direct effect on the blood vessels of the skin, causing them to open up. This explains both the characteristic flushed look of anyone who has had a few drinks and the permanent red nose and pink cheeks of the chronic alcoholic. In the latter case, the flushed appearance may in time prove to be permanent as the blood vessels gradually lose their ability to contract.

❷ Do even small amounts of alcohol make you flush?

Occasionally, severe flushing is seen when only small amounts of alcohol are consumed, in which case the flushing is highlighting an underlying medical condition. Hodgkin's disease, for example, is a form of cancer of the lymph glands that in the very early stages may be asymptomatic. However, a glass or two of alcohol in somebody with the disease can provoke acute and profound flushing, a sign that could be instrumental in helping the doctor make a diagnosis. Similarly, someone with a carcinoid tumour can experience sudden and unexplained flushing if the hormone serotonin secreted by the tumour mixes with alcohol in the bloodstream. A carcinoid is a small, relatively benign tumour in the lungs or intestine. Associated symptoms are diarrhoea and wheezing.

❷ Are you taking any medication?
There are a number of medications that can cause flushing as a side effect, including Diabinase, used to treat non-insulin-dependent diabetes, and cholesterol-lowering drugs and megavitamins containing niacin or nicotinic acid. Steroids, used in a number of serious medical conditions such as polymyalgia rheumatica, chronic asthma and rheumatoid arthritis, can also have this effect.

❷ Have you lost weight, become jittery and noticed increased sweating?
An over active thyroid increases the tick-over speed of the body so that everything, including the heart, works faster and harder. A flushed skin with increased sweating are common features, along with other symptoms such as bulging eyes, weight loss, diarrhoea, an increased appetite and an intolerance of hot weather.

❷ Are you permanently short of breath?
In chronic lung disease, the body responds to the problem of getting enough oxygen to the red blood cells through the lungs by making more red blood cells. This produces a flushing of the skin, particularly of the cheeks.

❷ Is the flushing associated with severe itching after a hot bath or with gout?
In certain blood conditions, for example polycythaemia, a flushed skin is caused by the bone marrow specifically producing excessive numbers of red blood cells. The extra red blood cells are broken down to form uric acid, which can then build up in the joints and lead to gout.

❷ Has the weight increased on your trunk at the expense of your arms and legs?
In Cushing's syndrome there may be a flushed appearance of the skin due to the excess amount of cortisone produced by the adrenal glands sitting above the kidneys. Fat will also accumulate on the body and the back of the neck, producing the so-called 'buffalo hump', although the arms and legs remain thin. Blood pressure tends to be elevated and there may also be obvious stretch marks in the lower abdomen and an increase in unwanted hair.

SUMMARY
FLUSHING AND BLUSHING

POSSIBLE CAUSE	ACTION
Emotional	Psychotherapy, hypnosis, beta-blockers.
The menopause	Consider hormone replacement therapy.
Fevers	Identify cause and treat appropriately.
Alcohol	Abstain or reduce consumption.
Hodgkin's disease	Chemotherapy and/or surgery.
Carcinoid tumour	Surgical excision.
Medication	With your doctor, identify and then discontinue or reduce dosage of drug responsible.
Overactive thyroid	Antithyroid drugs or surgery.
Chronic lung disease	Medical treatment of underlying condition.
Blood conditions (polycythaemia rubra vera)	Reduce number of red blood cells through radioisotope treatment.
Cushing's syndrome	If drugs are responsible, reduce dosage of steroids; if a tumour is responsible, surgery or radiotherapy.

ACNE

Acne is an inflammatory skin disease that affects the tiny pores covering the face, arms, back and chest and the oil-producing sebaceous glands attached to them. It is caused by an abnormal response in the skin to normal levels of the male hormone testosterone in the blood. Both men and women have a certain level of testosterone on board, but for reasons not yet fully known, people who suffer from acne are much more vulnerable to the effects of this hormone. Usually acne is self-limiting and will eventually correct itself, but in some cases it may take years or even decades, and there is no way of predicting how long it will take.

Acne develops when the ducts through which the sebaceous glands normally release their oil become blocked. This is because in acne sufferers the tough, outer layer of the skin consisting of piles of dead, leathery cells narrows the openings of the ducts, thereby preventing the release of the oil. As a result of this blockage, the oil-producing glands become swollen, leading to inflammation with reddening and the formation of lumps in the skin. Once bacteria get inside, whiteheads and blackheads soon form. Bacteria may then be released on to the surface of the skin, thereby infecting other glands and causing a vicious circle to be set up. Because there is a great deal of ignorance concerning acne, it is worth remembering the following facts. There is no direct link between acne and diet, although a good, balanced diet is always important and can affect the condition of your skin generally. It is a myth that chocolate and fried foods make acne worse. Acne is not caused by poor hygiene either, and in fact most people with acne wash much more frequently than those without the condition in an attempt to get rid of the excess oil produced by their skin, although normal, regular washing with mild soap twice a day is really all that is required.

TREATMENT

Treatment for acne involves topical creams and lotions that can be painted on or rubbed into the skin. These include benzoyl peroxide, which has a germicidal activity and therefore reduces the amount of bacteria on the skin. Antibiotics in cream or lotion form also reduce the level of bacteria in the skin and prevent their spread, whilst oral antibiotics usually taken in a low dosage over a period of several months can gradually eradicate the common bugs that make acne a great deal worse. For women taking the contraceptive pill, one brand known as Dianette contains alongside the normal, medium dose of oestrogen a drug called cyproterone acetate that combats the effects of testosterone in the body. Any woman requiring oral contraception and who also wants to have acne treated would therefore do well to ask their doctor for this one. Finally, there is a synthetic form of vitamin A known as isotretinoin used to treat very severe forms of acne where there is cyst formation and scarring. This is given only under hospital supervision, and courses of treatment last up to four months. Isotretinoin must be used with

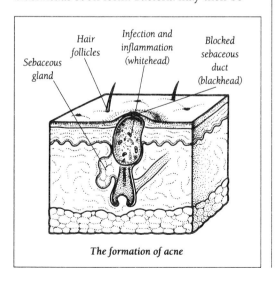

The formation of acne

great caution because of its side effects. Because it is harmful to unborn babies it must never be used if there is any possibility of pregnancy. It can also affect the function of the liver and the level of fats in the blood. Nausea, headaches and hair loss are also possible.

❷ *Do your spots get worse before your period?*

Many women notice that their acne deteriorates 2–7 days before their period starts, due to changes in the hormonal levels at that stage in the menstrual cycle.

❷ *Are you pregnant?*

Pregnancy can affect acne, either improving or exacerbating the condition as the result of hormone fluctuations.

❷ *Do you sweat a lot?*

Sweating can have a bad effect on acne. Up to about 15 per cent of sufferers find their acne flares up when they have been sweating a lot. Working in a humid atmosphere or going on holiday to very humid climates can have a similar effect. Regular washing and exercise are generally helpful.

❷ *Are you taking any medication?*

Some medicines can make acne worse. Certainly the oral contraceptive pill, steroids, anti-epileptic preparations and anabolic steroids can all produce acne and are worth avoiding if possible.

❷ *Do you regularly use cosmetics and/or hair oils?*

Cosmetics can make acne much worse by adding yet more grease to the surface of the skin, and even hair oils, especially the ones used to defrizz very curly hair, are best avoided. Some suntan oils can have a similar effect, so they too should always be used with caution by anyone with acne.

❷ *Do you wear tight clothes?*

Clothing should be loose and airy. Headbands, tight bra straps and collars can all cause spots in these areas.

❷ *Has your acne developed recently, long after puberty, when you have never been affected before?*

Some medical conditions can also be responsible for acne, particularly those associated with an increase in testosterone levels. Amongst the commonest are glandular disorders, for example acromegaly, in which there is an increase in the size of the hands, feet and lower jaw, and ovarian disorders. In abnormalities affecting the pituitary gland, the adrenal gland or the ovaries there are almost always associated symptoms, which can include visual disturbance, headaches, weight gain, period irregularity and high blood pressure, any of which might alert the physician to the true underlying problem.

SUMMARY
ACNE

POSSIBLE CAUSE	ACTION
Hormonal changes (puberty, menstruation, pregnancy)	Avoid overcleaning the skin. Topical creams or lotions, antibiotics. If very serious, isotretinoin under hospital supervision.
Sweating	The above, plus regular washing and exercise.
Medication	If caused by the pill, consider changing to Dianette. Otherwise, with your doctor identify and then discontinue or reduce dosage of drug responsible.
Cosmetics, hair oils, suntan oils	Avoid or change brand.
Tight clothing	Wear loose, airy clothes, preferably cotton.
Glandular disorders (acromegaly, ovarian disorders)	Cause and treat through medical, surgical or radiotherapy treatment.
Pituitary-gland disorders	As above.
Adrenal-gland disorders	As above.

SNORING

A widespread problem, snoring is caused by vibration of the soft back part of the roof of the mouth (the soft palate) and the uvula, the flap of tissue hanging down from the back of the throat when you look at your tonsils in a mirror. In sleep these muscles are completely relaxed and floppy, and when the tongue falls back towards them there is partial obstruction of the air-flow. Snoring will only ever occur if the amount of obstruction becomes critical, and for many people this never happens. In some people, however, a complete obstruction occurs temporarily, resulting in sleep apnoea syndrome. In this condition the sufferer will wake throughout the night, unable to breathe at all as the soft palate falls back against the back of the throat, preventing the inflow and outflow of air to the lungs. There are different types of sleep apnoea, which may or may not be linked to underlying medical problems, but the commonest form is obstructive sleep apnoea, affecting up to 1 per cent of men between the ages of 30 and 50. Such men are usually overweight and snore heavily. Severe sleep apnoea is potentially serious and in rare instances can result in high blood pressure, stroke and/or heart attacks.

In the past all manner of remedies have been tried, including strapping a sharp object to the snorer's back to make sleeping on the back so uncomfortable that the sufferer moves on to his or her side thereby allowing the tongue to fall away from the back of the throat and relieve the obstruction. More recently a nasal dilator called a Nozovent has been produced, which is designed to hold open the nostrils to allow a better inflow of air. Sleeping without pillows is also recommended, because when the head is tilted right back with the chin up the tongue is less likely to obstruct the airflow. Recent surgical techniques can remove or stiffen up the soft palate and uvula, though state-of-the-art laser techniques may less hassle. However, such techniques will not be available on the NHS for some time.

SUMMARY
SNORING

POSSIBLE CAUSE	ACTION
Simple snoring	Sleep on your side with no more than one pillow. Avoid alcohol, smoking and being overweight.
Severe snoring	In a child with enlarged adenoids or tonsils, surgical removal of these will help. In an adult, surgery to shorten the soft palate (uvulo-palato-pharyngoplasty, or UPPP).
Severe sleep apnoea	Continuous positive airway pressure (CPAP), in which compressed air is forced into the airway through a mask or tube inserted into the nostrils.

HICCUPS

Hiccups, which as most people will know are usually temporary and even mildly amusing, are caused by a spasm of the diaphragmatic muscle due to irritation of the nerves supplying the diaphragm. A variety of problems can cause this irritation, some more serious than others, in which case the hiccups may become long-standing and troublesome. In extreme cases, they may even be associated with a serious illness. Of the various remedies suggested for hiccups any or all of the following are worth trying, although they almost certainly will not work if there is an underlying physical problem. A shock or dramatic surprise can sometimes do the trick. Alternatively, you can hold your breath for as long as possible or drink iced water from the 'wrong' side of the glass. Eating granulated sugar is another possibility, as is breathing in and out of a paper bag. If these fail, you can try pulling your tongue out or pressing on your eyeballs. These may sound rather strange but they are all designed to prevent further hiccuping by stimulating the vagus nerve, which has a controlling effect on the depth and frequency of respiration. Because lung inflation 'stretches' the diaphragm, just as holding your breath does, hiccups may be dissipated in this way. However, the best way to deal with this important nerve is to massage the carotid sinus, which is situated at the side of the neck over the carotid artery. The danger with this, though, is that it can lower the blood pressure and cause fainting, so it should only be practised by a doctor and certainly never on both sides of the neck at the same time! In all other cases of hiccups, including those where there is an underlying physical cause, chlorpromazine is the drug most likely to be found effective.

❷ Have you been drinking and/or smoking?

Hiccups are common in smokers and in people who drink large quantities of alcohol, especially in conjunction with hot, spicy meals. There are a number of measures that can be carried out by the person with hiccups to remedy the muscular spasm (see above), but whatever you do, the hiccups will stop spontaneously in time.

❷ Have you had any recent chest or abdominal pain? Are you breathless or off your food?

Any form of irritation to the muscles of the diaphragm can result in hiccups. Above the diaphragm lie the lungs and their covering envelope, the pleura; infections there such as pneumonia and pleurisy can certainly produce this type of irritation of the diaphragm with resulting hiccups. Intestinal problems, including gall-bladder disease, inflammation of the liver and perforation of the stomach due to ulcers leading to the escape of air under the diaphragm, can have similar consequences. Hiccups are also common after surgical operations and often accompany pregnancy.

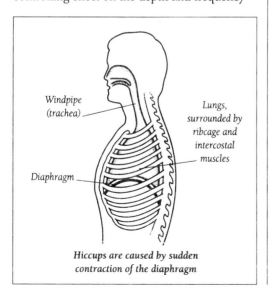

Windpipe (trachea)

Lungs, surrounded by ribcage and intercostal muscles

Diaphragm

Hiccups are caused by sudden contraction of the diaphragm

❷ Have you any muscle weakness, visual disturbance or headache?
Although rare, serious disorders of brain function, for example following a stroke or in the presence of benign or malignant tumours, can produce abnormalities of the nervous pathways responsible for the production of hiccups. This is, however, very unusual.

SUMMARY
HICCUPS

POSSIBLE CAUSE	ACTION
Diet, alcohol and smoking	Will settle spontaneously, but grandmother's remedies well worth trying.
Underlying physical disorders	Identify underlying problem and treat medically or surgically.
Nervous system disorder	Try chlorpromazine to stop hiccups. Consider surgical cutting of the phrenic nerve that produces hiccups as a last resort.

BAD BREATH

Although bad breath, or halitosis as it is known to the more academically minded, is something of an unpleasant joke to most of us, it can, very occasionally, represent the first sign of a serious underlying disease. Usually, though, it is due to some benign oral problem, which is why doctors often refer patients suffering from it to the dentist. Help is usually at hand, whether from the doctor or the dentist, but much depends on the original source of the problem, physiological reasons being the commonest. Understanding the various mechanisms whereby halitosis can occur is important. The production of normal saliva continues all day long, but is non-existent during sleep, which is why the cells that line the inside of the cheeks and gums and cover the tongue become drier during the night. The normal shedding of these surface cells allows a degree of biological breakdown during this period, and this is the reason for the characteristic odour of breath first thing in the morning. However, certain foods and drinks are capable of producing volatile fatty acids and other malodorous chemicals as they are broken down by the body and these odours can be given off from the lungs as you breathe out. Alcohol, garlic, pastrami and onions are prime examples, but spicy foods such as chili and curried dishes can also be culprits too.

When halitosis is not the result of diet, however, and when all the usual remedies like tooth-brushing and antiseptic gargles have been used to no avail, there are a number of questions you can ask yourself in a bid to discover the cause:

❷ *Did the bad breath come on suddenly?*
This suggests some kind of inflammation or infection inside the mouth, a dental abscess, or perhaps a slight temperature, often associated with a sore throat.

❷ *Do you suffer from toothache when you eat or drink anything hot or cold, bleeding gums when you brush your teeth, or a 'furry' tongue?*
Poor oral hygiene, dental plaque and caries, inflammation of the gums themselves (gingivitis) and hairy tongue, a condition often seen in heavy smokers, can all be responsible for bad breath.

❷ *Is your nose constantly blocked and/or do you have any discomfort in the cheekbone?*
People who are mouth-breathers as a result of chronic nasal obstruction, for example in sinusitis, inflammation of the adenoid glands, a foreign body in the nostril, nasal polyps or tonsillitis, should consider these conditions as the possible source of their problem. Mouth-breathing at night will cause a particularly dry mouth, increasing the putrefaction of the dead cells lining the mouth, with resulting bad breath. Your sense of taste and smell may also be affected. Much more rarely, growths within the larynx may do the same.

❷ *Do you suffer from a long-standing cough?*
Any chronic chest infection, including lung abscess, bronchiectasis and cancer of the lung, should be considered in long-standing halitosis. Trapped, infected mucus altered by contact with the air is the source of the odour. There may also be blood in the mucus.

❷ *Do you suffer from indigestion, swollen glands around the mouth or have trouble swallowing?*
Infections and inflammations of the salivary glands, inflammation of the lining of the stomach (gastritis), a hiatus hernia or any partial or complete obstruction of the gullet can cause halitosis.

❷ Do you feel generally unwell and have you noticed any weight changes?

A variety of more serious conditions including dehydration as a result of infections, kidney failure or diabetes may produce bad breath. Conditions such as leukaemia, Hodgkin's disease and other blood disorders can also have the same effect. Accompanying symptoms may include a high temperature and/or joint pains.

❷ Are you taking any medication?

Although many drugs can potentially lead to a strange odour on the breath, perhaps the commonest might be lithium, used in the treatment of manic depression, griseofulvin, used to treat fungal infections, and penicillamine, commonly prescribed for long-standing rheumatoid arthritis.

❷ Could you be imagining the bad breath?

Many people have something of a phobia about having bad breath and are particularly anxious in company. However, very occasionally the persistent and profoundly held conviction that halitosis exists where in fact it does not can be a forerunner of some mental disorders such as schizophrenia and depression.

SUMMARY
BAD BREATH

POSSIBLE CAUSE	ACTION
Poor oral hygiene	Regular, brushing of the teeth and tongue, occasional mouthwash, regular visits to hygienist.
Dental plaque and caries, gingivitis	Preventative treatment as above, regular dental visits, dental treatment.
Sinusitis	Infective: decongestants, antibiotics, possibly surgery. Allergic, steroid sprays, antihistamines.
Swollen adenoids	Consider surgical removal.
Foreign body	Removal.
Nasal polyps	Surgical removal.
Tonsillitis	If viral, symptomatic relief. If bacterial and fever is present, antibiotics.
Chronic chest infection (chronic bronchitis, bronchiectasis, lung abscess)	Antibiotics.
Cancer of the lung	Surgical, radio- and/or chemotherapy.

Continued . . .

SUMMARY
BAD BREATH

POSSIBLE CAUSE	ACTION
Inflamed, blocked or dry salivary glands	Antibiotics, surgery or steroids respectively.
Gastritis	Avoid alcohol and smoking. Antacids. Antibiotics if infection responsible.
Hiatus hernia	Dietary adjustment (eat little and often), antacids, keep weight down, surgery if severe.
Gullet obstruction	Surgery to bypass or remove blockage.
Dehydration	Fluid replacement.
Kidney failure	Medical treatment, including dialysis if necessary.
Diabetes	Control with diet, tablets or insulin.
Blood disorders (leukaemia, Hodgkin's disease)	Medical correction of underlying disorder.
Medication	With your doctor, identify and then discontinue or reduce dosage.
Imaginary	Stress management, counselling.

BODY ODOUR

It is possible simply to become accustomed to a bad smell, and some people are unaware that their body odour is offensive. In fact, sweat itself has no odour, but when it becomes stale and is acted upon by the normal bacteria on the skin's surface, it produces the characteristic smell of body odour, particularly in the armpits, genitalia and feet. The problem can be avoided by washing thoroughly every day with soap and using deodorant products. Some say a person's body odour is highly characteristic of the individual and a hint of it can be a sexual turn-on, but excessive amounts of body odour certainly do not appeal to everybody.

Excessive sweating can be so marked that it seriously affects the individual's capacity to work. Hyperhidrosis, to give it its proper name, is caused by an excess of the sweat-producing glands in various parts of the body, particularly the armpits, the palms of the hands and the soles of the feet, although usually only one area is affected. Someone who sweats excessively will also have an increased tendency to body odour. The application of aluminium chloride (a 25 per cent solution commercially known as Driclor) is effective applied on alternate nights and allowed to dry. A reduction of the dosage as soon as possible is desirable as prolonged use can result in an eczema-like reaction in the skin.

❷ *Have you lost weight and do you feel constantly hot?*
With an overactive thyroid gland, the presence of too much thyroxine hormone stimulates the body's metabolism to work faster than normal, leading not only to excessive sweating but also to weight loss, a fast pulse, intolerance of hot weather, an increased appetite, diarrhoea and possible bulging eyes.

❷ *Are you constantly tense and anxious?*
In anxiety states, the individual will be nervous and jumpy, and excessive sweating may be accompanied by a fine tremor of the hands and/or panic attacks.

❷ *Do you have a high temperature and feel tired all the time?*
Excessive sweating can be a result of the high temperature associated with chronic infections.

SUMMARY
BODY ODOUR

Possible Cause	Action
Heredity	Aluminium chloride solution. Beta-blocker drugs. In severe cases, surgery.
Overactive thyroid gland	Medical treatment with drugs. Radio therapy or surgery if neccessary.
Chronic infection	Identify and treat underlying conditions.

222

GENITAL ITCHING

Anybody who has suffered from unbearable itching down below will know how infuriating, inconvenient and embarrassing it can be. Basically the three main areas that commonly cause problems are the front and back passage (the vagina and rectum) and the genitalia themselves.

ANAL ITCHING

❷ *Is there intense anal itching?*

One of the earliest symptoms of worms is anal itching which can be intense. The diagnosis, which will be strongly suspected on clinical grounds, will be confirmed by sending off a sample of the patient's motions for microscopic discovery of the worms or their eggs. Treatment usually takes the form of oral piperazine, taken on two occasions, 14 days apart. The whole family should be treated, not just the individual concerned.

❷ *Is the itching accompanied by soreness and/or bleeding?*

Haemorrhoids, which are basically varicose veins in the anal area, can produce itching as well as bleeding, partly due to the inflammation and mucus production. Treatment consists of creams and ointments, suppositories, injection therapy or surgery.

❷ *Is there any discharge?*

This suggests the presence of a fistula, an abnormal channel of communication from the lining of the rectum to the outside. The discharge will be accompanied by inflammation, often with intense itching and sometimes pain too. Surgical treatment is required.

❷ *Is there any associated skin rash?*

Pruritus ani is a condition in which there is intense itching for no apparent reason. Often the skin is inflamed and sore and looks moist and red. There may have been a history of antibiotic treatment in recent days and weeks which has allowed the over-population of the area with fungal elements which may be causing the problem. Antifungal creams and ointments, with or without mild steroid cream, can be highly effective, although strong steroid creams should always be avoided as they can do more harm than good by causing long-standing thinning of the skin.

❷ *Have you been eating a lot of spicy food?*

Just as spicy foods can irritate the lining of the mouth, so they can irritate the back passage and should therefore be avoided by susceptible people.

❷ *Are you feeling particularly anxious about anything?*

People who are prone to tension and anxiety are also much more susceptible to itching around the back passage. The mechanism for this is not clearly understood, but the nervous system is closely associated with some of the functions of the skin and your mental state may therefore be reflected in what goes on elsewhere. Generally speaking the area needs to be kept clean and dry, with anti-fungal talc or mild steroid cream applied where appropriate. The anxiety itself needs to be alleviated by means of reassurance and education. Steroid preparations should never be overused.

VAGINAL ITCHING

❷ *Is there any discharge?*

Infection with the organism monilia, a condition commonly known as thrush, produces an itchy white discharge that generally speaking can easily be treated with antifungal creams or pessaries. Occasionally, however, reinfection from the bowel produces recurrent thrush, in which case oral medicine is required in addition to the creams. The diagnosis should always be made properly with vaginal swabs and culture of the organism in a laboratory, but many doctors guess at the diagnosis and treatment from the symptoms alone. Another common infection is trichomoniasis, which produces an even more itchy, yellowy-watery discharge with resulting inflammation and irritation of the skin.

❷ Are you or could you be going through the menopause?

When the level of circulating oestrogen diminishes during the menopause, effects include a decreased resistance to infection, dryness of the vagina, and an increased risk of trauma through intercourse. The problem is easily offset by hormone replacement therapy.

❷ Could you be reacting to toiletries?

Various perfumed soaps, bath oils and deodorants can irritate the sensitive lining of the vagina, resulting in intense itching and inflammation of the skin. Susceptible individuals should use a simple soap with no added ingredients.

❷ Have you lost weight and/or do you feel constantly thirsty?

Undiagnosed or uncontrolled diabetes is another common cause of itching in this area. Treatment of the infection and control of blood sugar are vital. When women who have not formerly realized they are diabetic develop vaginal itching, simple urine and blood testing will reveal the underlying problem.

❷ Is there a small crop of blisters on the skin?

Infection with the herpes virus commonly causes itching and tingling two days before the characteristic rash appears. Treatment involves acyclovir antiviral cream or tablets.

❷ Is the itching intense, particularly at night, with scabs and sores?

The scabies mite burrows beneath the skin, causing severe itching, particularly at night when the skin is warm. Pubic lice called crabs cling to the pubic hair and lay their eggs along it. Treatment for both conditions involves a special lotion.

❷ Is the doctor unable to find a cause?

Occasionally, perhaps due to anxiety or poor hygiene, there can be intense itching around the front passage for no obvious reason. The condition may respond to a mild hydrocortisone cream, to hormone replacement therapy.

AN ITCHING PENIS

❷ Has your sexual partner recently had any vaginal itching or discharge?

Fungal infections may produce thrush which can be transmitted between male and female partners if both are not treated. Men can carry thrush totally asymptomatically but itching is an occasional problem.

❷ Is the foreskin red, swollen and tender?

A bacterial infection can produce a swollen and painful red foreskin. Antibiotics are required.

❷ Is there a crop of blisters on the skin?

Infection with the herpes virus produces itching and tingling in the two days before the obvious blistering rash appears.

❷ Is there intense itching at night with scabs and sores?

This could be a result of infection with scabies or scabs – see under 'Vaginal Itching'.

SUMMARY
GENITAL ITCHING

Possible Cause	Action
Anal itching	
Intestinal worms	Oral piperazine.
Haemorrhoids (piles)	Creams and ointments, suppositories, injection therapy or surgery.
Fistula	Surgery.
Pruritus ani	Creams and ointments plus the occasional use of a mild steroid cream.
Spicy foods	Dietary advice.
Anxiety	Anxiety management, mild steroid cream.
Vaginal itching	
Infection (thrush, trichomoniasis)	Appropriate medication.
The menopause	Consider hormone replacement therapy.
Allergy	Avoid irritants. Mild steroid preparations.
Diabetes	Control blood sugar, treat infection.
Herpes	Acyclovir antiviral cream or tablets.
Scabies or pubic lice	Application of suitable insecticide lotion.
Nonspecific	Mild hydrocortisone cream, hormone replacement therapy.
Penile itching	
Bacterial infection	Appropriate antibiotics.
Thrush	Antifungal cream.
Herpes	See above.
Scabies or pubic lice	See above.

225

INCONTINENCE

Incontinence means passing water when you don't want to. Whether it's just a small drip staining the underclothes or a profuse and unstoppable flow, it is always uncomfortable and often embarrassing. It has been estimated that something like one in three women will experience this symptom at some point after the birth of a baby and that one in five women over the age of 65 suffer from it. Approximately three million people in Britain have incontinence problems, three-quarters of whom are female. The good news is that 90 per cent of cases are curable. Symptoms may be precipitated by coughing, sneezing or laughing, in which case the condition is often termed stress incontinence. Similarly, exercise such as lifting and bending can bring on the problem, as can love-making. Sometimes the sufferer may experience no warning whatsoever, but others may notice they need to get up during the night to empty their bladder more often, and that they need to go more frequently during the day. In more serious cases, the sufferer is totally unable or unwilling to go out socially for fear of not being able to find a loo in time, and there may be bed-wetting at night and constant dribbling during the day.

The underlying problem causing incontinence is weak pelvic floor muscles that are unable to control the outflow of urine from the bladder. Women suffer a great deal more than men because of their anatomy, in particular the shortness of their urethra – the tube from the bladder to the outside – compared to that of men. They rely much more heavily on the function of their sphincter muscles, the circular muscles that run round the urethra at the base of the bladder, which can be damaged and stretched during childbirth or through being overweight, although they can be retrained by exercise to overcome the problem.

❶ Are you passing urine more frequently? Is it bloodstained?
Any acute or chronic infection of the bladder (cystitis) can cause irritation and inflammation of the bladder neck with the urge to empty the bladder frequently, including at night. Incontinence and the passage of blood in the urine are not uncommon.

❷ Are you constipated?
Because the rectum is situated behind the bladder, any moderate degree of constipation causing retention of waste material can press on the bladder, increasing the risk of incontinence. Treatment of the constipation with diet and/or laxatives often solves the problem.

❸ Are you pregnant?
In pregnancy not only does the growing womb put great pressure on the bladder, but the female sex hormone progesterone softens and dilates the urethra, allowing urine to escape without warning and infection to ascend from below. Cystitis is also more likely, therefore, and the combination of these problems produces incontinence.

❹ Have you had particularly difficult labours?
During childbirth, the passage of the baby's head and shoulders tends to bruise the base of the bladder and the sphincter muscles in the mother, and temporary incontinence can result. Stretching of the ligaments around the base of the bladder almost always occurs, and this is why pelvic floor exercises should be so religiously taught and practised in the first few weeks after delivery of the baby.

❺ Are you taking any medication?
A number of drugs can increase the likelihood of incontinence, including tranquillizers,

sedatives, antihistamines, diuretics (water pills) and antispasmodics of the type used to treat heartburn.

❷ Do you have any backache, muscle weakness or numbness?

The function of the bladder and sphincter muscles depends on the integrity and function of the nerves in the spinal cord. Deep-seated problems of the nervous system, including multiple sclerosis, a slipped disc, Parkinson's disease and other abnormalities of the spinal cord itself should always be considered if any of the above symptoms are experienced, and especially if the incontinence itself is of a sudden and severe nature.

❷ Are you diabetic, or are any of your family diabetic?

Undiagnosed diabetes can often present the sufferer with a severe thirst and a need to pass copious amounts of urine, the result of a high level of sugar in the blood being excreted through the kidneys and taking large amounts of water with it. The patient often has to empty his or her bladder frequently, and occasionally incontinence is an associated feature. Long-standing diabetes can also affect the nerves supplying the bladder, with a similar effect. Bladder infections are also more likely in the presence of diabetes.

❷ Do you have any serious worries at the moment?

Occasionally incontinence can be a feature of depression and anxiety, in which case, the problem will respond to treatment of the underlying cause.

❷ Are you very overweight?

Just as childbirth, heavy exertion and constipation can stretch the pelvic-floor muscles and produce pressure on the bladder,

causing incontinence, so can being overweight. Any woman with incontinence who is overweight should therefore try to get her weight down as soon as possible before attempting to settle her incontinence by other means.

❷ Are you going through the menopause?

During this time of life, levels of circulating oestrogen diminish. As a result the pelvic-floor muscles tend to become laxer and less well supported, the vagina becomes dry, and the urethra more prone to inflammation and infection. Some degree of prolapse of the womb is not uncommon, causing kinking of the urethra in the front wall of the vagina, and incontinence can be a result.

Hormone replacement therapy has been shown to be highly beneficial in treating many of these conditions, but occasionally surgery does prove necessary.

❷ Do you have a poor urinary stream (men)?

Approximately one in three men over the age of 50 develop an enlarged prostate. In this condition, the increase in pressure on the urethra caused by the prostate gland leads to dysfunction of the normal sphincter muscles, so that incontinence may result. There is usually difficulty starting to pass a stream of urine (hesitancy), the stream is often of poor quality, and there may be dribbling and leakage after finishing. New medications are helpful, but surgery is highly effective. The condition is usually benign, but with increasing age the possibility of malignant changes in the prostate gland increases significantly.

❷ Is there laxity of the vaginal walls with a bulge at the front or back of the vagina?

Any descent of the uterus into the vagina as a result of weak pelvic-floor muscles alters the normal valve mechanism at the bladder base and may result in leakage of urine. Surgery can put right this condition, which is known as prolapse.

SUMMARY
INCONTINENCE

POSSIBLE CAUSE	ACTION
Cystitis	Urine sample to identify responsible organism. Appropriate antibiotics.
Constipation	Dietary modification, adequate fluid intake, laxatives.
Pregnancy	Exclude urine infection. Restrict fluids to six cups per day.
Childbirth	Practise pelvic-floor exercises after childbirth. 'Passive' pelvic-floor exercises with electrical stimulation if necessary (Faradism). 'Internal weight training' with aluminium weights covered in Perspex to retrain pelvic-floor muscles.
Medication	With your doctor, identify and then discontinue or reduce dosage of drug responsible.
Nervous system disorders	Identify cause. Medical treatment.
Diabetes	Diet, oral hypoglycemic tablets or insulin.
Psychological	Treat underlying disorder.
Being overweight	Dietary restriction and exercise.
The menopause	Consider hormone replacement therapy.
Enlarged prostate	Surgery, although medical treatment for early cases may be possible.
Prolapse	Incontinence pads and pants, vaginal rings or surgery.

WIND

Wind can be both embarrassing and uncomfortable for most people. However, although flatulence is almost always a benign and harmless temporary condition, there are occasions when it is a symptom of some more permanent and serious underlying disorder.

To help establish what the cause of the problem might be, ask yourself the following questions:

❷ Do you overeat, or eat a particularly high-fibre diet?

During my many years as a practising general practitioner I have found that most patients complaining of wind can be treated very simply with the recommendation that they eat less. Occasionally additional advice focusing on the type of foodstuffs they eat can be helpful, as certainly a diet very rich in fibre can produce a great deal of gas. Gas-forming carbohydrates particularly responsible for wind include cabbage and beans. Generally speaking, changing both the quality and quantity of one's diet, avoiding sweets and taking charcoal biscuits can dramatically improve the problem of flatulence.

❷ Do you suffer from stomach cramps and spells of constipation or diarrhoea?

Irritable bowel syndrome is one of the commonest complaints affecting the digestive system. It is associated with alternating constipation and diarrhoea, bloating, abdominal, cramp-like pains and flatulence. It tends to come and go, is much more common in women and consequently is often mistaken for gynaecological disease. The person affected is often of an anxious nature and the combination of symptoms and their long-standing nature is usually enough for a diagnosis to be made, although other more serious problems should first be excluded.

❷ Are you by nature tense and nervous?

Air swallowing (aerophagy) is a nervous habit, usually performed subconsciously, in which the individual gulps down pockets of air, thereby causing upper abdominal bloating and belching. The air isn't got rid of completely by belching or by being absorbed into the body, and wind is therefore the result of this disorder, which fortunately tends to be temporary in nature.

❷ Do you suffer from indigestion?

Anything that produces inflammation of the lining of the gullet or the stomach, for example ulcers and hiatus hernias can often be associated with wind. The wind is usually brought up via the northern route but not always by any means.

❷ Is the wind brought on by eating fatty foods?

Inflammations and disorders of the gall bladder, including stones and infections (cholecystitis), may be associated with indigestion, pain in the right upper corner of the abdomen, and wind.

❷ Are you over 50 and noticing significantly altered bowel habits and/or weight loss?

Although this is certainly not a common explanation for wind, it is nevertheless worth pointing out that various tumours of the digestive system, including in the gullet, the pancreas and the colon, can occasionally manifest themselves early on by wind. Altered bowel habits, particularly in the form of constipation or diarrhoea, generally accompany the wind. These symptoms in anybody over the age of 50 should be investigated as soon as possible. *See your doctor to discuss immediately.*

SUMMARY
WIND

Possible Cause	Action
Diet	Dietary modification. Avoid carbohydrates and sweets. Use charcoal biscuits.
Irritable bowel syndrome	Adjust amount of fibre in diet, antispasmodics, psychotherapy.
Air swallowing (aerophagy)	Counselling, relaxation therapy.
Indigestion	Antacids, dietary modification, H2 antagonist drugs to prevent acid production.
Gall-bladder disease	Medical or surgical treatment.
Cancer	Medical or surgical treatment.

ATHLETE'S FOOT

Athlete's foot, or tinea pedis, is certainly not confined to athletes, although they are particularly susceptible to contracting it because their physical exertions and constant showering and bathing mean that the skin of their feet is often moist and warm, providing the ideal environment for the fungus that causes the problem.

This is why swimming pools and showers are good places to pick up this condition in which not only are the feet smelly, but they can also itch, possibly with white patches on the skin between the toes. If the nails are affected by athlete's foot they will turn thick and yellow.

Preventing the environment from being attractive to the fungus is important, so wearing absorbent cotton socks with talc inside them, avoiding anything but well-ventilated leather shoes, plus daily washing followed by thorough drying are strategies worth trying if you are affected. Various anti-fungal preparations can also be applied. They come in powder or ointment form, and are effective when applied for a good two to three weeks after all the symptoms have cleared up. This ensures that all remaining fungal elements are thoroughly eradicated so that the condition does not recur.

9
THE NERVOUS SYSTEM

The central nervous system is a vast data bank capable of receiving, processing and delivering information. It is more complex than any computer and is infinitely more compact. One way or another it controls every function of all other parts of the body.

The central nervous system consists of the brain and spinal cord, both of which are made up of billions of intercommunicating nerve cells called neurones. Information enters the CNS through the sensory nerves, which bring in sensations such as taste, touch, smell and pain from the various sense organs. Information is then sent out from the CNS along motor nerves to the muscles in other parts of the body that control movement and the reflexes. The part of the nervous system that regulates automatic internal body functioning such as pulse rate, bowel activity and temperature control is called the autonomic nervous system.

The overriding function of the nervous system is that of self-preservation. It allows the body to respond to sensations such as pain and changes in temperature by taking appropriate avoidance action or making the necessary adjustments. Many responses are automatic, such as the reflexes, but others are stored and learned as part of the nervous system's ability to memorize and rationalize. Higher functions such as speech, mood, cognitive and abstract thought are even more complex.

Because the nervous system is so complex and so vital, any disorder affecting its anatomy or physiology has potentially far-reaching

effects. Each one of the billions of tiny cells that constitute the nervous system is subject to infection, injury, entrapment by adjacent structures, degeneration and new growths.

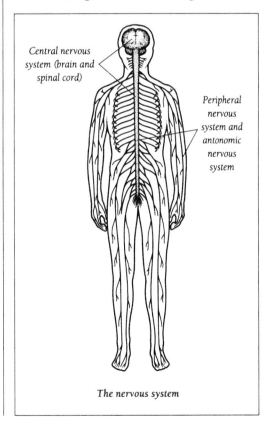

Central nervous system (brain and spinal cord)

Peripheral nervous system and antonomic nervous system

The nervous system

231

VISUAL PROBLEMS

Visual problems are disturbing and should always be reported urgently to a doctor. The ability to see depends on the smooth working of a very complex pathway that can be interrupted anywhere along its course.

To begin with, light passes through the clear front of the eye, the cornea, and then through the pupil, whose size is constantly changing depending on the available light intensity and the nearness of the object being observed. From there the light travels through the elastic lens within the eyeball itself, which relaxes and contracts in order to focus whatever image is being looked at on to the retina at the back of the eye. The retina registers the size and colour of the object and transmits this information along the optic nerves to the brain itself.

The thin covering over the surface of the eye, the conjunctiva, is there to protect the eye against assaults from the external environment, including viruses, bacteria, allergies and foreign bodies. The surface of the conjunctiva is lubricated with antiseptic tears produced by the lacrimal gland. These keep the eyeball from drying out and protect it from various infections. The control and co-ordination of the eye muscles, pupillary size and lens function are all controlled by the brain. Any abnormality affecting an individual part of these structures can lead to visual symptoms, and possible causes range from trivial, everyday problems like the viral conjunctivitis experienced when you have a cold, right through to much more serious ones such as retinal detachment, which may cause sudden partial blindness in one eye.

Any kind of visual disturbance should therefore be taken seriously with a visit to your doctor, who may refer you to an ophthalmologist, or eye specialist. When any pathology within the eye itself has been excluded, he or she may refer you to a neurologist, or nerve specialist, if disorders of the brain and nervous system are incriminated.

❷ Is the eye red and sore and does it hurt to blink?

Any irritation or inflammation on the front of the eye such as a speck of dust or a viral infection can produce watering of the eye and tenderness.

❷ Does very bright light bother you?

This symptom, known as photophobia may occur in local infection or inflammation of the eye, or when there has been acute injury. It is also a classic symptom of meningitis.

❷ Do you have 'floaters' in your field of vision?

Floaters are the shadowy shapes that move across our field of vision as we move our eyes. They are much more obvious when looking at a bright background such as a white wall or the sky and merely represent the debris of dead cells that have been shed from the eye's back wall. They are more likely in people over the age of 30 and are particularly common in people with short-sight.

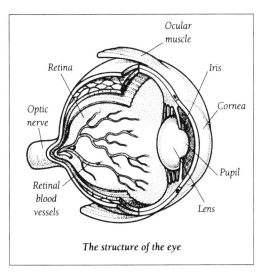

The structure of the eye

❷ Has your vision deteriorated as you have got older?

Just like our joints and our skin, which degenerate as the years go by, the back of the eyes become less sensitive too, resulting in failing sight.

❷ Has the pupil changed from being jet black to milky or opaque?

This change is caused by a cataract, a condition in which the lens of the eye becomes calcified and less elastic. As a result less light passes through and focusing is more troublesome leading to dim and blurred vision.

Modern surgery can easily restore vision very quickly.

❷ Have you recently developed tunnel vision?

You can see straight ahead very clearly, but you have blind spots at the periphery – on each side – of your vision. This is a symptom of glaucoma, the commonest treatable cause of blindness in Britain. *See your optician immediately.*

❷ Are your visual symptoms followed by a blinding headache?

Haloes around bright objects, zigzag flashes of light and blindness in half your field of vision all suggest the early stages of migraine, in which case they will soon be followed by the characteristic headache and nausea, with or without vomiting. Consult your doctor, and read the section on imgraine in this book.

❷ Are you experiencing bright flashing sparks or showers of light, followed by a 'curtain' crossing the field of vision?

These symptoms suggest a detachment of the retina, which requires *urgent* treatment with laser therapy to prevent further detachment and to replace the retina in its proper position.

❷ Are you over 60, and finding it difficult to read unless the print is magnified and very well lit?

In this condition, known as senile macular degeneration, part of the eye responsible for seeing anything straight ahead is altered. It is due to the ageing process, and although difficult to treat, vision may be improved by various visual aids such as glasses, contact lenses or magnifying classes. Consult your optician for advice.

❷ Are you currently taking any medication?

Blurred vision, spots in front of the eyes and the appearance of bright rings around coloured objects such as light bulbs or the headlights of oncoming cars may well be side effects of certain drugs.

Any drug that alters muscle tone can alter the action of the ciliary muscles that control the shape of the eye's lens. Antidepressants and drugs used to control bladder conditions are particularly likely to cause these problems.

❷ Does the blurred vision or blindness in one eye come and go?

These symptoms in someone over 60, especially if he or she has high blood pressure, suggest that the problem is a transient ischaemic attack, when a small blood clot travels around the bloodstream and lodges in the artery supplying the eye. A TIA is commonly the forerunner of a full-blown stroke. Young women in their thirties or forties who take the oral contraceptive pill and who smoke are also prone to strokes because of the increased susceptibility of their blood to clotting. Because treatment with anticoagulants and aspirin may prevent strokes, which can be disabling and sometimes fatal, from occurring, *anyone suffering from these symptoms should visit a doctor urgently.*

233

❷ Is there visual disturbance with loss of feeling or movement down one side of the body?

The commonest form of stroke affects half of one entire side of the body, including the ability to see on one side.

❷ Are you over 50, with a low-grade fever and have lost the sight of one eye?

If you also have generalized aching and stiffness in the muscles and a diminished appetite, your condition could be the result of temporal arteritis, in which there is partial blockage of the temporal artery. A biopsy is necessary, and steroids are *urgently* required to prevent possible permanent blindness.

❷ Have you had blurred vision as a diabetic?

Sometimes inadequate blood-sugar control can result in weak eye muscles. The condition is usually temporary.

❷ Have you had blurred vision with difficulty walking or balancing?

This certainly requires investigation by your doctor as it might be an early sign of multiple sclerosis or a benign or malignant growth within the brain itself.

❷ Has double vision occurred gradually?

Ballooning of certain arteries within the brain that lie next to the optic nerves can interfere with the function of those nerves and produce double vision and headaches.

❷ Are you over 60 with gradual blindness in one eye?

If you also have glaucoma, diabetes or raised blood pressure, the problem could be a clot in the main vein at the back of the eye (retinal vein thrombosis), a condition that requires *emergency medical treatment.*

❷ Have one or both eyelids become droopy?

When this occurs on one side only it usually represents an injury to a nerve, possibly due to a virus or even to a small stroke. A droopy lid affecting one eye only associated with a headache is more sinister, however, in that it might be the first manifestation of an underlying brain tumour. *These symptoms should be referred urgently to a neurologist.* When both lids droop, an allergy that has caused swelling of the tissue around the eye should be considered. In this case there will also be itching. If the drooping of the eyelids comes on very gradually, this suggests myasthenia gravis, a disorder in which there is a fault in the chemical transmitters that allow the muscles that lift the eyelid to contract. Other muscle groups may also be affected later. Medication or removal of the thymus gland at the base of the neck are usually effective.

SUMMARY
VISUAL PROBLEMS

POSSIBLE CAUSE	ACTION
Local eye problems (inflammation, infection, injury, allergy)	Antibiotics, anti-inflammatory eye drops, possible surgery.
Floaters	No treatment required.
Age	Regular visits to the optician and appropriate glasses.
Cataract	Surgical removal and implantation of artificial lens.
Glaucoma	Medication or surgery.
Migraine	Treat headache and nausea. Vision normally restore spontaneously.
Retinal detachment	Urgent laser treatment or surgery.
Senile macular degeneration	Visual aids can certainly help. Laser therapy is sometimes worth trying.
Medication	Discontinue or reduce dosage.
Transient ischaemic attack, stroke	Urgent anticoagulants, aspirin.
Temporal arteritis	Urgent steroid treatment.
Diabetes	Adequate control of blood sugar.
Meningitis	Urgent medical treatment.
Multiple sclerosis	Supportive therapy, steroid treatment, vitamin B injections.
Blood-vessel abnormalities within the brain	Medication or surgery.
Retinal vein thrombosis	Medical emergency requiring urgent hospitalization.
Myasthenia gravis	Antihistamines. Neostigmine or other anticholinesterose drugs. Surgical removal of thymus gland in some cases. Steroids.
Brain tumours	Surgery or radiotherapy.

235

HEARING PROBLEMS

Hearing problems are common. Approximately 25 per cent of all people over the age of 55 suffer from some degree of hearing loss, although it is important to note that most of these problems are avoidable, reversible, manageable or even eminently and easily curable. Many conditions can be improved by the use of modern hearing aids, which come in various shapes and sizes, most of them available on the National Health Service, with the type of aid recommended depending on the particular abnormality. To understand the nature of these various abnormalities, it is first of all important to be aware of how it is that we hear.

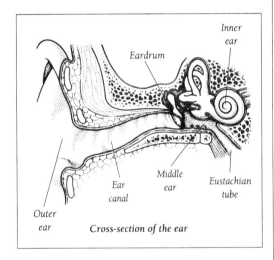

Cross-section of the ear

When sound waves enter the ear, they travel along the external ear canal towards the eardrum. The eardrum vibrates in response, and as it does so it moves three small bones situated in the middle part of the ear. These in turn send sound waves through the fluid-filled canals of the inner ear, stimulating the delicate hair cells responsible for transmitting sound along the auditory nerve to the brain. Problems in any of these areas can cause difficulties with hearing.

❷ Is the ear canal dry, flaky, itchy or painful?
This suggests that the outer part of the ear, the canal, may be blocked by an inflammatory skin condition, for example a boil or infected eczema.

Both of these are extremely common, and in fact cause more temporary problems with hearing than any other condition.

❷ Did the hearing loss occur suddenly, perhaps after cleaning your ears or swimming?
The build-up of thick wax can obstruct sound waves entering the ear. Simply syringing out the wax after softening it with special drops can produce the most welcome and immediate restoration of hearing.

❷ Do you have a cold, especially with earache?
In this case, the eardrum itself is inflamed with the infection.

❷ Have you been subjected to very loud noises or to sudden changes in atmospheric pressure recently?
Any form of acoustic or direct trauma can damage the eardrum. Rapid descent in an aeroplane or acute pressure changes experienced when diving underwater can also perforate the eardrum, seriously affecting its ability to vibrate and transmit sound normally to the acoustic nerve.

❷ Do you suffer from frequent colds or nasal congestion?
Colds or acute or chronic sinusitis can lead to a build-up of fluid behind the eardrum. The drum itself is not inflamed, but everything sounds muffled because the presence of the fluid impedes the three little bones responsible for the onward transmission of sound waves.

❶ *Does deafness run in your family?*
In the hereditary condition known as otosclerosis, which runs strongly in families, the three bones in the middle ear – the stapes, the malleus, and the incus – fuse together so that they are no longer able to move and transmit sound waves to the inner ear.

❷ *Has your hearing deteriorated with age?*
The commonest of the inner-ear disorders is presbyacusis, the medical description for hardness of hearing associated with simple old age. In this case, the nerve impulses are simply not transmitted as efficiently as was once the case, making it difficult to pick out a conversation in a crowded, noisy room, for example. Hearing aids can boost the sound and restore hearing to adequate and sociable levels.

❸ *Do you work in a very noisy environment? Do you like your personal stereo at full volume?*
Certain occupations can make you susceptible to hearing loss. Workers in the aeronautics industry can experience acoustic damage, as can anyone not adequately protected against the noise of gunfire, for example in the army. Similarly, younger people these days are more likely to suffer problems as the result of the constant use of loud personal stereos or of dancing too close to the powerful speakers at discos or pop and rock concerts.

❹ *Did the hearing loss begin with giddiness and ringing in the ears?*
With Ménière's disease sufferers experience a sudden onset of severe vertigo accompanied by nausea and vomiting. The attacks last several hours, with the patient having to stay in bed for two or three days. The return to work is usually delayed because the patient remains unsteady whilst walking. Deafness is

experienced during an attack, but hearing recovers over a period of days, although there may also be ringing in the affected ear (tinnitus), often worse before or during the attack. Some patients become progressively deaf as the disease progresses, although the progress of the disease is variable. Nobody knows what causes it, although excessive fluid and salt intake, overwork and emotional upsets are all possible causes. The disorder usually affects people in middle age.

❺ *Did deafness on one side occur suddenly with numbness or weakness on one side of the body?*
This would suggest the possibility of a stroke, due either to a blood clot or a haemorrhage.

❻ *Did the problems begin after a mumps infection?*
Infections are worth considering since direct bacterial infection from the outside or from the mumps virus can permanently damage the sensitive nerve endings in the inner ear, resulting in significant loss of hearing.

❼ *Is the hearing loss in one ear only, and was it preceded by noises in that ear?*
Nerve damage can occur as the result of a benign tumour on the acoustic nerve itself (acoustic neuroma), or through hardening of the arteries to the hearing part of the inner ear or to the brain itself. With an acoustic neuroma there may be strange noises heard in one ear, which becomes progressively deaf. Surgery, I am pleased to say, can cure this condition.

❽ *Did you have any pre-existing medical conditions?*
Hearing loss can sometimes be due to disorders far removed from the ear itself, for example, an underactive thyroid gland, rheumatoid arthritis, diabetes or kidney problems.

237

❷ *Are you currently taking any medication?*
Certain drugs, including high doses of aspirin, antibiotics of the streptomycin group and quinidine, a heart drug, should be considered as possible causes of hearing problems.

SUMMARY
HEARING PROBLEMS

Possible Cause	Action
Chronic inflammation of the skin	Remove pus and debris. Treat with antibiotics and anti-inflammatory agents.
Wax	Soften wax and syringe out.
Acute infection of eardrum	Antibiotics.
Perforated or scarred eardrum	Spontaneous resolution or surgery.
Fluid behind eardrum	In chronic cases: long-term antihistamines or drain fluid through eardrum surgically. In acute cases: for example after a cold, fluid is spontaneously reabsorbed.
Otosclerosis	Hearing aid or stapedectomy operation.
Presbyacusis	Hearing aid.
Noise damage	Avoidance, protective earmuffs, hearing aid.
Ménière's disease	Reduce fluid and salt intake, stop smoking and overworking, surgery.
Trauma	Possible surgery.
Infection	Medical treatment.
Stroke, hardening of the arteries	Anticoagulants or aspirin.
Acoustic neuroma	Surgery.
Pre-existing medical condition	Treat underlying cause.
Medication	With your doctor, identify and then see whether you can cut down or change the responsible drug.

LOSING YOUR SENSE OF TASTE OR SMELL

Smell and taste are sensations that travel to the brain along independent nervous pathways. However, the two are clearly linked. Any loss of your sense of smell can adversely affect your sense of taste, even though the underlying problem may only directly affect the former. Usually the cause is a temporary virus infection, but there are a number of other possibilities that must be considered.

❷ Do you have a cold?

The common cold is associated with the production of excessive amounts of nasal discharge and mucus and with congestion of the membrane lining the nose and sinuses. The mucus is Nature's way of dealing with the germs, which are wrapped up in this sticky substance so that white blood cells can work on them and kill them off. However, the mucus also prevents the smooth passage of air past the nerve endings that transmit the sensation of smell, which as a result is temporarily lost. Similarly, furring of the tongue caused by excessive mouth breathing or by smoking can jeopardize the ability of the taste buds to relay the flavours of what we eat and drink.

❷ Do you have nasal congestion with a frontal headache and/or pain behind the cheekbones?

Acute and chronic sinusitis can both cause the sense of smell to be lost by directly interfering with the olfactory nerves that lie in the ceiling of the nasal passages and which may be obstructed by mucus.

❷ Are you over the age of 65?

Just as the reflexes gradually become slower with advancing years, so does the sensitivity of your sense of smell. This is a normal process and is not therefore part of any disease.

❷ Do you smoke?

Smoking certainly reduces your ability to appreciate delicate tastes and aromas. The same tarry deposits that clog up the lungs coat the sensory nerve endings in the nose and on the tongue, making them function poorly.

❷ Is one nostril usually blocked?

Nasal polyps are teardrop-shaped growths of a benign nature that arise from the membrane lining the nose. They can grow larger and larger, in which case they can block the airway completely, producing congestion of the nose, and mouth breathing. They are often associated with losing your sense of taste and smell.

❷ Have you been using decongestants regularly for a long time?

Decongestants work by shrinking the little blood vessels in the lining of the nose in order to stop them from leaking fluid. When used for two or three days only, they are fine, but if they are used every day over a long period of time they cause permanent paralysis of the blood vessels, which as a result are no longer able to constrict, causing permanent swelling and leakage of fluid. The nasal passageways remain continuously blocked, therefore, with a consequent reduction in the sensitivity of the sense of smell. For this reason chronic use of decongestants should be avoided.

❷ Have there been any recent headaches, unsteadiness and/or double vision?

Very, very occasionally a brain tumour may be responsible for interruption of the nervous pathways that take the sense of smell from the nose to the brain. In this case, however, there will usually be other symptoms such as personality changes and headaches, in which case you should see your doctor *urgently*.

SUMMARY
LOSING YOUR SENSE OF TASTE OR SMELL

POSSIBLE CAUSE	ACTION
Virus infections	Symptomatic relief only.
Sinusitis	Antihistamines or antibiotics, symptomatic relief.
Smoking	No treatment required. Preferably give up, otherwise cut down.
Polyps	Surgical removal.
Decongestant abuse	Surgery to strip the swollen membrane lining the nose.
Brain tumour	Surgery or radiotherapy.

DIZZINESS AND VERTIGO

For many people the words dizziness and vertigo mean one and the same thing. However, as both symptoms are extremely common, it is worth defining them properly. Dizziness usually means a sensation of impending loss of consciousness; it is often described as feeling light-headed, 'swimmy', or as if you are going to fall down at any moment. People suffering from vertigo, on the other hand, will feel as though either they themselves or their immediate surroundings are spinning around. Whereas dizziness is usually caused by problems in the circulation, vertigo is usually the result of an abnormal function of the balance mechanism situated in the inner part of the ear, and is often associated with other symptoms. If vertigo comes on very suddenly it is accompanied by nausea and vomiting, often with profuse sweating. If the onset is more gradual, however, it may be described by the sufferer simply as 'poor balance', since various compensatory mechanisms come into play to soften the severity of symptoms.

❷ Do you have or have you recently had a heavy cold?

By far the commonest cause of vertigo is a viral illness of a trivial nature that within a few days leads to the onset of giddiness, nausea and sickness. The symptoms are the result of the virus spreading to the inner ear where the balance mechanism is situated. The condition, known as labyrinthitis, normally settles within a week to ten days with bedrest and medication.

❷ Is there any deafness or discharge from the ear?

Any kind of discharge, perforation of the eardrum or infection in the middle-ear cavity can lead to balance disorders with attendant vertigo. An examination of a person with this symptom should therefore include a good look at the outer ear and the eardrum for signs of such problems.

❷ Do you suffer from palpitations or undue fatigue and pallor? Do you have a heart murmur?

Abnormal heart rhythms, valvular heart disease and low blood pressure can lead to dizziness, as can anaemia and migraines. The common factor in all these conditions is a reduction in the amount of oxygen being delivered through the circulation to the brain.

❷ Does the vertigo occur when you look up or over your shoulder?

Arthritis in the neck, otherwise known as cervical spondylosis, can lead to giddiness and vertigo. The neck contains two small arteries that run up through the vertebrae to supply the back of the brain, the cerebellum, with blood. The cerebellum is necessary for maintaining an upright posture and balance, which is why in this common arthritic condition sufferers often experience vertigo when looking upwards or over their shoulder, for example when reversing into a parking space.

❷ Are you taking any medication?

Vertigo can be provoked by numerous drugs, notably certain diuretics, aspirin, quinine, chloroquine and some antibiotics.

❷ Does the vertigo come and go with ringing in your ears and advancing hearing difficulties?

Ménière's disease is a condition in which there is recurrent vertigo associated with ringing in the ears (tinnitus) and progressive loss of hearing. The condition comes and goes and because of the associated symptoms is usually unmistakable. Attacks last from a few minutes to several hours. It is uncommon before age 50.

❷ *Have you experienced any double vision, weakness in the limbs or numbness?*

Anything that affects the normal anatomy or physiology of the brain may provoke vertigo or dizziness. Concussion after a knock on the head can do this, but so too can more serious disorders such as brain tumours or multiple sclerosis. Usually, however, there will be other symptoms and signs to suggest that some more central and deep-seated problem is causing the dizziness or vertigo.

❷ *Are you feeling particularly anxious or depressed for any reason at the moment?*

Vertigo is not unlikely in anxiety states or following an emotional shock as the rapid overbreathing (hyperventilation) often associates with these conditions can bring on this symptom. It is also commonly seen in depression in which case it is often long-standing and constant.

SUMMARY
DIZZINESS AND VERTIGO

POSSIBLE CAUSE	ACTION
Viral infection	Bedrest and antihistamines.
Ear problems	Identify cause and treat.
Circulatory problems (abnormal heart rhythms, valvular heart disease, low blood pressure)	Discover cause and treat.
Cervical spondylosis	Anti-inflammatory medication, cervical collar, physiotherapy, gentle manipulation.
Medication	With your doctor, identify drug responsible and then discontinue or reduce dosage.
Ménière's disease	Supportive care. There is no definitive cure at present.
Nervous system disorders (concussion, brain tumour, multiple sclerosis)	Identify cause and treat appropriately.
Emotional	Reassurance, counselling, medical treatment for underlying cause.

FAINTING

Fainting means a temporary loss of consciousness, for which there are a number of possible causes, including a sudden reduction in blood pressure, epilepsy, heart-rhythm disorders, and rarely, a temporary cut-off of the blood supply to the brain, known as a transient ischaemic attack, or TIA for short. Distinguishing between the various causes is important, as the treatment for each is entirely different. Simple, or vasovagal, fainting describes a sudden, brief loss of consciousness due to temporary interruption of the blood supply to the brain, and there is hardly ever any underlying brain disease or abnormality related to the blood vessels supplying the brain. The faint itself occurs very suddenly or over a few seconds and is often preceded by blurred vision, dizziness, cold extremities and sweating. There may be enough warning for the sufferer to take evasive action such as sitting or lying down, but otherwise the patient becomes intensely pale and limp and sinks to the ground sighing, sweating, and, occasionally, vomiting. Attempts by well-meaning observers to sit or hold up the patient do a lot more harm than good by delaying restoration of the blood supply to the brain and muscle twitching and seizures can occur as a result. The best way of restoring the circulation is to get the head as near to the ground as possible in order to counter the effects of gravity which make it harder for the heart to pump blood to the brain. This is why it is always far better to let the patient sink to the floor, because although rare the resulting convulsions can certainly confuse the diagnosis. It is also worth remembering that an eyewitness description can be tremendously helpful in distinguishing a seizure from a faint. In simple fainting the person slides to the ground and remains completely limp. In a seizure, the patient is usually quite rigid to begin with and then may jerk or twitch, bite his or her tongue and/or become incontinent.

❷ Did the faint occur after getting up suddenly or jumping out of a hot bath?

Simple fainting is the result of a sudden drop in blood pressure and can be caused by something as simple as coughing or straining, for example trying to empty the bladder when it is obstructed by an enlarged prostate, or even by getting up quickly from a chair in a hot room or jumping out of a hot bath. Similarly, when you drink alcohol with a meal, blood is diverted to the intestine for digestive purposes and consequently there is a drop in blood pressure elsewhere. Emotional states are also common precipitating factors for simple faints.

❷ Are you taking any medication?

A vast array of medications can produce a fall in blood pressure followed by fainting. All drugs taken to reduce blood pressure can cause fainting, of which the commonest would be all the treatments used as can diuretics, used to rid the body of extra water. Anti-angina preparations such as glyceryl trinitrate, tranquillizers, beta-blockers, antidepressants, digoxin, and levodopa, used to treat Parkinson's disease, can all cause similar problems.

❸ Do you often experience palpitations, or have a heart murmur or suffer from chest pain?

When the heart rate is too slow, that is below 50 beats per minute, the blood supply to the brain will be inadequate and fainting can result. Drugs such as digoxin and beta-blockers can have this effect, but it also occurs spontaneously in a condition known as a complete heart block, in which the heart does not beat nearly fast enough due to interruption of the nerve impulses to the heart muscle itself.

243

On the other hand, when the heart beats too fast, say over 200 beats per minute, it cannot beat efficiently at each contraction and the blood pressure may fall as a result. Again, the conducting tissue within the heart is at fault. *This requires urgent correction.* Valvular heart disease and heart attacks can also lead to circulatory problems and fainting.

❷ *Has there been any abdominal pain or blackness of the motions?*

Blood loss from any site, whether from an open wound on the outside or from a peptic ulcer in the stomach, can produce a drop in blood pressure sufficient to cause fainting. Dark motions in the days preceding the faint make the possibility of internal bleeding likely as blood lost into the stomach quickly turns to a jet-black colour when mixed with the motion. *See your doctor urgently.*

❷ *Was the faint preceded by hunger pangs, sweating and irritability?*

These are the characteristic symptoms of very low blood sugar (hypoglycaemia), normally seen in diabetics who have taken too much insulin or not had enough carbohydrate in their normal daily diet, but very occasionally in non-diabetic people. Usually, the body automatically controls the level of glucose in the blood within narrow limits. However, it does now seem that a small minority of the population are susceptible to abnormally low dips in blood sugar under certain circumstances. The condition is not serious, although it can cause fainting, with the attendant risks of injury. Accompanying symptoms also include altered behaviour and palpitations.

❷ *Do you get easily anxious or panicky and then tend to breathe too fast?*

Some people when they become anxious or upset unconsciously breathe more rapidly (hyperventilate). Over the course of several minutes this lowers the amount of carbon dioxide in the blood, which in turn alters the calcium content, leading to pins and needles in the hands and feet and light-headedness, followed by fainting.

Actual fainting can be prevented by asking the person to breathe in and out of a paper bag. This allows them to breathe in the carbon dioxide they are exhaling so that it is re-absorbed back into the body.

❷ *Was the faint followed by sudden paralysis and/or slurring of speech?*

With a stroke there is an alteration of the blood supply to the brain. If there is severe hardening of the arteries, the chances of a blood clot completely obstructing a blood vessel are great. If blood pressure is significantly raised, the chance of a weak point in the blood vessel bursting and causing haemorrhage is similarly increased. Clots are more common over the age of 60, in smokers, in people who don't take enough exercise, and in those with certain kinds of heart disease. Haemorrhage tends to occur in people with uncontrolled high blood pressure.

Of all strokes, about 85 per cent are due to clots and 15 per cent to haemorrhage. In both cases in addition to the loss of function in part of the body, for example weakness or numbness in an arm or leg, there may well be fainting at the outset.

❷ *Did the faint occur after turning the neck to one side?*

Built into the carotid artery, which is located in the carotid sinus just below the jawbones, are sensitive pressure sensors.

Occasionally, pressure caused by something as gentle as turning one's neck, can produce a drop in blood pressure, causing fainting.

SUMMARY
FAINTING

POSSIBLE CAUSE	ACTION
Simple faint	Lie patient flat and allow spontaneous recovery. Try to identify trigger factor(s).
Medication	With your doctor, identify and then discontinue or reduce dosage of responsible drug.
Heart or circulation disorders	Consult with your doctor about stopping any drugs responsible. Use drugs to modify heart rate. Appropriate medical or surgical treatment for heart attack, heart failure or valvular heart disease.
Haemorrhage	Identify source of bleeding. Treat medically or surgically and replace blood.
Hypoglycaemia (low blood sugar)	Administer emergency glucose. Stringent blood-sugar monitoring if diabetic.
Hyperventilation	Try to avoid overbreathing. If necessary, counselling. Breathe in and out of paper bag.
Stroke	Supportive care, anticoagulants if indicated, physiotherapy.
Carotid sinus pressure	No treatment except to loosen any restrictive neckwear. Resolves spontaneously.

SEIZURES

A seizure is caused by a sudden burst of electrical activity within the brain. This can happen for a variety of reasons and can manifest itself in a number of ways. Seizures may happen once in a lifetime, in which case there may be a temporary chemical or electrical imbalance with the brain, or they may be recurrent, in which case there is usually a more permanent underlying abnormality. Recurrent seizures are known as epilepsy. Any kind of seizure, whether it is happening for the first time or has been experienced before, is dramatic and alarming to all concerned, although sometimes less so for the victim, who, in the majority of cases, has lost consciousness and is therefore unaware of what is going on. Sometimes the sufferer will drop to the ground, hurting him- or herself in the process, and become rigid and pale. After this generalized stiffening of the arms and legs there may be uncontrollable jerking of all four limbs, frothing at the mouth and possibly urinary incontinence. This is known as a grand mal seizure, and is commonly seen in the majority of cases of adult epilepsy. These seizures are often preceded by an aura, or warning sign, such as a strange hallucination of smell or taste. Some people also notice that their seizures are triggered by bright lights, loud noises, stress or fatigue. The recovery phase is quite lengthy, with the sufferer disorientated and drowsy for several hours after the seizure, in contrast to a simple faint, in which case the individual promptly recovers as soon as he or she is horizontal, preferably with head down and feet raised. However, in other cases there may be no loss of consciousness at all. In *petit mal* epilepsy, experienced mainly by children, there is simply a loss in concentration for a few moments, which may be passed off as simple day dreaming. Alternatively, there may be a focal seizure in which consciousness will not be lost, but there will be uncontrollable jerking in one part of the body such as the thumb or the wrist. In the mildest form of seizure there may be hallucinations of vision, hearing or smell with no affect on consciousness or muscle contraction. In each case, however, there is an underlying abnormality of brain function caused by unpredictable electrical discharges in the brain cells themselves. If the discharge is restricted to one small area of the brain, the symptoms may be mild and located in one part of the body only, but if the discharge spreads across the whole of the brain substance, full-blown *grand mal* seizure will ensue.

It is important, for example, to check that the patient has not simply fainted through a sudden drop in blood pressure, or become giddy and stumbled as a result of medication used to treat high blood pressure. It is also important to rule out an abnormal heart rhythm, especially in an elderly person. To establish whether a true epileptic seizure has taken place, therefore, thorough questioning of an eyewitness is necessary. Often, after medical investigation, a precise cause can be found for seizure. However, the majority of recurrent seizures are not proven to be related to any detectable underlying disorder, a condition known as idiopathic epilepsy. Further investigation can also ascertain whether anticonvulsive therapy will be required. To obtain a driving licence there has to be freedom from seizures whilst awake during the day for more than two years with or without anticonvulsant medication.

❷ *Is there a family history of recurrent seizures (epilepsy)?*
In the majority of people suffering from idiopathic epilepsy (epilepsy of unknown cause) there is a history of the condition in close relatives.

THE NERVOUS SYSTEM — SEIZURES

❷ Is there a history of meningitis or treated brain tumour?

Meningitis and encephalitis are infections that produce inflammation in the covering layers of the brain and spinal cord. This too can produce scarring and the electrical discharges that trigger seizure.

❷ Has the patient ever been knocked out or had any significant head injury?

Any of these would make the possibility of recurrent seizures (epilepsy) more likely. In a large number of epileptics there is a history of head injury of some kind; usually there is an interval between the acute injury and the onset of seizure symptoms. It is also worth enquiring into the patient's birth history because if labour was particularly quick, if it was a breech delivery, if forceps or other instruments were used or if there was an initial failure to cry, then significant brain damage may have occurred. It only takes a small scar in the brain substance to cause ongoing recurrent seizures.

❷ Did slurring of the speech and weakness down one side of the body or face precede the seizure?

A stroke is caused by interruption of the blood supply to part of the brain, the result of a blood clot or haemorrhage. There is an initial inflammatory reaction in the dying brain tissue that can trigger a seizure at the time of the stroke and a further, slower reaction whereby the injured brain cells form scar tissue which is capable of producing convulsions at any time in the future by irritating the surrounding functioning nerve cells.

❷ Is the patient over 25 years of age?

In people over the age of 25 who have never previously had one, a seizure is more likely to be the result of a newly developed underlying condition. Because of this, these individuals

require particularly thorough investigation, especially as there is an increased possibility of a brain tumour being responsible. In the under-25-year-old age group a diagnosis of idiopathic epilepsy (that is, of no known cause) is much more likely.

❷ Was the seizure localized, affecting only part of the body?

Localized seizures are often associated with an abnormality in one part of the brain and are more likely to be seen with a tumour or following a stroke, when only one small area of the brain is affected by pressure or by lack of blood flow respectively.

❷ Was the seizure generalized, affecting the whole body?

Someone suffering a generalized seizure will experience jerking of the limbs, loss of consciousness, and will also bite his or her tongue. Generalized seizures are common after serious injury or as the result of chemical imbalances of the blood, as seen with alcohol and other kinds of drug abuse.

❷ Is the patient taking any medication or drugs or drinking heavily?

Medication to treat depression, asthma and tuberculosis can all cause seizures, as can the usually innocent penicillin when it is given to an individual allergic to it. Seizures are also commonly experienced by drug abusers, particularly those using amphetamine ('speed') and those coming off illegal drugs cold turkey. In the majority of one-off seizures the trigger factor is alcohol, perhaps the most abused drug of all in this country.

❷ Is the person diabetic and on insulin?

Most insulin-dependent diabetics will at some stage in their lives suffer from abnormally low blood sugar caused by an accidental overdose of insulin. When there is too little glucose in the blood, the brain cannot function normally and a seizure may follow the other symptoms of confusion, irritability, fast pulse, sweating and loss of consciousness.

❷ Does the patient have an irregular heartbeat or suffer chest pain on exertion?
Because the brain requires a normal blood supply for proper functioning anything that disrupts the blood supply, for example a fall in blood pressure or an abnormal heart rhythm, can result in a seizure, which is why this is a not uncommon complication of an acute heart attack, when the heart muscle fails to pump blood properly to the brain.

❸ Has the patient experienced any unexplained fatigue lately?
This suggests the possibility of kidney or liver disease. These organs are responsible for the eradication of various toxins in the body and when they fail, the toxins build up and can trigger a seizure.

❹ Did the seizure occur after prolonged and unprotected exposure to the sun?
A combination of dehydration and direct irritation of the brain tissue itself as the result of overheating can cause a seizure.

SUMMARY
SEIZURES

POSSIBLE CAUSE	ACTION
Recurrent seizures of unknown cause	Long-term anticonvulsant therapy.
Meningitis/encephalitis	Medical treatment with antibiotics if necessary.
Head injury	Anticonvulsant therapy. Anyone suffering a significant head injury, particularly a fractured skull, should be warned of the possibility of seizures.
Stroke	Supportive and anticonvulsant therapies. Stroke sufferers should be warned of possibility of seizures occurring in the future.
Brain tumour	Radiotherapy or surgery.
Alcohol	Avoid this common trigger factor in susceptible individuals or modify intake.
Drugs	Avoid further drug abuse, but beware of 'cold turkey'. Gradual methods of withdrawal, psychotherapy and counselling through drug rehabilitation centres are recommended.
Medication	With your doctor, identify and then discontinue or reduce dose of drug responsible.
Diabetes	Emergency glucose. Long-term control of blood sugar. Avoid overdose of insulin.
Heart attack	Careful monitoring of heart and blood-pressure, medical treatment.
Disorder of kidney or liver	Treat underlying problem and remove toxic substances from blood.
Heart-rhythm disorder	Medical treatment for underlying cause.
Seizures of any kind	Adequate fluid replacement, paracetamol in children or aspirin in adults, tepid sponging of the skin, lowering the surrounding temperature.

TREMBLING AND SHAKING

People can shake for a variety of reasons but will do so most often when they are tired, under pressure or anxious. We all know the expression 'shaking with anger', and frustration and irritation are two additional sources of shaking that most of us have experienced at one time or another. Vigorous exercise can have the same effect. Whatever the cause of the shaking or trembling, however, the presence of anxiety and tension will always make it worse, so much so that doctors often make the mistake of attributing the shaking to emotional factors, whereas some underlying disorder may actually be responsible. Even when there is some physical disease process at the root of it all, reducing the level of anxiety and worry can improve the symptoms.

To establish the cause of the problem, ask yourself the following questions:

❷ Are you especially tense and anxious?

Shaking is normal, predictable and acceptable when it is obviously caused by high emotion, stress, fear or worry. Before examinations or before physical competitions it is quite normal to experience all the effects of increased adrenaline in the bloodstream, and in conjunction with the tremor there may be a fast pulse, palpitations, nausea, sweaty palms and diarrhoea. Adequate relaxation or stress counselling can be very effective in reducing these physical situations. However, when they are particularly bad and are brought on by certain situations such as flying or giving an after-dinner speech, the physical symptoms can be reduced by taking a beta-blocker type of drug such as propranolol, which abolishes the physical symptoms without causing any sedation. Less potent medication comes in the form of aromatherapy, and essential oils such as lavender can be very helpful.

❷ Is the shaking better when you are resting?

As its name suggests, familial or essential tremor runs in families and several members of the same family may experience this kind of tremor, which is not evident at rest, as in Parkinson's disease, but becomes prominent when reaching out for something. It usually starts in the sufferer's twenties or thirties, and either clears up on its own later or gets worse with advancing age. It can affect one or both hands, and sometimes causes occasional involuntary movement of the head. Familial tremor is not a disease, nor is it a sign of an underlying condition. The main risk to sufferers is that because they find alcohol can settle the tremor, it encourages them to drink regularly every day. In the long-term, of course, this is not a good idea, since any habitual drinking can lead to problems in other respects.

❷ Is the trembling worse when you are resting?

The tremor of Parkinson's disease is characteristically present when the person is resting, and is made better by reaching out for something. Thus even when the patient is standing still or sitting, he or she will exhibit the classic tremor of the hands, as well as the typical 'pill-rolling' action in which the forefinger is rubbed against the thumb. In addition to the tremor, which can also affect the head and neck, there may be generalized muscular rigidity, which can make walking problematical, and which sometimes causes a stooped posture. Initiation of movement, for example beginning to climb a flight of stairs, is difficult, and there is also an absence of facial expression and a tendency to dribble from the corner of the mouth. These symptoms are unmistakably those of Parkinson's disease. The disease usually begins in the sufferer's sixties or seventies and becomes increasingly common and severe as the years go by. It is occasionally seen in younger people in their twenties or thirties as a result of head injury or drug abuse.

❷ Are you taking any medication?
A number of medications can cause tremors, which generally speaking settle down when the drug is stopped. Examples include lithium, used to treat manic depression, and other kinds of antidepressants. Theophylline, used in the treatment of asthma, phenytoin, used in the treatment of epilepsy, and prochlorperazine, used to control nausea and dizziness, can also produce these involuntary movements, especially in the elderly. Alcohol and the caffeine contained in tea and coffee can have the same effect.

❷ Do you feel constantly hot and have you lost weight?
An overactive thyroid gland stimulates the body generally, causing overactivity of all the organs, including the digestive system, the circulation and the nervous system. The result is anxiety, jumpiness, weight loss, increased appetite, intolerance of heat, diarrhoea, tremor of the hands, and quivering of the tongue when it is poked out.

❷ Are you drinking too much alcohol?
Anyone who wakes up in the morning with the shakes and reaches for the whisky bottle to control them is well on the way to alcoholism. Such physical dependence on alcohol is bad news, and the tremor induced by withdrawal from alcohol is a very good reason indeed to consult the doctor urgently for further help.

❷ Are you diabetic and checking your blood sugar regularly?
If the blood-sugar level of a diabetic falls very low (hypoglycaemia), the result can be a tremor with generalized weakness and increased sweating. This is always the result of an overdose of insulin therapy or other hypoglycaemic, so diabetics should always be on their guard against this. Associated symptoms include irritability, hunger pangs, palpitations and altered behaviour patterns.

❷ Do you shake much more noticeably when performing fine movements?
The part of the brain responsible for controlling fine movements is situated behind the brain stem and is called the cerebellum. When it is affected in such conditions as multiple sclerosis or in very rare instances of tumour, sufferers will experience the characteristic 'intention tremor', in which the shake becomes much worse when the limb is extended to perform a certain function. For this reason, a common test employed by doctors is the finger–nose test, when the patient is asked to reach out and touch the doctor's finger and then bring it back to touch his or her own nose. In cerebellar conditions, the tremor becomes much worse as the sufferer's finger approaches the doctor's finger or his or her own nose. Other symptoms include double vision, numbness and/or muscle weakness in the arms or legs.

❷ Could it be old age?
There's no doubt that the simple matter of ageing increases a physiological tremor. It affects the head and hands in particular in the over seventies, but is of no great significance and does not warrant treatment.

❷ Has the individual suffered any sudden weakness or numbness in the limbs and/or slurring of speech?
When a stroke occurs, there can be weakness or paralysis down one side of the body together with tremor.

❷ Do your skin and eyes have a yellow tinge and/or do you have a swollen abdomen?
Jaundice and a swollen abdomen are both characteristic of liver failure. In this case, the tremor is of a flapping type, when the outstretched arms exhibit a flapping of the hands due to alternating flexion and straightening of the wrists.

SUMMARY
TREMBLING AND SHAKING

POSSIBLE CAUSE	ACTION
Physiological	No treatment required other than reduction of anxiety.
Familial or essential tremor	Reassurance.
Parkinson's disease	Medication. Brain surgery may be possible in the future.
Medication	With your doctor, identify and then discontinue or reduce dosage of drug responsible.
Overactive thyroid	Medication, surgery or radiotherapy.
Excess alcohol	Abstinence.
Diabetes	Stringent control of blood sugar. Always carry glucose for emergency use.
Multiple sclerosis	Supportive therapy.
Increasing age	Reassurance.
Stroke	Supportive care, anticoagulants if indicated, physiotherapy.
Liver disorders	Treatment of underlying cause.

WEAKNESS

The symptom of weakness anywhere in the body is particularly worrying as it threatens mobility and independence. It may be generalized, affecting the whole body, and in fact general fatigue and loss of strength are extremely common symptoms attributable to illnesses ranging from the common cold through to rheumatoid arthritis and AIDS. Equally, there may be no underlying physical disorder whatsoever and the weakness may be manifestation of a psychological problem such as depression. Weakness can also be localized, affecting a particular part of the body, and the pattern of the disability is in fact very important when making a diagnosis as weakness that is experienced equally on both sides of the body until usually have a quite difference cause from weakness that is well localized and asymmetrical. Weakness in a particular part of the leg, for example, frequently accompanies a slipped disc where the cartilaginous disc between the vertebrae in the lower back is pushing against the nerve roots emerging from the spinal cord, compressing them. The squeezed nerves cannot then function properly, producing weakness and loss of power in the muscles supplied by that nerve. Another common example is the localized weakness affecting the whole of one side of the body following a stroke. In both these cases the weakness comes on suddenly. In multiple sclerosis and motor neurone disease, however, the onset is usually much more gradual, a factor that can help the doctor reach the correct diagnosis.

Wherever it occurs, weakness is a symptom that should never be ignored. With nerve compression, for example, urgent treatment can effect a complete cure, whereas negligence and loss of time increased the likelihood of permanent nerve damage and ongoing disability. To help determine the underlying cause of your symptoms, ask yourself the following questions:

GENERALIZED WEAKNESS

❷ Have you recently had an infection that seems to be lingering on?
Infections ranging from the fairly trivial in the case of a temperature with a common cold right through to glandular fever, ME, tuberculosis and brucellosis can all produce generalized weakness with aching muscles. Associated symptoms include a cough, swollen glands and weight loss.

❷ Do you feel short of breath and look particularly pale?
Anaemia caused by lack of iron, vitamin B12 or folic acid is likely to produce all these symptoms in addition to generalized weakness.

❷ Do you become breathless on exertion and are your ankles swollen, particularly last thing at night?
A build-up of fluid in the circulation together with congestion of the lungs due to weak heart-muscle action may be responsible for weakness, especially if there is general tiredness and lethargy as well.

❷ Do you feel cold all the time and have you gained weight?
If your whole body has slowed down, both mentally and physically, and you also feel weak, your thyroid gland could be under-active. Associated symptoms also include constipation, coarse, thinning hair and a thickening of the skin of the lower leg.

❷ Do you feel excessively thirsty?
Undiagnosed diabetes with a very high blood-sugar level causes weight loss, fatigue, weakness, thirst and large amounts of urine to

be passed. The diagnosis can be confirmed by a simple urine test or blood test.

❷ **Has your skin turned darker in some areas and do you feel faint on standing?**
Amongst other things, the adrenal glands produce the body's natural steroids, so that in a condition such as Addison's disease, in which the glands are underactive or hardly work at all, the result can be severe muscular weakness. Scattered pigmentation appears at various sites and blood pressure also drops. Unless it is treated, the condition becomes life-threatening. Nowadays, however, cortisone replacement therapy has a dramatic and lasting effect.

❸ **Is the weakness accompanied by a low-grade fever, anaemia and weight loss?**
These symptoms suggest rheumatoid arthritis or systemic lupus erythematosus, a chronic inflammatory disorder affecting the 'connective' tissue of the body, that is those cells that form the scaffolding and framework of the various organs, holding them firmly together. In its severest form it can affect most parts of the body, including the joints and kidneys. There are usually other signs such as a facial rash and joint problems to suggest the true nature of the underlying problem.

❹ **Is there severe weight loss and pallor? Is there any localized pain or discomfort?**
The effects of cancer on the body are far-reaching and include the breakdown of protein from the muscles. As a result, in the advanced stages of several forms of cancer there will be severe weight loss and muscle wasting.

❺ **Is there any upset of the bowels?**
When the intestine is unable to absorb nutrients from the diet properly, the resulting malnutrition will cause weakness. Usually the underlying problem will be suggested by

intestinal symptoms as diarrhoea, pale motions, abdominal bloating and/or wind.

❻ **Are you taking any medication?**
Medication can alter the fine balance of the minerals in the muscle tissue, causing weakness. Diuretics or water tablets commonly do this because potassium tends to be lost as water is expelled from the body. If potassium levels fall significantly, severe muscle weakness can occur. This is common in the elderly and when steroid treatment that has been taken for long periods of time is stopped.

❼ **Does muscle weakness run in the family?**
There are a number of other, rarer, conditions that can produce generalized wasting and weakness, including muscular dystrophy, of which there are many types, all varying in the age of onset and in severity. In the autoimmune disorder myasthenia gravis, antibodies are produced that damage the receptors in muscle tissue that normally respond to nerve-cell signals by contracting.

❽ **Does the weakness mainly affect the eye muscles?**
Sufferers find that their muscles become fatigued quite painlessly after continued exercise and that the eye muscles are particularly affected, but that the problem recovers after rest. The condition is more common in women than in men and often starts around the age of 30. Treatment involves drugs that make available more of the chemical transmitters to nerve cells.

❾ **Does the weakness occur from time to time after a high-carbohydrate meal?**
This is characteristic of familial periodic paralysis, which can also come on following rest after prolonged exercise.

LOCALIZED SYMMETRICAL WEAKNESS

Here we are talking about weakness affecting one part of the body but usually on both sides.

❷ Has there been any back pain or loss of height recently?

Damage to the spinal cord leading to weakness in the back can be caused by trauma or by collapsed vertebrae compressing the cord, perhaps as a result of thinning of the bones, as in osteoporosis, or the hollowing out and erosion of the bones seen in various forms of cancer. Certain viruses can also affect the spinal cord right across its width, resulting in weakness of the body below that point. The pain will usually be experienced in the centre of the back, but depending on which nerves in the spinal cord are compressed, the weakness can be felt in any part of the lower body.

❷ Is the weakness in the feet or hands?

Inflammation of the long nerves in the body (neuritis) can affect the muscles in the body's extremities, for example in the toes and feet. This can occur in long-standing diabetes, in chronic alcohol abuse, in vitamin deficiencies and in lead poisoning.

❷ Is there any family history of muscle weakness?

Inherited disorders of the muscles come in various shapes and forms, one of which, Duchenne muscular dystrophy, involves weakness in the same muscle groups on both sides of the body. Classically there will be elevated levels of certain chemicals in the bloodstream, produced as the result of muscle breakdown, and this normally leads to the diagnosis. This condition usually develops in childhood, from the age of four, but some forms of muscular dystrophy become symptomatic in the late teens.

❷ Have you been diabetic for many years?

Long-standing diabetes may alter the normal function of the nerves, producing what is known as a polyneuropathy, or disorder of many nerves at a time.

Very stringent control of blood-sugar levels tends to minimize these complications, but diabetics will always be particularly prone to this condition.

However, it can also be seen in people exposed to toxins and poisons, those with autoimmune diseases or vitamin deficiencies, and alcoholics.

❷ Has there been any progressive weight loss or other seemingly coincidental symptoms?

Different cancers behave in different ways in the body, some of them producing hormones and chemicals which have far-flung effects on other parts of the body. Polymyositis is one example of this, where there the underlying problem causes pain and weakness in any isolated muscle group in the body.

ONE-SIDED (ASYMMETRICAL) WEAKNESS

Here we are talking about weakness affecting just one side of the body.

❷ Have you been fully immunized against polio?

Polio is an acquired form of weakness that generally follows infection with the polio virus, often causing a high temperature. Those who have never been immunized against polio or people whose resistance has waned and who travel to parts of the world where polio is still rife are especially vulnerable. For this reason, booster immunizations every ten years are recommended.

❷ Does the weakness affect one small area of the body only?

Compressed nerves, for example in the neck due to an extra rib or to osteoarthritis in the spine, can classically produce weakness in the hand or in one area of the arm. In carpal tunnel syndrome, sufferers experience weakness of the small muscles in the hand as the result of a constricting band of fibrous tissue at the wrist.

❷ Have you hurt your back through heavy or awkward lifting?

A slipped disc in the spine can move backwards against the nerve roots emerging from the spinal cord causing weakness in the muscle of the legs. This is in fact an extremely common condition, often seen in general practice and in orthopaedic wards in hospitals.

❷ Did the weakness come on suddenly, accompanied by confusion and/or slurred speech?

Strokes can damage the part of the brain responsible for initiating movement on the other side of the body. Depending on the site of the damage there may be muscular weakness on the affected side or loss of sensation. In very serious strokes there may be both. Generally, the weakness will begin very suddenly.

❷ Did the symptoms begin very slowly?

When weakness comes on gradually, an abscess in the brain tissue should always be suspected, as should bruising between the brain and the skull from a head injury. Benign and malignant tumours may occasionally be responsible, although these are far more rare.

❷ Did the weakness last no more than 24 hours?

Usually referred to by the medical profession as 'transient ischaemic attacks' (TIAs), these are small blood clots that travel through the blood vessels supplying the brain, producing all the symptoms of a stroke but totally resolving themselves within 24 hours. They are best treated with anticoagulants or other medication such as aspirin to prevent the tiny platelets in the blood from sticking together.

❷ Are you under 35 and have developed double vision and/or sudden localized weakness in an arm or leg?

Multiple sclerosis can produce a wide variety of symptoms in the nervous system and the onset of any new weakness in one limb in a younger patient should at least raise the possibility of multiple sclerosis. Usually there are visual symptoms that the person concerned notices to some degree, and there may be altered sensation in certain parts of the body, but creeping weakness in one or other arm or leg is one of the commonest symptoms.

❷ Has there been any weight loss and trembling of the muscles?

Motor neurone disease is a rare and progressive condition that has no known cure. Weakness of the muscles with loss of muscle bulk and a fine 'trembling' of the muscle fibres called fasciculation are characteristic of this disorder. It is now thought to be the result of exposure to the polio virus in years gone by, which for reasons not yet known later produces death of the nerves that allow normal muscle function. It always occurs over the age of 50 and more commonly over the age of 70.

❷ Is the muscle weakness restricted to one small area?

In mononeuritis, there is inflammation of individual nerves due to chemical damage or assault by the body's own antibodies. Possible causes include diabetes and polyarteritis nodosa, an autoimmune disorder where there is widespread damage to certain blood vessels.

256

SUMMARY
WEAKNESS

POSSIBLE CAUSE	ACTION
Generalized weakness	
Infection	Identify underlying infection and treat accordingly.
Anaemia	Treat cause and correct anaemia.
Heart failure	Diuretics, treat underlying cause.
Underactive thyroid gland	Thyroid replacement hormone.
Diabetes	Regulate control of blood sugar.
Underactive adrenal gland (Addison's disease)	Cortisone replacement.
Autoimmune disease (rheumatoid arthritis, systemic lupus erythematosus)	Identify type. Medical treatment.
Cancer	Symptomatic relief, surgery, radiotherapy, chemotherapy.
Malabsorption	Dietary modification, food supplementation.
Medication	With your doctor, identify and then discontinue or reduce dosage of drug responsible.
Muscular dystrophy	No curative treatment. Keep muscles as active as possible. Physiotherapy. Surgery to 'move' or 'lengthen' shortened tendons.
Myasthemia gravis	Medical treatment. Surgery. Steroids.
Localized symmetrical weakness	
Familial periodic paralysis	Avoid heavy exertion and high-carbohydrate meals. Potassium supplements following on attack.
Spinal problems	Identify site of problem and cause. Medical or surgical treatment.

Continued . . .

SUMMARY
WEAKNESS

POSSIBLE CAUSE	ACTION
Neuritis	Adequate control of diabetes, reduce alcohol consumption, treat lead poisoning.
Muscular dystrophy	Medical treatment.
Cancer, polymyositis	Surgical treatment plus radiotherapy and chemotherapy, steroids if appropriate.
One-sided (asymmetrical) weakness	
Polio	Physiotherapy.
Compression of individual nerves	Remove source of compression, physiotherapy, surgery.
Slipped disc	Medical or surgical treatment.
Stroke	Control high blood pressure, anticoagulation if appropriate, physiotherapy, supportive care.
Compression of brain tissue	Identify cause, medical or surgical treatment.
Transient ischaemic attacks	Anticoagulants, drugs to prevent stickiness of platelets, investigate extent of hardening of the arteries, artery bypass surgery.
Multiple sclerosis	High-potency steroids, vitamin B12 injections, supportive therapy.
Motor neurone disease	Physiotherapy, supportive care
Mononeuritis	Identify underlying cause, appropriate treatment, physiotherapy.

ALTERED SENSATION (PINS AND NEEDLES AND NUMBNESS)

Elsewhere I have stressed the importance of pain in alerting us to underlying problems or dangers. Equally significant, however, is any alteration to or loss of this ability to feel, as this can signify a number of conditions from the benign to the more serious, all of which require further investigation and possibly treatment.

For the body to be able to experience such sensations as pain, heat, cold, tingling and itching, and if necessary to act upon them, it relies on the nervous pathway that connects the surface of the skin to the brain. When this is working as it should, sensations felt on the surface of the skin are transmitted from the nerve endings that lie in and under it, along the nerves to the spinal cord. From there the message is carried to another set of nerves to the brain, which then tells us what to do. Any disorder affecting the nerve endings, the nerves, the spinal cord or the brain itself, will therefore affect the sufferer's ability to feel and/or act upon that feeling, either by producing a tingling sensation, or by causing complete numbness.

For example, nerve endings in the skin may have been destroyed by surgical operations where the nerves have been cut through, or by the formation of scar tissue as the result of burn injuries sustained in the past. With a first-degree burn intense pain will still be felt because all the nerve endings remain intact and fully functional. In a third-degree burn, however, otherwise known as a full-thickness burn, the nerve endings are destroyed, so that although in the long term the injury is far more serious, there is no pain.

Conditions affecting the nerves that transmit sensation from the skin to the spinal cord include shingles, arthritis, which puts pressure on the nerves and a slipped disc in the spine.

Nerves in the spinal cord can be interrupted by viral infections, injury, for example a broken neck, and tumours. Disorders in the brain itself producing altered sensation include skull fractures, strokes and abnormal growths.

SENSATION DISORDERS AFFECTING ONE SIDE OF THE BODY

These are far more common than both sides being affected simultaneously. When considering the mechanics of altered sensation, it is important to realize that generally one side of the brain controls the opposite side of the body, that is the left side of the brain controls the right side of the body.

THE WHOLE OF ONE SIDE

❷ *Did the numbness occur very suddenly?*
A stroke is the commonest cause of sudden loss of sensation in the whole of one side of the body and is due either to a clot in the blood vessels supplying part of the brain or to a haemorrhage. It is particularly common in the elderly, who often have a degree of hardening of the arteries and high blood pressure. Control of these two things by means of screening examinations can do a great deal to prevent disabling or even life-threatening strokes. Where there is evidence of high blood pressure, this must be reduced with medication, whilst anticoagulants can be used to decrease the chance of thrombosis in susceptible individuals. A diet low in saturated fat, abstinence from smoking, regular exercise, and for diabetics a good control of blood sugar are also highly recommended.
Younger women who take the oral contraceptive pill and smoke are also particularly at risk, so regular monitoring of their blood pressure and advice regarding smoking are important.

❷ Was the numbness preceded by flashing lights and a one-sided headache?
Occasionally severe migraine can produce similar symptoms to a stroke, with loss of sensation down one side of the entire body, but if this is the case, it will almost always be preceded by the typical visual symptoms of a migraine, together with headaches, nausea and vomiting. The symptoms are totally reversible and recovery generally occurs within a matter of hours.

❷ Did the numbness develop gradually over a few days or weeks?
A gradual loss of sensation in the whole of one side of the body may be associated with rare brain tumours, but these are often accompanied by a progressive headache and a number of other symptoms such as visual disturbance, loss of balance and/or convulsions.

ONE SIDE OF THE FACE ONLY

❷ Have you recently had a painful, blistering rash on one side of your face?
The herpes zoster virus that causes shingles affects the nerve that normally transmits sensations from the skin of the face and forehead to the spinal cord and then to the brain. The virus is identical to that of chicken pox, which, after the typical infection earlier in life, lies dormant in this nerve. It can be reactivated many years afterwards, often after an injury or during some other infection, when it produces tingling followed several days later by a painful rash on one side of the face.

❷ Do you visit your dentist regularly?
Although rare, severe dental problems such as neglected abscesses or fractures, can erode and damage the facial nerves, producing altered sensation in part of the face.

❷ Has there been any injury?
Facial injury involving fractures can occasionally damage or slice through nerves, resulting in loss of sensation.

❷ Have you had any visual problems?
Multiple sclerosis can cause alteration of nerve function almost anywhere in the body, including loss of sensation in the face. This diagnosis should always be considered when other symptoms characteristic of the condition are felt in various parts of the body, for example tingling, twitching and muscle wasting.

THE ARM ONLY

❷ Is the whole arm affected?
When the whole arm is affected and it is not simply due to the blood supply being cut off through sleeping on it awkwardly, the abnormality most likely to be causing the problem is either a stroke or multiple sclerosis. In the former the onset is sudden, in the latter gradual.

❷ Is only part of the arm affected?
When only part of the arm is affected, this suggests that an individual nerve, and there are many supplying the arm, is being compressed or irritated. Common causes of this include arthritis in the neck or a slipped disc in the same area pushing backwards against the particular nerve.

❷ Are the symptoms mainly in the hand?
In carpal tunnel syndrome a tight band of tissue on the inside of the wrist compresses the median nerve running from the forearm to the hand. This is a particularly common problem, especially for women and during pregnancy. Symptoms are generally experienced first thing in the morning. Tapping with a forefinger in

the middle of the inside of the wrist can often bring on the symptoms (Tinel's sign) and there is tingling or numbness in the thumb and the index and middle fingers. Treatment involves cortisone injections to alleviate the pressure on the nerve, or surgery to remove the fibrous band constricting it. If the condition has come on during pregnancy, however, it often clears up spontaneously following delivery.

THE LEG ONLY

❷ Is the whole leg affected?
The whole of one leg can become numb or tingly as the result of a stroke or problems high up within the spinal cord.

❷ Has the numbness started very gradually in the toes, slowly moving further up the leg?
This suggests peripheral neuropathy, or a problem affecting the very distant nerves of the body, that is, in the body's extremities, perhaps as a result of vitamin deficiency, diabetes, or from toxins in the body such as excess alcohol or metal poisoning. Occasionally, the condition is also seen in the presence of certain tumours.

❷ Is only part of the leg affected?
When only part of a leg is affected, as in sciatica, it is highly likely to be due to a slipped disc or to a small benign lump called a neurofibroma on the individual nerve.

❷ Is only the front of the thigh affected?
Pregnant women in particular retain a lot of fluid in their bodies and this can lead to compression of the nerve that runs through the groin into the front of the thigh. Because of this it is quite common for pregnant women to experience a patch of numbness in the front of the thigh, a condition known as meralgia paraesthetica. It also affects overweight people.

THE LEG AND THE ARM

❷ Did the numbness occur suddenly?
Very occasionally a stroke can cause sensation disorders in one arm and one leg only, with nothing in between, although it is more common for the whole of one side to be affected.

❷ Have you also had visual problems?
Multiple sclerosis can affect many different sites in the body and must therefore be excluded as a possible cause of sensation abnormalities in an arm and a leg on either or both sides of the body.

❷ Did the symptoms begin gradually, accompanied by severe headaches and/or seizures?
Whilst it is possible for the gradual onset of sensation disorders in an arm and a leg to be due to a tumour, this is thankfully very rare indeed. However, other symptoms would include the onset of seizures, blurred vision and headaches.

SENSATION DISORDERS AFFECTING BOTH SIDES OF THE BODY
These are generally far more rare than disorders affecting one side of the body only.

❷ Have there also been visual problems?
Although possible, multiple sclerosis is a very rare cause of this condition.

THE WHOLE OF BOTH LEGS

❷ Have you recently hurt your back through heavy or awkward lifting?
A disc that has slipped backwards against the spinal cord can press on the nerves, producing sensation disorders in both legs.

❷ *Have you also experienced any visual problems?*

Multiple sclerosis is characterized by the patchy degeneration of nerves at widespread and often unrelated regions within the body. If there is malfunction of the nerves in the spinal cord, both legs may suffer abnormal sensation.

❷ *Have the symptoms appeared gradually in a previously healthy person?*

Benign or malignant growths affecting the spinal cord and brain must be thought of where there is slow onset of sensation disorders in both legs.

PART OF BOTH LEGS FROM THE TOES UPWARDS

❷ *Do you take enough vitamins? Are you exposed to any poisons at work?*

Abnormal nerve function (polyneuropathy) in distant parts of the body can produce sensation disorders in part of both legs from the toes upwards. This may be due to poisoning from alcohol or other toxins, but diabetes and some of the chronic rheumatic disorders such as systemic lupus erythematosus and polyarteritis nodosa could also be responsible.

❷ *Have you also had any visual problems?*

Tingling or partial numbness in part of both legs could be the result of nerve damage caused by multiple sclerosis.

❷ *Could your diet be lacking essential vitamins?*

A serious deficiency of folic acid or vitamin B may result in problems within the spinal cord and sensation disturbance in this area. A diet with plenty of green leafy vegetables, wholegrains, fish, meat and liver is important.

COMPLETE LOSS OF SENSATION BELOW THE NECK

In this situation there is severe disruption of the spinal cord below the fifth vertebrae in the neck.

❷ *Is neck movement very restricted? Has there been any previous neck injury?*

Occasionally in severe osteoarthritic and rheumatic conditions, and in disc problems in the neck, there can be pressure on the spinal cord with resulting sensory changes.

❷ *Has the onset of symptoms been gradual?*

This together with very rigid legs points to a spinal-cord tumour as a possible cause.

262

SUMMARY
ALTERED SENSATION

POSSIBLE CAUSE	ACTION
Whole of one side	
Stroke	Lower blood pressure, anticoagulants, aspirin, physiotherapy.
Migraine	Pain relief, antinausea treatment.
Tumour	Surgery or radiotherapy.
Face only	
Herpes infection (shingles)	Acyclovir tablets or cream.
Dental problems	Dental surgery.
Injury	Surgery.
Multiple sclerosis	Medical care and supportive therapy.
Arm only	
Stroke	See above.
Multiple sclerosis	See above.
Compressed nerve (osteoarthritis, slipped disc)	Surgery.
Carpal tunnel syndrome	Surgery or cortisone injection.
Leg only	
Spinal cord problems (slipped disc, injury)	Surgery or traction.
Stroke	See above.
Peripheral neuropathy	Medical treatment.
Tumour	Surgery.
Slipped disc	Rest, physiotherapy, epidural or surgery.
Neurofibroma	Surgery.
Meralgia paraesthetica	No treatment until after childbirth. Otherwise, cortisone injection and weight loss.

Continued . . .

SUMMARY
ALTERED SENSATION

POSSIBLE CAUSE	ACTION
Leg and arm	
Stroke	*See above.*
Multiple sclerosis	*See above.*
Tumour	*Surgery.*
Whole of both legs	
Slipped disc	*See above.*
Multiple sclerosis	*See above.*
Tumour	*Surgery.*
Part of both legs	
Polyneuropathy	*Medical treatment.*
Multiple sclerosis	*See above.*
Vitamin deficiency	*Medical treatment.*
Below neck	
Spinal cord compression	*Surgery.*
Tumour	*Surgery.*
Multiple sclerosis	*See above.*

FACIAL PARALYSIS

Paralysis of the facial muscles can occur gradually or suddenly. In most instances sufferers will notice within a matter of hours, often during their sleep, that they cannot move the muscles on one side of their face, so that they have a crooked smile, they dribble saliva from the corner of the mouth on the affected side and they cannot close their eyelids fully. They can't puff out their cheeks and keep their lips tightly together on the bad side and they may not be able to wrinkle their forehead. In many respects the sudden onset of facial paralysis is a good sign as it tends to suggest the benign nature of the underlying problem. Viral infections of the nerves controlling the muscles of the face are responsible for such sudden onset paralysis, whereas more serious problems tend to account for the more slower onset problems. In the latter, headaches or seizures often accompany the facial symptoms.

❷ Did the crooked smile develop suddenly?

Bell's palsy is the name given to a benign form of facial paralysis. The condition is usually temporary, lasting a period of usually about six weeks, and tends to improve spontaneously, although it often leaves about 10 per cent of sufferers with permanent weakness. It appears to be triggered by a virus infection of the nerves supplying the facial muscles, and the early administration of steroids may limit the degree of paralysis and hasten recovery. Bell's palsy is the commonest cause of paralysis on one side of the face and often causes a great deal of alarm as the effects are very obvious. There are never any arm or leg symptoms with Bell's palsy, as there often are with a stroke or a tumour, and an important distinction is that someone with Bell's palsy will be unable to close the eye on the affected side or wrinkle the forehead.

❷ Has there been slurred speech, numbness or weakness in arms or legs?

A stroke is caused by a clot formation in or bleeding from a blood vessel supplying part of the brain. When this occurs, that particular part of the brain dies and the nervous pathways that instruct the muscles to move are interrupted. This can affect the face alone, but more often than not the arm and leg on the same side are affected too. The patient may also have difficulty speaking. Possible warning signs during the preceding few days or weeks include headaches, short-lived drooping of the corner of the mouth and/or speech difficulties. Such transient ischaemic attacks should always be thoroughly investigated by your doctor. High blood pressure should be reduced with appropriate medication, whilst anticoagulants and/or aspirin may be used to prevent clot formation in arteries furred up with cholesterol deposits.

❸ Did the facial weakness come on gradually over a few days or weeks, and was there any visual disturbance?

Occasionally, the gradual onset of facial paralysis with or without symptoms in the same arm or leg may be associated with an underlying brain tumour, although this is a far less likely cause than either Bell's palsy or a stroke. In fact brain tumours are relatively rare, accounting for only 10 per cent of all malignancies. They are more common in children and around the age of 50. There is often associated headaches and possibly the new symptom of seizures. In these instances, blood pressure is usually normal and there is no obvious hardening of the arteries. Like strokes, brain tumours are potentially life-threatening. *See your doctor urgently.*

SUMMARY
FACIAL PARALYSIS

POSSIBLE CAUSE	ACTION
Bell's palsy	Early treatment with steroids, physiotherapy to passively exercise the paralysed muscles. Usually resolves within six weeks.
Stroke	Anticoagulants, control of blood pressure, supportive care.
Tumour	Surgery and/or radiotherapy.

MEMORY LOSS, CONFUSION AND BEHAVIOURAL PROBLEMS (DEMENTIA)

This combination of symptoms is relatively common, especially in the elderly, and it is vital not to dismiss them as incurable. There is no doubt that Alzheimer's disease is generally over-diagnosed, and the 'senile' label is best avoided until other causes have been ruled out. In fact, about 20 per cent of people with symptoms apparently identical to those of senile dementia turn out to have one of those conditions the doctors can do something about, especially if treated early on, when further deterioration can be prevented. Generally speaking, when memory loss and confusion occur suddenly the prospects of treatment are very good, but this is often not the case if they appear more gradually.

❶ Are you feeling stressed and/or overtired?

From middle age onwards any failure to recall immediately a name or telephone number can be worrying. The truth is that this happens to all of us and is simply a sign of a momentary lapse in concentration. Either the information doesn't register properly in the memory to begin with, or else its storage or recall lets us down. This kind of benign forgetfulness is temporary and is not caused by any underlying disorder. There are no changes to the personality or intellect, and nor are there any signs of anxiety or depression. However, stress and/or fatigue could just be Nature's way of reminding us to slow down.

❷ Are there any changes to the personality and intellect?

Ten per cent of people over 65 and 20 per cent of those over 75 have some degree of dementia with Alzheimer's disease accounting for about 80 per cent of all cases. Classic symptoms are a failure in short-term memory so that telephone numbers, addresses, shopping items and recent conversations are completely forgotten. There is also intellectual deterioration and personality and behaviour may change drastically too. People affected are often found living alone in squalor, unable to dress or feed themselves. They run a high risk of accidental injury from the misuse of kitchen appliances or from domestic fires and overall they are a considerable handicap to themselves. Relatives may be informed by the police or social services that they have wandered off at strange times of the day or night, only to forget where they live or the correct route home. To date there is no effective treatment and sufferers depend on adequate social support and eventually residential care.

❸ Are the symptoms accompanied by a high temperature?

Children and adults with high temperatures can become delirious as a result of their fever, and this effect is particularly pronounced in the elderly, even when the fever is not that high. Pneumonias, urine infections, strokes, heart attacks and liver and kidney disorders can therefore come to everybody's attention with the symptoms of memory loss and confusion, but toxic damage as a result of mercury or manganese poisoning should also be considered as this too can lead to behavioural problems.

❹ Do you feel cold all the time and have you gained weight?

When the thyroid gland slows down so does the body generally. Symptoms include a slow pulse, coarse, thinning hair and constipation, and on a mental level there can often be marked slowing down of intellectual function together with confusion.

❷ Are there any symptoms of headaches, visual disturbance and/or seizures?

Any physical brain abnormality can produce the generalized symptoms of confusion and memory loss, but often there will be other signs such as headaches or epileptic seizures to help the doctor identify the nature of the problem. Possible causes include infections such as meningitis and encephalitis, aneurysms (ballooned areas of blood vessels supplying the brain) and tumours.

❷ Does the person concerned eat an adequate diet with enough fresh food?

A poor diet can lead to a serious deficiency in the B group of vitamins, resulting in memory loss and confusion if left untreated for any length of time. The problem is particularly common among elderly people, especially those who live alone with few savings and no family, unable to look after themselves properly and refusing all offers of help from the various social-services support agencies. They may rely heavily on canned food, which tends not to be rich in minerals and vitamins, and are therefore very susceptible to developing such psychological problems. However, this form of dementia is eminently reversible.

❷ Is there a problem with excessive alcohol consumption?

Many people will have experienced waking up in the morning after the night before not being able to remember exactly what they did the previous evening, nor how they got home. This kind of memory loss, the result of acute alcoholic stupor, occurs largely because the events never 'registered' in the first place, and any loss of short-term stored memory in such cases is temporary. However, the loss of memory in chronic alcohol abuse is quite a different matter altogether. When large amounts of alcohol are consumed on a daily

basis there will be gradual but significant deterioration of the memory, resulting in a severe social and psychological handicap. This is a serious sign of alcoholism and if left untreated may lead to profound psychiatric disturbance.

❷ Does the person concerned feel miserable and tearful all the time?

Memory loss may be one of the first signs of true clinical depression as confusion, lack of concentration and disorientation are frequently seen in depressed people, although they may not even be obviously tearful or morbid. In elderly people especially depression can certainly mimic true dementia.

When elderly patients who have been diagnosed as suffering from dementia are given antidepressants, as many as ten per cent will make a swift and full recovery.

❷ Is the person concerned taking any medication?

Many different drugs, whether prescribed by a doctor or used illegally, can cause symptoms of mental aberration, including memory loss and behavioural problems. Examples are sedatives, anticonvulsants, steroids, antidepressants, digoxin, barbiturates and lithium. Illegal substances such as solvents, LSD and ecstasy can have similar effects or worse.

❷ Has there been any recent head injury?

Head injuries that occurred days or even weeks before the onset of symptoms may be responsible for memory loss. In fact, as many as 50 per cent of all people developing dementia-like symptoms as the direct result of blood-clot formation between the brain and the skull (subdural haematoma) never recall the actual injury. X-rays may not be all that helpful because there won't necessarily be a fracture of the skull, but CAT scans have aided the diagnosis tremendously. Treatment consists of strong steroid drugs that help to reabsorb the collected fluid from around the brain; surgery may be necessary to remove the blood clot.

❷ Did the symptoms begin during cold weather?

The gradual loss of body temperature slows down mental functions, leading to confusion and eventually a dementia-like state. The effects of hypothermia (chronic exposure to cold temperature) are particularly common in the elderly, who do not have as much fat under their skin to keep them warm as younger people do, and who may well have problems affording heating bills during very cold weather. The danger increases if the person concerned also suffers from an underactive thyroid gland, which slows down the tick-over speed of the body. The two together can be life-threatening.

❷ Has there been repeated injury to the head?

The 'punch drunk' syndrome, otherwise known as 'boxer's dementia', is the result of suffering repeated blows to the head and is therefore frequently seen in amateur and professional boxers who have fought one bout too many. Symptoms include memory loss and confusion but there may also be loss of balance, slurred speech and tremor. It is indistinguishable in most respects from Parkinson's disease.

❷ Is the person concerned exposed to carbon monoxide or heavy metals either at home or at work?

Inhalation of carbon monoxide gas or chronic exposure to heavy metals including mercury and lead can often lead to dementia-like symptoms.

❷ Has anyone in the family been diagnosed as having Huntington's chorea?

A rare condition known as Huntington's chorea can affect adults for the first time during their late twenties, causing progressive and inexorable loss of intellect. There is usually a family history, but regrettably there is no effective treatment available at present.

❷ Has the person concerned just had a convulsion?

People prone to epileptic seizures experience loss of memory for up to an hour or more following a convulsion. This is a result of the generalized electrical discharge that has occurred throughout the brain during the convulsion and does not cause any permanent loss of higher mental function or memory.

❷ Is the ability to walk affected?

Otherwise known as hydrocephalus, fluid on the brain can be present at birth or may develop later in life in adults secondary to some other problem such as meningitis or a previous head injury. In this condition, there is interference to the normal flow of cerebrospinal fluid in the various hollow chambers within the brain substance and the resulting increase in pressure in these chambers leads to progressive brain-cell damage. Together with memory loss and confusion there is often an abnormal gait and a tendency to fall over frequently. When detected early, however, by means of a brain scan, this is one of the many treatable conditions responsible for dementia-like symptoms.

A 'shunt' operation can be performed in which any excess fluid within the brain can be safely drained away into the circulation through a narrow tube. This alleviates any undue pressure on the delicate brain cells and prevents any further deterioration in cerebral function.

❷ Have there been any short-lived episodes of slurred speech and/or weakness in the arms or legs lately?
Symptoms of dementia that seem to wax and wane and produce gradual deterioration in mental function can often be the result of tiny strokes affecting the brain. Very often patients retain a fair degree of insight into what is going on and there is no personality change.

However, they may be moody and their ability to walk in a co-ordinated and smooth fashion is often affected. The condition is associated with hardening of the arteries and raised blood pressure and for this reason is seen more commonly in smokers and diabetics. Investigation with CAT scans can be very helpful.

SUMMARY
MEMORY LOSS, CONFUSION, AND BEHAVIOURAL PROBLEMS (DEMENTIA)

POSSIBLE CAUSE	ACTION
Benign forgetfulness	Reassurance.
Alzheimer's disease	Supportive and social care.
Infection	Identify underlying cause and treat appropriately.
Under-active thyroid gland	Thyroid replacement treatment.
Nervous system disorders	Look for infection, arterial swelling or tumour and treat appropriately.
Malnutrition	Identify and correct the deficient dietary component with dietary adjustment, tablets or injections.
Alcohol abuse	Abstinence.
Depression	Counselling, psychotherapy, electroconvulsant therapy (ECT) in restricted cases.
Medication	With the doctor, identify and then discontinue or reduce dosage of drug responsible.
Head injury	Rule out a blood clot on the brain, but if present treat with steroids and/or surgery. Otherwise, counselling and psychotherapy.

Continued . . .

SUMMARY
MEMORY LOSS, CONFUSION, AND BEHAVIOURAL PROBLEMS (DEMENTIA)

Possible Cause	Action
Hypothermia	Restore body temperature.
Punch drunk syndrome	Treatment as for Parkinson's disease.
Environment	Remove all toxic substances from the working environment.
Huntington's chorea	Supportive care.
Epilepsy	Anticonvulsants for epilepsy, but no specific treatment for memory loss, which is temporary.
Hydrocephalus	Reduce cerebrospinal fluid pressure through a 'shunt' operation.
Mini-stroke	Reduce blood pressure, low-fat diet, stop smoking, possibly anticoagulants or aspirin.

ANXIETY

Anxiety is an emotional state in which there is a general sensation of fear and apprehension. Usually it is a response to stressful events, but it can also occur without any such provocation, in which case it may take the form of completely unpredictable panic attacks ranging from the mild to the incapacitating. Those people who have an anxious nature will suffer from generalized and persistent anxiety all their lives. In fact, small amounts of anxiety can be useful, keeping us alert and helping concentration. The trouble starts when it becomes excessive, when we develop physical symptoms and cannot think straight, at which point it becomes a handicap. But psychological stress is not the only underlying cause of anxiety. There are a number of physical disorders that very commonly prove to be responsible.

❶ Are you under a lot of pressure?

Many people thrive on pressure, but others can be upset by it. Life events such as redundancy, divorce, separation, bereavement, illness and overwork are common sources of stress and certainly impinge on most people's lives at some stage. Often, sufferers are not initially aware of the tension they are under because they automatically employ coping mechanisms that effectively mask the symptoms. It is only when these mechanisms fail or are overwhelmed that physical symptoms break through and come to the individual's attention. Such symptoms include tremor, palpitations, sweating, overbreathing, nausea, dizziness and chest pain.

❷ Do you have any overriding phobias, for example are you frightened to go out in public?

Phobias are anxieties and fears that are out of all proportion to the provoking stimulus or the demands of the situation. They cannot be controlled by the sufferer nor reasoned away. They are usually so bad that the individual affected avoids the problem at all costs, a course of action that seriously jeopardizes his or her quality of life. In agoraphobia, there is a fear of crowds, so that shopping, going out in public, or using lifts or public transport are all avoided. Some people never leave the safety of their own homes. Other phobias may be specific to one particular thing such as spiders, heights or the dark, whilst social phobias mean that any situation where the person concerned could be observed by others, such as in a restaurant or theatre, will be stringently avoided. Whatever the type of phobia, however, the anxiety produced is powerful and all-consuming.

❸ Are you a woman in your late 40s or early 50s?

During the menopause certain psychological and physical symptoms are common. In about 20 per cent of cases there are fairly severe symptoms, the commonest being hot flushes, irregular vaginal bleeding and weight gain. Insomnia, irritability, depression and anxiety can also occur, but certainly not invariably. Any woman who becomes anxious for the first time in her life should therefore consider the possibility of hormonal causes and arrange for blood tests to be taken by her doctor to see whether the menopause has started. If it has, hormone replacement therapy may very well be dramatically effective in reducing any anxiety.

❹ Has anyone close to you died recently?

Bereavement makes people anxious. It can also temporarily make them hypochondriacal. It reminds us, sometimes quite brutally, that we are all mortal. It is therefore not at all uncommon for a woman whose husband has recently died of a heart attack, for example, or for a man whose wife has died of cancer to become preoccupied with the possibility of the same thing happening to them. These kinds of cardiac neuroses and cancer phobias are seen all the time in general practice and require patient and sympathetic handling. They are really no more than stress and phobia combined and a thorough physical examination and counselling are usually all that is required.

❷ *Do you suffer from palpitations and have you lost weight for no apparent reason?*
An overactive thyroid gland leads to symptoms of both physical and mental overactivity. Endless energy and anxiety are therefore accompanied by weight loss, muscle wasting, palpitations, tremor and an intolerance of hot weather.

SUMMARY
ANXIETY

POSSIBLE CAUSE	ACTION
Stress	Counselling and reassurance, stress management, psychotherapy, relaxation techniques, complementary medicine, short-term tranquillizers as a last resort.
Phobia	Behavioural therapy, antidepressant drugs, training in social skills for social phobias.
The menopause	Reassurance and explanation, hormone replacement therapy.
Hypochondriasis	Counselling and reassurance. Full medical examination, behavioural therapy.
Overactive thyroid gland	Medicines to reduce thyroid-hormone production. Surgery to remove part of gland or radioactive iodine in older patients.
Impotence	Psychosexual counselling and/or sexual prothesis. Hormone treatment still highly controversial.

DEPRESSION

Depression can be part of a normal reaction to some traumatic life event such as illness or bereavement, but it can also emerge out of the blue. The disturbance in the way the person concerned feels may last just a day or two, or for several weeks or months at a time.

The main sign of depression is a permanently low mood from which the individual concerned cannot be cheered up. Instead, he or she finds it impossible to derive any enjoyment from life and sees the whole world as pointless, bleak and without pleasure. Thought processes often slow down, and there will be little or no interest in work or current affairs. Depressed people also talk less and more slowly. They often feel guilty about trivial things, feel themselves to be worthless, and are reluctant to talk about their problems out of embarrassment and low self-esteem. They often sleep badly, waking early in the morning with thoughts of gloom and despondency, and because the appetite is usually lost, weight can drop. There is often also a reduction in sexual interest. In severe depression there may be hypochondriacal delusions or even ideas of suicide, and sometimes real attempts at self-harm are made. There are also a number of physical conditions that can predispose someone to this problem.

❷ Are you feeling anxious, panicky or preoccupied?

Depression can be accompanied by anxiety or can accompany phobias, schizophrenia, obsessive compulsive behaviour or even anorexia or bulimia, the two eating disorders.

❷ Has your weight changed and do you feel tired all the time?

Hormonal disorders caused by an under-active adrenal, thyroid or pituitary gland (at the base of the brain) can result in depression.

❷ Has your skin become very pale?

Anaemia can cause not only pallor, breathlessness and fatigue but can also produce depression. For this reason, anybody with depression should undergo a full physical examination, including blood tests and other investigations to exclude the possibility of physical conditions such as this.

❷ Has disability brought about the depression?

It is not at all uncommon for people with Parkinson's disease or those who have had a stroke to become depressed. This is largely because of the effects of the illness on their quality of life and independence, but in some conditions such as multiple sclerosis, for example, a definite element of depression appears to be part and parcel of the actual illness itself.

❷ Has there been a recent infection?

Most people who have overcome a bad case of flu or glandular fever will have experienced the long-drawn-out episode of depression lasting several days or weeks that can follow. ME, previously and rather unkindly referred to as 'Yuppie flu', is a particularly long-standing form of depression thought to be associated with a previous viral infection, and is otherwise known as post-viral fatigue syndrome. Along with the depression, it tends to be characterized by severe aching of the muscles on even the slightest exertion. Viral hepatitis and AIDS can also lead to depressive symptoms.

❷ Is there any existing serious disease?

Partly as a consequence of knowing you have a terminal disease, and partly as a result of the disease itself, various cancers that may or may not have spread to other sides of the body can produce an intense and ongoing depression.

❷ Have you experienced any recent trauma, such as an injury or an operation?

Depressive symptoms are not at all uncommon following operations or head injuries, even minor ones resulting in concussion.

❷ Are you taking any medication?

Many medications have been found to bring on depressive symptoms, including steroids, sulphonamide antibiotics, contraceptives, digoxin, isoniazid, used in the treatment of tuberculosis, alcohol, barbiturates and medicines used to treat high blood pressure.

SUMMARY
DEPRESSION

POSSIBLE CAUSE	ACTION
Psychiatric disorders	Counselling, supportive psychotherapy, occupational therapy programmes and social intervention. Also drug therapy and ECT.
Hormonal disorders	Medical treatment to replace the missing hormones.
Anaemia	Identify cause and treat appropriately.
Nervous-system disorders	Treat underlying condition, antidepressant therapy.
Infection	Sympathetic and supportive care, magnesium supplements for ME, rest, antidepressant therapy.
Cancer	Treatment of underlying condition, anti-depressants.
Injury, surgery	Explanation, preoperative counselling, supportive care.
Medication	With your doctor, identify and then discontinue or reduce dosage of drug responsible.

SLEEPING PROBLEMS

Most people spend about a quarter of their lives asleep. Those who do not would like to. It seems an awful waste of time when there is so much to do, but the truth is we all need a proper amount of sleep to stay really healthy. Sleep is a kind of recovery exercise for the brain and body, and without it we feel irritable, lethargic and unhappy. Physically our reactions are slower and we suffer headaches and stress. In severe cases genuine ill health can result. In fact, as a GP, I know that 15 to 20 per cent of patients in doctors' surgeries have sleep-related problems. So great are the difficulties, and so complicated the causes, that 88 separate classifications of specific sleep disorders now officially exist.

HOW MUCH SLEEP DO WE NEED?

This varies a great deal and depends on the individual. Einstein reputedly thrived on four hours' sleep a night, as does Lady Thatcher, but other people need a full ten hours. Small babies enjoy about 16 hours' deep sleep a day. Their grandparents, on the other hand, may sleep for only four to five hours, of which a much smaller proportion is deep sleep.

INSOMNIA

Insomnia is the long-standing failure to obtain enough sleep for proper daytime functioning. There are a number of possible causes, so if you are trying to get to the root of your problem, ask yourself the following questions:

❷ *Are you taking naps during the day?*
No one should be surprised to have problems sleeping at night if he or she is catnapping during the day as this reduces the need for sleep at night and upsets the normal circadian rhythm whereby we stay active and alert by day and sleep at night. Elderly people frequently

suffer from insomnia as a result of daytime catnapping, so much so that occasionally their day/night routines become completely confused. Nevertheless, those who lead particularly hectic lives and are lucky to get their heads down for six hours or less at night, can greatly benefit from 40 winks during the day. Those with sleeping problems should also avoid lying-in in the morning, since this can upset proper sleeping routine and make you less tired when it comes to going to bed.

❷ *Do you work very long hours?*
You are not a machine. You cannot expect to work flat out all day, then throw the switch and conk out. Your busy mind needs time to slow down and relax. Your muscles need to relax. Adrenalin needs to soak away. This means no work or hassle of any kind for a couple of hours before bed. So, instead of reading that report or attempting to cram in a bit more revision before that examination, try a good novel, watch television, do some yoga or have a massage, or, better still, why not have a cuddle with a loved one?

❷ *Do you take enough exercise?*
Physical exercise dramatically improves the quality of sleep – ask any athlete. However, all sorts of activities are just as effective. Whether it is bowls, golf, dancing, jogging or simple walking, the benefits can be rapidly felt. Try to get plenty of fresh air and establish a simple daily workout routine that suits you.

❷ *Do you have irregular sleeping habits?*
Normal sleeping biorhythms are reinforced by routine and upset by irregular bedtimes. Shift workers, people doing overtime and teenagers out on the town every other night are therefore particularly likely to suffer from insomnia. Not only do they feel tired, but the difficulty experienced getting to sleep and then staying

asleep sdisturbs the value and quality of that sleep. Whether you are five or 50, a sleep routine can work wonders. A hot bath followed by a bedtime milky drink, a quick read of that novel and then lights out really works.

❷ *Are you eating just before bed?*

Whilst a good breakfast can set you up for the day, a large, indigestible meal late at night can stop you sleeping by heating up the body and making the heart beat faster. If you can, allow at least three hours between finishing your supper and bed.

❷ *Do you drink a lot of tea and/or coffee, especially in the evenings?*

Many people don't realise that the caffeine contained in these will prevent them from sleeping at night. Cola drinks, red wine, chocolate and cheese can all do the same.

❷ *Do you smoke and/or drink alcohol?*

Even small quantities of tobacco and/or alcohol are likely to keep you awake. Smoking excites the nervous system and stops you sleeping. Alcohol makes you drowsy at first, but then wakes you up in the middle of the night as the effect wears off.

❷ *Is your bed uncomfortable?*

You spend up to a third of your life in bed, so invest in a decent one and replace it when necessary. Joint pains, backache, neck stiffness and muscle tension commonly interrupt people's sleep if their sleeping posture is bad.

❷ *Are you regularly disturbed by noise?*

Crying babies, a partner's snoring, loud music or busy traffic are not conducive to sound sleep. Equally, bright daylight can keep you awake. So fix dark curtains or blinds, keep doors closed and use earplugs if you have to.

❷ *Is your bedroom well ventilated?*

You need to be warm without being suffocated to get a good night's sleep. So open those windows and snuggle down.

❷ *Are you kept awake by discomfort?*

Any disorder causing pain can keep you awake, common examples being various forms of arthritis and neuralgia. In men, prostate difficulties can interrupt sleep by making you need to empty your bladder frequently during the night. Heart and lung conditions are also likely to interfere with a proper night's sleep.

❷ *Are you taking any medication?*

Certain medicines can cause insomnia. Painkillers, certain antidepressants, drugs used to treat asthma, high doses of thyroid hormone and amphetamines ('speed') are all common culprits. Also, anyone who has been taking sleeping tablets regularly and then abruptly stops can expect to develop 'rebound insomnia'.

NARCOLEPSY

Narcolepsy is a rare syndrome characterized by uncontrollable sleeping bouts during the day, often accompanied by episodes of collapse due to complete loss of muscle strength. Other features include sleep paralysis, when the sufferer has the sensation of being awake but is totally unable to move, and hallucinations. It is estimated that in Britain about 40,000 people suffer from some form of narcolepsy, about 18,000 of which have actually been diagnosed. Once the diagnosis has been confirmed, sufferers can learn to recognize situations that are likely to be sleep-inducing. They can also learn to recognize warning signs and therefore avoid dropping off in dangerous circumstances. Medication has to be taken for life and doctors use stimulants as well as antidepressants to deal with the problem.

SUMMARY
INSOMNIA

POSSIBLE CAUSE	ACTION
Catnapping	Don't have a lie-in, try to avoid catnapping during the day.
Working long hours	Ensure adequate relaxation. Don't take your work home with you; if necessary, write down any worries still in your mind before going to bed.
Not enough exercise	Try to get into the habit of regular aerobic exercises, speeding up the pulse and rate of breathing for a minimum of 15 minutes at a time.
No routine	Try to re-establish a sleeping routine and avoid shift work if possible.
Eating too late	Try to ensure the last meal is only of moderate size and finished three hours before bedtime.
Caffeine	Cut down on caffeine-containing drinks such as tea, coffee and colas.
Smoking and drinking	Reduce or stop if possible.
An uncomfortable bed	Invest in a new one.
Too much noise	Use earplugs if you have to.
Poorly ventilated bedroom	Try to ensure fresh air and warmth.
Physical disorders	Treat underlying condition, especially pain, appropriately.
Medication	With your doctor, identify and then see whether you can cut down or change the responsible drug.

11
SEXUAL PROBLEMS

Some people live for sex, some people are dying for it, and a few people can live happily without it. But for the vast majority of us, sex is a natural and important part of a loving relationship. Good sex should be safe, enjoyable, private, free from worry, and above all fun. It can be one of the greatest morale boosters, making us feel attractive and desirable, it can relieve tension, and it is one of the best ways to end a row. But when things do go wrong, it can cause an enormous amount of misery and have far-reaching effects on both partners. About 20 per cent of patients visiting their doctor do so for sex-related problems, and it's very important that you never feel too embarrassed to consult your GP or a Relate counsellor if you are concerned about some aspect of your life.

I N TRUTH there are relatively few sexual relationships where everything is considered perfect, but most problems sort themselves out within a short space of time. Difficulties only become serious when there are repeated failures to achieve or maintain normal sexual intercourse. Problems can occur during the desire, arousal or orgasm phases of intercourse, with some difficulties common to both men and women and others experienced by one sex only.

IMPOTENCE

Very simply, impotence is the failure to obtain or maintain an erection. (It should not be confused with infertility, which is the inability to produce children.) Many people regard erection as an easily obtained reflex reaction, and indeed the processes that allow it to happen are largely automatic. But the ability to achieve and sustain an erection depends on many factors, and when any one of them ceases to function normally, problems can occur.

The process is initiated by sexual desire. Higher centres in the brain activate nerves that allow the blood vessels in the penis to open and fill up the erectile spongy tissue inside with blood. Tiny muscles around other blood vessels contract, closing down the veins that usually carry blood away and thereby allowing the erection to be maintained. The male hormone testosterone also has a part to play. This hormone is produced by the testicles and is carried about in the bloodstream. Lack of it for any reason diminishes libido and adversely affects erection.

Most men suffer from impotence at some stage in their lives, and generally it is the result of stress, anxiety in the early stages of a new relationship, or too much alcohol. In these situations, the problem is usually temporary and will resolve itself spontaneously. Sometimes, however, impotence becomes recurrent and persistent, in which case there is a risk that long-standing sexual problems will follow, and treatment is therefore usually sought. Impotence also tends to be an increasing problem with advancing age, and it has been estimated that approximately 7 per cent of men aged 50 complain of impotence, rising to 55 per cent by the age of 70. Whilst in younger men impotence is usually related to anxiety, the older you are, the more likely it is that there is a physical cause.

➊ Do you feel particularly anxious?

If circumstances are not conducive to relaxed sexual intercourse, perhaps through fear of being discovered, of infection or of recurring heart problems, or because of embarrassment, your performance can suffer. This is also true at the start of a new relationship, when you may worry about being judged by your partner. If this worry should interfere with normal erection there will be increased anxiety the next time intercourse is attempted and so a vicious circle is established. This can also occur later on in a long-standing relationship if your partner is more demanding than you are, and you feel that your virility or masculinity are in question.

➋ Are you feeling particularly stressed and/or overtired?

There is no doubt that these two lifestyle factors can produce impotence and adequate time to switch off from hassles and problems is important. Taking sufficient leisure time, holidays and physical activity, as well as giving yourselves enough quality time for a good sexual relationship, are recommended.

➌ Are you drinking too much alcohol?

In small quantities, alcohol allows people to lose some of their inhibitions. Because it can have a relaxing effect, it can be a potent enhancer of sexual drive. But too much alcohol can cause erection difficulties, whilst long-term drinking of excessive amounts of alcohol can have more far-reaching effects such as alcoholic cirrhosis, which not only produces testicular atrophy (wasting) but also a reduced sperm count and a deficiency of the male hormone testosterone. However, the liver is capable of regeneration even when it has been considerably damaged, and recovery will prevent any further atrophy of the testicles and therefore any further drop in testosterone levels.

➍ Do you have any pre-existing medical condition?

Disorders such as diabetes, multiple sclerosis, spinal-cord injury and hardening of the arteries can all lead to a failure of the reflexes involved in obtaining an erection. If the nerves are damaged, for example in multiple sclerosis or spinal-cord injury, the only permanent treatment is a prosthesis, which can be implanted into the shaft of the penis and inflated manually when required. Temporary erections can be brought about by injecting a substance called papaverine into the shaft of the penis. The sufferer can do this himself once he has learnt the simple technique from a urologist.

➎ Are you a heavy smoker?

Smoking accelerates hardening of the arteries, including those blood vessels necessary for producing an erection. In certain cases, therefore, giving up smoking may help to restore sexual function.

➏ Are you taking any medication?

Certain drugs may produce temporary impotence, particularly those used to control high blood pressure and drugs used in the treatment of depression. It's always worth asking your doctor whether the medication you are taking could be responsible for the symptom, and if so, it may be discontinued or the dose reduced.

● *Have you lost your sex drive?*

In most instances loss of libido in men is due to fatigue, stress, illness or boredom. Despite popular belief, true hormonal deficiency is rare.

Some private clinics specializing in the treatment of impotence claim good results using male sex-hormone injections for the treatment of the male menopause, but this is highly controversial. Most authorities do not recognize the male menopause since there is no appreciable diminution in the levels of sex hormones in the blood, such as occurs in the female menopause, and also because most medical studies on the subject have failed to show any benefit from the administration of such hormones to men with the symptom of impotence. Nor are the (possible) long-term side effects of such hormones on the liver and heart fully understood.

SUMMARY
IMPOTENCE

POSSIBLE CAUSE	ACTION
Performance anxiety	*Make sure that surroundings are appropriate, ensure adequate relaxation, talk to partner about any anxieties, psychosexual counselling if necessary.*
Stress and fatigue	*Ensure adequate relaxation, sleep and exercise.*
Alcohol abuse	*Stop drinking.*
Chronic illness	*Medical or surgical treatment for underlying cause, penile prosthesis or papaverine injections as appropriate.*
Smoking	*Stop.*
Medication	*With your doctor, identify and then discontinue or reduce dosage of responsible drug.*
Hormone deficiency	*Treat underlying cause. Use of testosterone analogues is highly controversial.*

PAINFUL SEX

It is unfortunate that the natural and usually highly pleasurable act of sexual intercourse should so often be a painful experience. Nevertheless, there are a number of conditions, both psychological and physical, that can cause discomfort, irritation or pain, some of which affect both sexes alike, others affecting one sex only. Men can experience pain on erection or when sexual intercourse actually takes place, whilst women can feel superficial pain at the entrance to the vagina or may only experience it deep inside with full penetration. Some women only suffer from it at certain times of their menstrual cycle. For both sexes, particular lovemaking positions can cause problems.

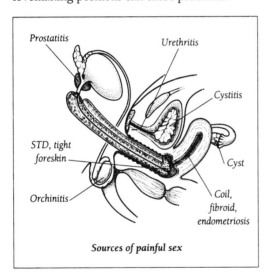

Sources of painful sex

MEN

❷ Is it difficult or painful to retract the foreskin?

A tight foreskin that cannot be fully retracted can cause sex to be painful, particularly if the narrow flap of tissue on the undersurface of the head of the penis is short, making it stretch and split on penetration. This may sometimes rupture and bleed, or, alternatively, small splits can appear in the foreskin itself, allowing an infection to develop.

❷ Is the tip of the penis tender, swollen and red?

A simple infection caused by bacteria getting into the tip of the penis and foreskin can lead to a condition known as balanitis, which is characterized by swelling, redness and discomfort. It certainly makes intercourse painful and requires treatment with antibiotics and salt baths.

❷ Does your sexual partner also have symptoms (discomfort and/or discharge)?

Thrush can be transmitted from the female partner to the man, and although symptoms are often mild and transient, some men experience redness, irritation and pain on intercourse. A male thrush carrier is also capable of reinfecting his female partner, even though her original symptoms may well have settled following a course of antithrush pessaries or tablets. For this reason, men and women should always be treated together when either has a thrush infection.

❷ Have you had an itching sensation followed by a crop of tiny, open blisters?

Herpes produces a burning, tingling sensation, followed a few days later by an outbreak of a crop of small blisters that rupture and ooze on to the surface of the skin. At this stage it is particularly painful, and antiviral acyclovir ointment or tablets are helpful. This is a transmittable disease and intercourse should be avoided until the blisters have completely healed up.

❷ Does your female partner use an intra-uterine coil (IUCD)?

If so, the threads that hang down from the cervix may occasionally produce discomfort in the male partner. If this is the case, the threads may need to be cut shorter by a doctor or gynaecologist.

❷ Has there been any previous discharge or kidney stone? Is the urinary poor and does it hurt to urinate?

Previous infection or damage from the passage of a kidney stone may result in the narrowing of the urethra, the tube that runs through the shaft of the penis to allow the carriage of semen and urine. When the stricture is significant, pain may be experienced on intercourse and dilatation through surgical procedures is required.

❷ Do you use spermicidal cream or jelly or penile lubricants?

Very occasionally a severe allergy to spermicidal cream or jelly can produce soreness, redness and itching of the penis. Avoiding these substances will resolve the problem.

❷ Does your penis bend painfully to one side during erection?

In this condition, known as Peyronie's disease, a small area of fibrous, scar-like tissue develops on one side of the shaft of the penis, preventing it from expanding normally on erection. As a result when erection occurs, a distinct bend appears in the penis, which may prove painful on penetration. Doses of multivitamins are often tried, although these are rarely very effective. If Peyronie's disease becomes advanced, surgery may be carried out, resulting in a shorter but straighter penis and no pain.

❷ Do you practise rectal sex?

If so, you can develop pain from piles, fissures (splits in the lining of the rectum), or from other consequences of trauma. Adequate lubrication is helpful.

WOMEN

Women can experience painful sex for a number of reasons, but contrary to popular belief it is never due to incompatibility with penile size. All women can deliver the head of a child successfully and no man is ever that well endowed. There are, however, other causes to consider.

❷ Do you feel particularly worried?

Just as men can experience impotence as a result of psychological problems, so stress and anxiety can lead to difficulties for women. Inexperience, fear of pregnancy, and ambivalent feelings towards your partner can all inhibit proper preparation and readiness for lovemaking, causing physical symptoms, including vaginal dryness and muscle spasm, that can make sex not only painful but at times impossible. Enough time for relaxation and extended foreplay are important, but relaxed and comfortable surroundings are also recommended.

❷ Is vaginal dryness a problem?

This has a number of possible causes but is most usually related either to anxiety or to the hormonal changes that accompany the menopause, although some women simply produce less natural lubrication than others. Whatever the cause, the resulting soreness during sex can be reduced by the simple application of lubricants such as KY jelly or Replens, and if necessary the prescription of hormone replacement therapy in some shape or form.

❷ Have you recently given birth?

Where there has been trauma to the skin and muscles of the pelvic floor, there may be considerable discomfort and pain for some days and weeks afterwards. This is in fact an extremely common cause of sexual difficulties and the doctor needs to put aside adequate time at the usual six-week postnatal examination to enquire about any problems and to prescribe appropriate treatment if necessary. Occasionally an episiotomy (a cut made at the side of the vagina during delivery to allow passage of the baby's head) may heal as an area of tight scar tissue that does not stretch easily during intercourse. Usually gentle stretching, either manually or through gentle intercourse, will put this right, but lubrication is most useful and occasionally the scar itself has to be 'revised' surgically.

❷ Do you have any kind of abnormal discharge?

Infections can be superficial or deep. At the edge of each of the vaginal lips is a large gland called a Bartholin's gland, which may become inflamed if a bacterial infection begins within it. A distinct lump may be felt at the edge of the lips and may discharge infected material. Antibiotics are effective in the early stages but occasionally surgical drainage is required. Thrush is another common infection which usually produces a creamy-white cheesy kind of vaginal discharge that can irritate and produce pain on intercourse.

❷ Have you noticed a crop of painful open blisters at the opening of the vagina?

The herpes infection produces clusters of small, painful blisters preceded by a tingling, burning sensation and tends to be recurrent. Antiviral creams, ointments or tablets may reduce the frequency and severity of attacks, which tend to become less frequent as time passes. Intercourse should be avoided whilst the blisters are active.

❷ Is there vaginal discharge together with abdominal pain?

Sometimes infections can produce inflammation of deeper structures such as the fallopian tubes, in which case there may be pain on deep penetration and possible long-term infertility. Full investigation followed by adequate antibiotic treatment are essential.

❷ Do you use vaginal deodorants, bubble bath, scented soaps or talc?

Any of these synthetically made cosmetics could be setting up an allergic reaction in the delicate tissues around the vagina, resulting in irritation and discomfort.

❷ Do the muscles around your vagina tighten up in the earliest stages of lovemaking?

In this condition, known as vaginismus, the sufferer experiences a powerful contraction of the muscles around the vagina and sometimes of the inner surface of the thighs as well. There is usually a strong psychological reason for this totally involuntary reaction, which makes sex painful and sometimes impossible. It could be something as common as general stress and tension, but it could also be the result of long-standing feelings of guilt about sex or a consequence of childhood sexual abuse or adult rape. The condition is not in fact all that uncommon and the good news is that with vaginal dilators and psychosexual counselling a woman can learn to overcome the problem and in the future enjoy normal, loving, painless sex.

❷ Did the problem arise when making love for the first time?

The hymen hardly ever causes obstruction to intercourse since the appearance of normal menstrual flow each month is evidence that this membrane at the entrance to the vagina is no longer intact. However, in rare instances it may remain fairly tough, in which case minor surgery can be performed to overcome the problem.

❷ Have you developed swollen veins around the vagina during or following pregnancy?

Occasionally, varicose veins around the back passage or even around the vagina itself, developing towards the end of or after pregnancy, can cause difficulties. In most instances the varicose veins clear up after the birth of the baby, but in persistent cases surgical or injection treatment may be necessary.

❷ Is there deep pain inside during intercourse and does it coincide with your period?

Endometriosis is caused by movement of the cells that normally line the uterus along the fallopian tubes into the abdominal cavity itself, producing small amounts of bleeding coincidental with period times. This causes a sticking-together of the abdominal organs and because of these 'adhesions' there may be pain on deep penetration. The condition will be obvious to the doctor when he or she examines the patient. An operation called laparoscopy, in which a narrow telescope is used to view the inside of the pelvic cavity is often carried out to confirm the diagnosis, after which hormone treatment can be very successful.

❷ Is there pain deep inside during intercourse and is your lower abdomen swollen?

Ovarian cysts can be temporary or permanent, benign or malignant. If the cyst is of significant size, it may be responsible for pain on deep penetration. This possibility should always be borne in mind and investigated by a gynaecologist.

SUMMARY
PAINFUL SEX

POSSIBLE CAUSE	ACTION
Men	
Tight foreskin	Adequate lubrication, gradual stretching through frequent but gentle intercourse. Circumcision occasionally required.
Infection	Antibiotics, salt baths.
Sexually transmitted disease	Identify exact cause, medical treatment.
Coil threads	Trim threads.
Stricture	Surgical dilatation.
Allergy	Avoid causative substance.
Peyronie's disease	Megavitamins or surgery.
Rectal sex	Identify problem, medical treatment.
Women	
Anxiety and stress	Proper sexual technique, adequate relaxation, relaxing surroundings, lubrication.
Vaginal dryness	Treat with lubrication or hormone replacement therapy.
Following childbirth	Adequate lubrication, gentle foreplay. Surgical revision of episiotomy scar if necessary.
Infections	Identify underlying organism and treat with antibiotics.
Allergy	Identify and avoid causative substance.
Vaginismus	Psychosexual counselling, lubrication, vaginal dilators.
The hymen	Very occasionally minor surgery required.
Varicose veins	Injection treatment or surgery.
Endometriosis	Hormonal treatment or surgery.
Ovarian cysts	Surgery if necessary.

PREMATURE EJACULATION

For men, this is the commonest sexual problem of all. It is particularly likely early on in a relationship and is generally triggered by anxiety and tension. The man is unable to prevent himself from reaching his climax too early and the problem is often associated with impotence.

However, in long-standing cases and where relationship difficulties are setting in, the squeeze technique, originally devised by Dr James Semans and further embellished by Masters and Johnson, can be taught by psychosexual counsellors with a very high success rate. In this, the couple avoid intercourse for several weeks but learn to prolong foreplay, during which the female partner stimulates the male partner's penis manually. Each time he is on the verge of climax, she squeezes the penis firmly at the tip, which immediately abolishes the feeling of imminent climax. In time, when ejaculation can be delayed long enough, partial and then full sexual intercourse may be permitted, and eventually normal intercourse can take place on a regular basis. Very occasionally, premature ejaculation may be the result of an underlying physical problem, for example a disorder of the nervous system or inflammation of the prostate gland, but on the whole it is a problem seen in younger men with relatively little sexual experience.

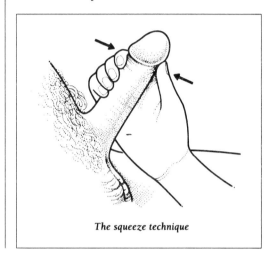

The squeeze technique

SUMMARY
PREMATURE EJACULATION

POSSIBLE CAUSE	ACTION
Anxiety, inexperience	Squeeze technique. A small amount of alcohol, local anaesthetic cream, and/or wearing a condom will reduce sensitivity.
Inflammation of the prostate gland	Antibiotics.
Nervous-system disorders	Identify disorder responsible. Appropriate medical or surgical treatment.

287

DIFFICULTIES WITH ORGASM

Difficulties experiencing orgasms can occur even when there is perfectly adequate desire and arousal. In fact, many women find they are unable to reach a climax through sexual intercourse alone, and require manual or oral stimulation. It has also been estimated that 10 per cent of women never reach an orgasm at all. Men too can experience difficulties as a result of psychological or physical problems.

❷ Are you relaxed?

Climax requires as much input from the mind and the emotions as from physical stimulation. If there is no link between the two, orgasms are often never achieved. Such difficulties often require psychosexual counselling. It always helps to involve one's sexual partner in this.

❷ Do you need to change your sexual technique?

For women there appear to be at least two separate components to orgasm, namely the muscular contractions associated with clitoral stimulation and those associated with vaginal penetration. Because all women respond to a variety of sexual techniques differently, only by experimenting will the individual discover what best brings her to orgasm. Some women, for example, will only achieve orgasm sitting astride their partner, whereas others achieve it through oral stimulation or straightforward intercourse in the missionary position.

❷ Have you any existing medical problems?

If nerves are damaged by a physical illness such as diabetes and multiple sclerosis, problems with normal climax may occur.

❷ Are you taking any medication?

Some medicines, notably beta-blockers to lower blood pressure and antidepressants, can occasionally cause problems with climax. Consult your doctor to see if this is the problem; simple discontinuation of the drug responsible should reverse the problem.

SUMMARY
DIFFICULTIES WITH ORGASM

Possible Cause	Action
Psychological problems	Psychosexual counselling.
Physical disorders	Medical treatment of underlying problem.
Medication	With your doctor, identify and then consider cutting down or changing the drug responsible.
Inadequate sexual technique	Counselling, advice regarding communication and foreplay. Experimentation with different sexual positions and with manual and oral clitoral stimulation. Use of vibrators. Psychosexual counselling.

INFECTIONS, BEDBUGS AND BODY LICE

There are a number of common infections that can occur in the genital area in both men and women. They can cause a range of symptoms, and common ones include itching, tingling, burning and pain. In addition, there may be discharge, bleeding, lumps and/or the urge to empty your bladder more often than usual. Bedbugs and lice can also produce similar symptoms, and although they are not infections as such, they are generally, albeit not invariably, passed on through close physical or sexual contact.

❷ Is there a white vaginal discharge that leaves red, sore, itchy areas beneath?

Vaginal thrush is an extremely common condition, one which 70 per cent of women will develop at some time during their lives. It is caused by a fungus called Candida albicans that lives naturally in the vagina at all times and only produces problems when the normal bacteria–fungus balance of the vagina is altered. This can happen during courses of antibiotics given for some other infection such as a sore throat, in pregnancy, or when taking the oral contraceptive pill. Diabetics are also more prone to developing thrush due to the higher sugar content of their blood. There is usually a vaginal discharge, which is white, thick and lumpy, and a sore, dry, red, itchy vagina. It may burn or sting to pass water and sexual intercourse can be uncomfortable. Men can carry thrush on the tip of their penis but tend not to get too much in the way of symptoms. As a result, unless both partners are treated at the same time, the man is likely to reinfect the woman again later. Treatment consists of creams, pessaries or tablets, all of which eradicate most of the thrush organisms so that the normal balance of bacteria and fungus in the vagina can be re-established.

❷ Is there a clear watery discharge in either partner?

Chlamydia is a bacterial parasite and is probably the most common sexually transmitted disease in the world today. Sometimes there may be no symptoms, not even irritation, but usually there is a discharge. A more frequent need to pass water is often reported and the diagnosis is only confirmed by identifying the organism from a swab test sent to the laboratory. The danger of chlamydia for women is that occasionally it can affect the fallopian tubes, leading to chronic infection and infertility. It is therefore important that the infection is identified and treated with antibiotics.

❷ Has a tingling sensation preceded a crop of painful, tiny blisters?

Genital herpes is caused by the herpes simplex virus and is characterized by clusters of blisters on either the vaginal lips or the shaft of the penis. It is often preceded by the warning signals of tingling, burning or aching. Some people also feel generally unwell, as if they have flu. The symptoms tend to be recurrent and the person is infectious to other people through sexual contact whilst the blisters are open and weeping. Treatment consists of antiviral cream or tablets, which not only reduce the severity and duration of each attack, but enables the body to reduce the number of recurrences.

❷ Are there any fleshy lumps growing in the genital area?

Genital warts can be seen and/or felt anywhere around or inside the vagina, cervix or back passage. Men tend to get them on the penis, on or under the foreskin. As time goes by they gradually enlarge, causing itching. They are common and are becoming even more so. In women, they are also associated with an increased risk of cervical cancer. Treatment involves either painting the warts with a special kind of paint called podophyllin or using burning or freezing techniques under local anaesthetic.

❷ Is there a yellowy-green discharge in either partner?

Gonorrhoea is one of the oldest sexually transmitted diseases and produces a fairly heavy greeny-cream discharge from the urethra that in women can sometimes spread to the uterus and fallopian tubes, causing abdominal pain and a temperature. Men often complain of pain when they pass urine and a similar offensive discharge. They too can have complications, which can include swelling and pain in the testicle area and in some instances a form of arthritis. Antibiotics are required, together with medical supervision to ensure that the illness has completely cleared up.

❷ Is there a particularly offensive-smelling vaginal discharge?

Gardnerella is responsible for a particularly smelly type of vaginal discharge that can be grey and frothy. Treatment involves appropriate antibiotics under specialist supervision.

❷ Is there a painful ulcer in the genital or mouth areas together with swollen glands in the groin?

Like gonorrhoea, syphilis is an age-old type of sexually transmitted disease that is a lot less common than it used to be. Nevertheless, there are still about 1,500 cases recorded every year in this country. Symptoms include an ulcer, either on the shaft of the penis or near the vagina. It is not painful but very infectious during sexual contact. The glands in the groin may also enlarge and unless treated the infection will continue to spread to other sites in the body. Antibiotics are effective but must be given in the very early stages to prevent the infection from causing very significant damage to other parts of the body, for example heart disease or degeneration within the brain tissue.

❷ Is there a frothy, green-looking vaginal discharge?

Trichomoniasis is a parasite that lives in the deep folds of the vagina and is usually sexually transmitted. There may be no symptoms at all, or there may be an obvious infection with swelling and a frothy, green, unpleasant-smelling discharge that on occasions may be bloodstained. There may also be an increased need to urinate, necessitating urgent trips to the loo to empty your bladder. Antibiotics and specialist supervision are necessary.

❷ Is the skin below the pubic hair especially itchy in bed at night?

Intense itching of the pubic area, especially when warm in bed at night, may result from infestation with scabies (bedbugs) or pubic lice (crabs). They are passed on from person to person and although sexual contact need not occur, fairly close contact is necessary. For example, sharing clothes, towels or bedding is enough to transmit the bugs. Treatment is fairly straightforward with special lotions that are generally rubbed on to the area after a warm bath. Clearly all family members and close sexual contacts should be treated where appropriate.

SUMMARY
INFECTIONS, BEDBUGS AND BODY LICE

POSSIBLE CAUSE	ACTION
Thrush	Antifungal cream, pessaries or tablets.
Chlamydia	Antibiotics.
Herpes	Antiviral agents.
Genital warts	Podophyllin paint. Burning or freezing treatment (diathermy or cryotherapy).
Gonorrhoea	Antibiotics.
Gardnerella	Antibiotics.
Syphilis	Antibiotics.
Trichomoniasis	Antibiotics.
Scabies and pubic lice	Insecticide lotions.

INFERTILITY

Infertility is a sign that something is not working as it should. It is defined as the inability to conceive after trying for more than 18 months, although some authorities believe that people over 30 should reduce this to 12 months. A woman's fertility usually peaks between the ages of 24 and 27, whereas men generally remain fertile well into their eighties. It has been estimated that approximately one in six couples have problems conceiving, and infertility can be either primary (they have never had children) or secondary (they have previously had one or more children but are now having difficulties).

A large number of delicate processes need to occur without interference for a couple to be fertile and difficulties at any step of the way can lead to infertility. Firstly, there need to be enough sperm, which must be of good enough quality, to fertilize the egg. Then the egg has to be released by the ovary and find its way into the fallopian tube. The sperm then needs to be able to penetrate the outer layer of the egg and fertilize it, after which the fertilized egg has to move downwards, through the fallopian tube, to implant itself in the lining of the uterus, which must be prepared to take it. Finally, the implanted egg must burrow into the lining of the uterus and allow the embryo to grow. It is a complex process, and there are a number of common problems that can get in the way and lead to difficulties. The good news is that in 50 per cent of cases help is to hand and the problem can be put right.

❷ Do you smoke or drink heavily and/or are you under a lot of stress?

It has now been proven beyond doubt that lifestyle factors can have serious consequences on normal fertility. Men and women can both be affected by heavy smoking and drinking as well as inadequate or poor nutrition and high levels of stress. Pollutants in the atmosphere have also been incriminated in cases of unexplained infertility. Recent studies showing a general fall in the sperm count of young men compared to a decade ago have suggested that such environmental factors may well be responsible for infertility.

❷ Do you have regular periods?

Regular periods depend on a number of hormonal factors, not least the monthly release of an egg from the ovaries. In fact, failure to produce an egg each month accounts for the majority of infertility cases in women. Failure to ovulate can occur for many reasons. The ovaries themselves may be damaged from external injury or internal abnormalities such as endometriosis. Sometimes they may be abnormal from birth, containing no eggs whatsoever. Emotional and psychological upset can also disrupt the regular ovarian menstrual cycle. Finally, hormonal and chemical factors are often the underlying problem. Women who experience these problems and who suffer from anorexia nervosa, or who are gymnasts or athletes fall into these last two categories. Signs of ovulation include breast tenderness and fullness, sharp pain on one side of the abdomen midway through the cycle, and an increase in the normal symptomless vaginal discharge. There may also be a slight temperature change just before ovulation, but often this is too small to notice. Absence of these signs when previously they have been regularly present may be a sign of ovulatory failure. However, they may not be present in women who consistently ovulate. Happily, 90 per cent of cases of failure to ovulate can be corrected with special fertility drugs, and even when ovulation is not possible, surgical techniques can take eggs directly from the ovary and have them fertilized with sperm outside the body.

❷ Have you had any treatment on your cervix for abnormal smears or had your cervix sewn up after a difficult birth?

A narrowed or scarred cervix, or the presence in the cervix of unfavourable mucus that prevents the passage of the sperm into the uterus, may be the underlying cause of infertility. Previous surgery or laser treatment are occasionally incriminated but all of these problems are potentially correctable.

❷ Have you recently had heavy and irregular periods?

Uterine fibroids are muscular lumps in the wall of the uterus and can be large enough to interfere with fertility. Most fibroids are removed by surgical excision of the entire womb (hysterectomy), but if the fibroids are small and still affecting fertility, they can be excised by themselves in an operation known as a myomectomy. However, subsequent restoration of fertility cannot be guaranteed.

❷ Have you previously suffered from any sexually transmitted disease, especially where there was vaginal discharge and lower abdominal pain?

In moderate to severe cases, pelvic infection or pelvic inflammatory disease (PID) can lead to blockage of the fallopian tubes, thereby obstructing the passage of the egg from the ovary to the lining of the uterus. Microsurgery is usually required to overcome this problem and is becoming increasingly successful.

❷ Is there a lot of backache with the periods?

This usually long-standing condition can cause inflammation and kinking of the fallopian tubes and/or it can interfere with normal ovarian functions. Endometriosis may be asymptomatic and only discovered when infertility is investigated. In other cases it may cause lower abdominal pain, irregular vaginal bleeding and deep-seated pain on intercourse. Surgery or hormone treatment may be required to put it right, although quite often in vitro fertilization techniques will be required to correct the infertility side of things.

❷ Have you previously had a miscarriage or an abortion?

Occasionally a previous miscarriage or therapeutic abortion can lead to infertility problems by introducing infection or by damaging the cervix. However, with better surgical techniques of the last decade these problems are now relatively rare.

❷ Are the veins at the top of the testicles swollen and congested?

Varicose veins here can increase the temperature of the testicles thereby reducing their efficiency in manufacturing sperm. This is a potentially reversible problem.

❷ Have you noticed any persistent headaches or have your testicles become smaller (atrophy)?

Sperm production is dependent on the hormone testosterone, produced by the testicles, and on gonadotrophic hormones, produced by the pituitary gland at the base of the brain. These could be affected by liver disease or pituitary tumours respectively, causing a low sperm count. The problem is potentially reversible.

❷ Has a sperm count revealed poor-quality sperm?

Even if the number of sperm is adequate, the quality may not be. This can occur with infections of the genitourinary system, including tuberculosis, mumps and sexually transmitted diseases, or there may be blockage of the vas deferens, the tube that takes the sperm from the testicle to the outside, for reasons other than infections, for example direct trauma. Alternatively, there may be circulating antibodies that cause clumping of the sperm, which then become unable to function properly.

SUMMARY
INFERTILITY

POSSIBLE CAUSE	ACTION
Lifestyle	Stop smoking, reduce alcohol consumption, avoid stress, regular physical activity.
Failure to ovulate	Medical treatment and/or in vitro fertilization.
Cervical problems	Medical or surgical treatment.
Fibroids	May be removed surgically.
Pelvic infection	Antibiotics if acute, microsurgery if chronic with blocked tubes.
Endometriosis	Surgical treatment. In vitro fertilization if necessary.
Previous miscarriage or abortion	Medical or surgical treatment for complications.
Testicular atrophy	Hormonal treatment may stimulate sperm production if adequate testicular tissue remains. One normally functioning testicle is perfectly compatible with full fertility. Surgery or radiotherapy for pituitary-gland tumour.
Infection	Antibiotics.
Blockage of vas deferens	Microsurgery.
Sperm clumping	Steroids.

12

THE SKIN

The skin is the largest organ of the body. It protects the body's internal structures from external harm, and prevents the potential invasion of harmful foreign organisms such as bacteria and viruses. The hard outer layer can resist the action of all but the most powerful acids and alkalines, whilst continual friction and rubbing mean that the cells of the skin itself, as well as our nails and hair, are continually being replaced.

The skin has four other main functions: sensation, storage, absorption and heat regulation. Through the sensations of touch, pain and temperature, sensory endings within the skin warn us against the presence of painful stimuli thus protecting us from injury. The skin and subcutaneous tissues act as a store for water and fat. In fact, the fatty tissue under the skin is one of the main fat depots within the body. The skin also absorbs ultraviolet radiation from the sun, which is useful in the formation of small quantities of vitamin D. Finally, the skin is essential for regulating a constant body temperature independent of the temperature of the external environment. When the body needs to cool down, the skin can promote heat loss by conduction, convection, radiation and the evaporation of sweat on its surface. On the other hand, when heat needs to be conserved, blood vessels within the skin will shut down so that further heat loss will be minimized. Sweating stops and the tiny muscles controlling the hairs on the skin will stand erect, a throw-back to our more hairy ancestors who in this way trapped a layer of warm air over their skin.

The skin consists of a tough superficial layer called the epidermis, and a deeper layer containing blood and lymphatic vessels called the dermis. Finger- and toe-nails consist of a tremendously thickened clear layer of the epidermis. The dermis contains the elastic fibres that endow the skin with its flexibility. It is these elastic fibres that degenerate in old age, when the skin becomes noticeably wrinkled and lined. Hairs are found everywhere except on the palms of the hands, the soles of the feet, and parts of the external genitalia. Each hair follicle is lubricated by a sebaceous gland that produces oil to soften the skin. The skin also contains the sweat glands.

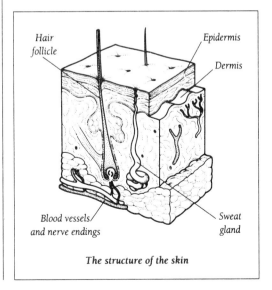

The structure of the skin

COLOUR CHANGES

There are a number of conditions that can affect the normal colour of the skin, either in a generalized fashion or in patches. Any such changes may represent a surface disorder such as a fungal infection or eczema, or be a reflection of changes occurring from within. Some conditions may even be inherited. In albinism, for example, there is an inherited and generalized melanin deficiency that produces pale skin and white hair, whilst phenylketonuria is another genetic condition where individuals have reduced melanin levels, causing them to be particularly pale-skinned and fair-haired.

INCREASED PIGMENTATION

The basic colour of your skin is determined by the amount of melanin, the skin's dark pigment, which is produced by special cells called melanocytes. The more melanin present, the darker the colour. This depends on heredity, but exposure to sunlight will increase the amount of melanin produced. Melanin has a protective action against the harmful effects of the sun's rays. It does not prevent loss of elasticity and the ageing effect of sunlight, but it does reduce the chances of cancer developing as a result of overexposure to solar radiation. Malignant melanoma is hardly ever seen in people with black skin, but in blond, red-haired and/or fair-skinned individuals its incidence is increasing at an alarming rate as more and more people take holidays in sunny climates and experience sunburn as a result of failing to use adequate protection in the form of sunblock creams. Malignant melanoma is a serious form of cancer responsible for a high proportion of deaths from cancer in the 25-40-year-old age group. However, there are a number of other causes of increased pigmentation, so ask yourself the following questions:

❶ Do you suffer from any red, itchy or flaky areas of skin?

Patches of dark skin can follow episodes of psoriasis, fungal infections, eczema or a condition known as pityriasis versicolor, which tends to produce patches along the lines of the ribs on the front and back.

❷ Are you taking the contraceptive pill, pregnant, or going through the menopause?

The hormonal changes that occur in pregnancy, during the menopause and as a result of taking the oral contraceptive pill can cause a condition known as chloasma, in which dark patches appear on the cheeks and forehead. Pregnant women can also develop a dark line called the linea nigra from the navel downwards, and the nipples and areola usually darken too.

❸ Do you use cosmetics?

Some cosmetics and perfumes contain chemicals which can cause photosensitivity in susceptible people. When this happens, your skin will react to sunlight more strongly so that tanned facial patches occur. These generally fade with time.

❹ Have you any freckles or moles that have recently changed shape, colour or size?

Any change in a pigmented mole should always be regarded with suspicion and reported at once to your doctor.

Change can be defined as any of the following: simple enlargement; the appearance of new and separate pigmented areas around the original mole; bleeding and irritation or alteration of the colouring over the surface. Generally speaking, most of these changes are only likely to be noticed in moles larger than the size of the blunt end of a pencil.

❷ *Has there been any weight change and general darkening of the skin?*

Addison's disease which is caused by underactivity of the adrenal gland, commonly produces darkening of the skin in conjunction with severe fatigue and weakness, weight loss, nausea and vomiting. In Cushing's syndrome, an overactive adrenal gland leads to darkening of the skin, together with increased weight, high blood pressure and a tendency for fat to collect around the base of the back of the neck.

❷ *Are there a number of flat, coffee-coloured patches anywhere on the skin?*

In the inherited condition known as neurofibromatosis, coffee-coloured areas, otherwise known as *Café-au-lait* patches, develop on the skin. There will also be small lumps on the nerves, and these may or may not give rise to symptoms of tingling pain.

❷ *Is the pigmentation confined to the body creases?*

If there are areas of dark, thickened, velvety skin, especially in the body creases, a diagnosis of acanthosis nigricans is likely. This is associated with a number of underlying conditions, including tumours that require specialized treatment.

❷ *Do you have varicose veins?*

Long-standing varicose veins around the feet and ankles can gradually leak blood pigments out into the overlying skin. Since these pigments contain iron, which darkens when deprived of oxygen, deep discoloration can take place over the course of time.

PATCHES OF PALE SKIN

❷ *Do you have, or have you ever had, any dry, flaky patches on the skin?*

It is very common for children who have had patches of eczema or fungal infection to have pale areas of skin on their faces. The same thing occurs in psoriasis in adults, as well as in pityriasis. What happens in these conditions is that when the skin scales flake off, they take melanin with them.

❷ *Are there areas of widespread loss of pigment?*

In the condition known as vitiligo, areas of skin stop producing melanin because for reasons not yet fully understood, circulating antibodies destroy the melanocytes. Vitiligo is associated with other autoimmune conditions such as thyroid disease and pernicious anaemia.

GENERALLY PALE SKIN

❷ *Are you breathless and tired?*

When the skin is generally pale, as opposed to being light only in small patches, the most usual cause is anaemia. This means that the concentration in the blood of the oxygen-carrying pigment, haemoglobin, is below normal. The pallor is particularly marked in the creases of the skin, the lining of the mouth and the undersurface of the eyelids. However, the degree of pallor does not accurately reflect the degree of the underlying anaemia.

BLUE SKIN

A bluish colour to the skin and lining of the mouth – otherwise known as cyanosis – is generally due to large amounts of deoxygenated haemoglobin circulating in the blood. The blueness is often most marked in the fingernail beds, lips and tongue.

❷ *Is the skin blue only in cold weather?*

In cold weather some people with no underlying condition turn literally 'blue with cold'. This is due to slowing down of the blood flow through the skin and does not indicate any significant problem.

297

❷ Do you have a heart murmur or get breathless when lying flat? Did you suffer from rheumatic fever as a child?
Any of these could indicate heart failure or valvular heart disease. Either condition can interfere with the heart's ability to pump blood around the body efficiently, leading to a sluggish circulation and blue tinges to the lips, face, nose and tongue.

❷ Are you or have you been a heavy smoker? Do you cough up phlegm every winter and are constantly breathless?
Even if the heart is functioning normally, if the lungs are unable to absorb enough oxygen from the air because of chronic lung disorders such as emphysema, chronic bronchitis or lung cancer, the blood will not be fully oxygenated and will remain a darker colour. It is this darker colour that gives the skin a bluish tinge.

YELLOW SKIN (JAUNDICE)
Jaundice is an unmistakable symptom. Not only does your skin develop a yellowish tinge, but so do the whites of your eyes. In fact, it is important to check that the whites of the eyes are yellow, because very occasionally doctors do see a condition known as carotenemia, which is caused by an excess intake of carotene in the diet, the result of consuming large amounts of concentrated carrot juice, leafy green vegetables and oranges. True jaundice is characterized by the presence in the tissues of the body of a yellow pigment called bilirubin. To help identify the nature of your underlying problem, ask yourself the following questions:

❷ Has jaundice come on suddenly?
This suggests an acute infection such as viral hepatitis, a gallstone obstructing the outflow channels from the liver, or some condition that is causing the acute breakdown of healthy red blood cells in the circulation such as malaria.

❷ Do you have a high temperature accompanied by pain in the upper-right corner of the abdomen?
This is highly suggestive of infection or inflammation of the gall bladder or possibly of a gallstone.

❷ Have you eaten any suspicious food lately, or recently travelled in the Third World?
You may have been picked up infectious hepatitis that has temporarily inflamed the liver. You can look forward to overcoming this on your own within about six weeks.

❷ Have you ever used illegal drugs intravenously?
The sharing of contaminated needles is one of the major reasons why hepatitis B is so common in today's society. Hepatitis B is a more potent and threatening infection of the liver than infectious hepatitis and in some instances can produce severe liver damage. *See your doctor urgently.*

❷ Have you had a blood transfusion recently?
Despite the screening of blood and blood products, the transmission of a third type of hepatitis known as 'non-A non-B' hepatitis is still a possibility, particularly in poor countries, and may result in jaundice.

❷ Have you had the jaundice before and does it come and go?
This suggests an inflammation of the gall bladder or the movement of gallstones within it or within the drainage ducts.

❷ Is the jaundice associated with very pale motions?
An obstruction to the outflow of bile pigment from the liver can result in the pigment failing

to reach the intestine, where it is responsible for the normal colouring of motions. This combination of symptoms therefore highlights the possibility of a gallstone completely blocking the various channels to the intestine. If in addition you have lost weight for no obvious reason, this suggests the possibility of something more serious such as a cancer and requires *urgent referral to a doctor.*

❷ *Have you taken any medication recently?*

Many drugs can cause jaundice, whether by breaking down healthy red blood cells earlier than they should, by affecting the liver itself, or by causing inflammation and obstruction to the outflow channels once the bilirubin has left the liver. A few examples include steroids, particularly anabolic steroids, some antibiotics, especially Erythromycin, some anti-depressants, some anti-cancer treatments, methyldopa which is used in the treatment of high blood pressure, rifampicin, used in the treatment of tuberculosis, some oral anti-diabetic tablets, some antithyroid preparations and, occasionally, the oral contraceptive pill.

❸ *Is the jaundice fairly long-standing and does it seem to be progressive?*

This suggests a slower process such as cirrhosis where the long-standing abuse of alcohol has caused scarring of the liver so that it is no longer able to handle normal amounts of bilirubin. Also worth considering are various malignancies that can either cause obstruction of the outflow of bile or damage the liver itself, for example cancer of the pancreas.

❹ *Is there any swelling of the abdomen?*

This can be caused by cirrhosis, where the liver tends to swell, or by free fluid present within the abdomen, perhaps as a result of an underlying malignancy somewhere within the abdomen.

BLACK SKIN

Completely black skin, particularly at the peripheries such as the fingers, toes and earlobes, is due to gangrene. In this condition underlying tissues die due to inadequate blood supply, which may be cut off as the result of extreme cold (in which case it is known as frostbite), blockage of the arteries due to general hardening and/or clot formation, infection, or direct pressure on or haemorrhage from blood vessels. It is usually preceded by severe pain. Bacterial infection may also develop, causing redness, swelling and weeping around the blackened area.

Gangrene is a medical emergency requiring urgent surgical treatment.

SUMMARY
COLOUR CHANGES IN THE SKIN

POSSIBLE CAUSE	ACTION
Psoriasis	Steroids, coal-tar preparations, ultraviolet light therapy.
Fungal injection	Antifungal agents.
Eczema	Oils, emollients, emulsifiers, mild steroids, Chinese herbal medicines.
Pityriasis versicolor	Moisturizing cream if itchy.
Chloasma	Stop oral contraceptive pill, treat menopausal symptoms. Colour changes reverse after pregnancy or stopping oral contraceptives.
Moles that enlarge or irritate	Urgent referral to doctor. Biopsy, excision or chemotherapy if malignant.
Hormonal changes	Treat underlying hormone imbalance.
Cosmetics	Change brand.
Addison's disease	Steroid supplementation of underactive adrenal glands.
Cushing's syndrome	Surgical treatment for overactive adrenal glands.
Neurofibromatosis	No treatment.
Acanthosis nigricans	Identify underlying condition and treat.
Varicose veins	Elastic stockings. Sclerotherapy. Surgical stripping of veins.
Bruising from other sources	Identify underlying cause and treat appropriately.
Patches of pale skin	
Local inflammation (eczema, fungal infection, psoriasis, pityriasis)	See above.
Vitiligo	Identify autoimmune disorder and treat.

Continued . . .

SUMMARY
COLOUR CHANGES IN THE SKIN

POSSIBLE CAUSE	ACTION
Generally pale skin	
Anaemia	Identify type of anaemia and treat.
Blue Skin	
Cold weather	Warmer clothing. Vasodilator drugs if peripheral circulation poor.
Heart disease	Medical treatment with diuretics for heart failure. Surgical treatment of valvular abnormalities.
Lung disease	Stop smoking. Medical treatment for chronic bronchitis, asthma, emphysema and bronchiectasis. Surgical or medical treatment for lung cancer.
Yellow skin	
Hepatitis	Bedrest, fluids, dietary restriction.
Gallstone	Medical treatment to dissolve stone; more usually surgery.
Gallbladder infection or inflammation	Antibiotics, pain relief, surgery when infection settled.
Medication	With your doctor, identify and then discontinue drug responsible.
Cirrhosis of the liver	Medical treatment.
Cancer	Medical and/or surgical treatment.
Malaria	Hospitalization for antimalarial treatment.
Black skin	
Gangrene	Emergency surgical treatment necessary.

DRY, FLAKY SKIN

Disorders of the skin attract some degree of social stigma because they are often visually obvious and cosmetically unattractive. In days gone by they were associated with contagious disease and lack of personal hygiene, but even though these myths have largely been exploded, the psychological effects of disfiguring skin conditions should never be underestimated.

❷ Is the skin itchy, thickened and cracked? Does it run in the family?

People suffering from eczema will have itchy, uncomfortable skin that generally looks dry, scaly and cracked. It is extremely common and affects babies and adults alike, although the majority of children with eczema grow out of it. Eczema is associated with asthma and hay fever and is certainly more likely if other members of the family are affected. Symptoms include dryness and flaking of the skin with cracking, red, angry areas leading to blistering, crust formation, pain and discomfort. Flare-ups of irritation tend to occur after exposure to particular trigger factors. These commonly include biological washing powders, perfumed soaps, bubble baths, chemical cleansers, woollen clothing, feathers, animal hair or feathers, and dietary components such as food colourings and preservatives and dairy products.

Recently, Chinese herbal medicine has been shown to be effective in treating eczema, even in certain cases where the condition is widespread and severe and where all standard treatments using powerful steroids and emollients have failed. It has been adopted in conventional treatment centres within the NHS, for example Great Ormond Street Children's Hospital, but close supervision is required as side effects may include detrimental effects on liver function.

❷ Are the skin patches covered in silvery scales with red areas beneath?

Psoriasis is a common skin condition affecting approximately 1 to 2 per cent of the population at some stage. It usually starts between the ages of ten and 30 and it can vary from just a few patches to covering almost the entire body. Sufferers notice red, circular patches on the skin that are covered with silvery-white scales. The patches can be from half an inch across to five or six inches. There will also be slight itching and irritation. The knees, elbows and scalp are most commonly affected, and on the scalp it is often mistaken for severe dandruff. However, close observation of the scalp shows that the scales are coming from localized areas, unlike dandruff, when the condition is much more general. The fingernails may become thickened, with tiny little pits and indentations, and the nail itself may lift away from the underlying nail bed. Occasionally, a type of arthritis resembling rheumatoid arthritis is associated with these symptoms, but this is not common.

Psoriasis responds to a variety of creams and ointments and also quite well to exposure to ultraviolet light.

❸ Are there a number of reddish-brown patches on the skin of the trunk area?

Nobody understands what causes pityriasis rosea, which mainly affects young adults and starts with a solitary patch called the herald patch. This is soon followed by other, scaly patches, usually on the trunk, which have a slightly raised edge and are reddish brown in colour. It often occurs within a few days of a mild sore throat, so infection is thought to have something to do with it. The disorder is usually symptomless apart from the rash, although there may occasionally be some irritation. The disorder clears up by itself within two to three months.

❸ *Are there just one or two roughly circular patches on the skin, with well-defined edges?*

Ringworm commonly affects the feet, hands, groin and, at times, the whole body, and is due to a number of different fungi. Although contagious, these fungal infections are not as infectious as is generally believed, and are certainly very slow-growing. The fungi live in the hard outer layers of the skin and don't affect the deeper living layers of the skin at all. The skin patches are red with a scaly, itchy top, and in between the toes there may be white patches with sogginess and peeling.

SUMMARY
DRY, FLAKY SKIN

POSSIBLE CAUSE	ACTION
Eczema	Avoid trigger factors, diet, moisturizers and emollients, steroid creams, Chinese herbal tea.
Psoriasis	Coal-tar preparations, steroids.
Pityriasis rosea	Mild hydrocortisone cream if itching is intense.
Ringworm	Antifungal preparations.

RASHES

Rashes can appear in a number of forms.

RASHES WITH BLISTERS

➊ Did you have red, blotchy spots on your face that have now turned yellow and crusty?

The red rash of impetigo turns to watery blisters, usually around the nostrils and mouth but also affecting the scalp and arms. The blisters enlarge and rupture, leaking a straw-coloured fluid and forming the characteristic yellowish-red, itching crusts. The disorder is due to a bacterial infection and in its mild form responds to antibiotic creams or ointments, or, in more widespread cases, oral antibiotics.

➋ Do you have clusters of tiny, painful blisters?

Shingles is caused by the herpes zoster virus and begins with a mild, flu-like illness. A day or two later a rash forms at any site on one side of the body and is followed by a cluster of small, painful blisters that dry, crust and then heal, leaving tiny scars. Occasionally there may be sharp, intense pain at the site of the original blisters, even when they have completely disappeared, and this is due to irritation of the underlying nerve in which the virus lay dormant. This is called post-herpetic neuralgia.

➌ Does the rash consist of raised, itchy pimples?

The spotty rash of chickenpox can turn into blisters that eventually burst and crust over. Adults will be affected more seriously than children and may have a severe generalized rash accompanied by headache, backache, chills and a high temperature.

RASHES WITH BLOTCHES

By blotches, I mean not a generalized rash, but distinct red or pink patches.

➊ Was the rash preceded by a severe cold?

Measles is always accompanied by snuffles, coughing, a high temperature and rosy areas around the cheeks. Then the characteristic brownish-pink spots appear all over the body, particularly on the face and neck. With new national policies of vaccination against measles (MMR), we should see less of it in the future.

➋ Is the rash very faint and did it begin behind the ears?

In contrast to true measles, german measles or rubella may be so mild that the rash is never even noticed. Alternatively it may begin with a slightly sore throat, followed by the appearance of pale rosy-coloured blotches all over the body, starting behind the ears. It can also be accompanied by slightly swollen lymph glands and sometimes stiffness of the joints. Adults will be affected more seriously than children and can develop severe headaches, irritability, lassitude and arthritis.

➌ Is the rash accompanied by neck stiffness and vomiting?

Any person with a high temperature who develops a severe headache with neck stiffness should be considered as a possible candidate for meningitis. If photophobia – discomfort looking at bright lights – is also present together with nausea and vomiting, the diagnosis becomes even more likely. In meningococcal meningitis there may also be a blotchy red rash that tends to turn a characteristic purply-black over a day or two, the result of the affect this particular bacteria has on the blood vessels in the skin. *Anyone suffering from this kind of rash together with these other symptoms should be treated as an acute medical emergency requiring urgent hospital admission and treatment.*

❷ Is the person concerned bedridden with a high temperature and suffering from confusion?

Septicaemia, or blood poisoning, occurs when a bacterial infection is severe and the bacteria is present in large numbers in the circulation. This is similar to the situation in meningococcal meningitis and the same red rash that turns purply-black may appear on the skin in this case.

OTHER RASHES

❶ Are there skin patches covered in silvery scales with red areas beneath?

The usual psoriatic rash consists of circular red areas of skin topped with a silvery scale of piled-up skin that flakes off very easily. It commonly affects the elbows, knees and scalp, although it can be more widely distributed over the whole body. It can also affect the nails, where it forms pits the size of the end of a pin.

❷ Are you taking any medication?

Any drug given for almost any condition is capable of producing an allergic skin rash, and all sorts of rashes are possible. So, when a rash develops on the skin for the first time, it's always worth asking yourself what medications you may have been given at any time during the previous ten days.

❸ Do you have a sore throat?

Scarlet fever is usually accompanied by a high temperature and a sore throat with a white, furry tongue. There may also be nausea and vomiting. The body rash tends to be fairly widespread and blanches when the skin is squeezed. The rash may itch, especially in the latter stages of the illness when the skin peels and flakes. Scarlet fever is also characterized by a flushed face, except around the mouth area, which remains pale, a phenomenon known as circumoral pallor.

❹ Do you have a tender, red rash on your face?

Erysipelas is a bacterial infection that gets into the tissues just under the surface of the skin on the face. It causes a raised rash, anything in colour from a dull red to scarlet, with a distinct advancing margin. Accompanying symptoms are a high temperature, intense headache, swollen face and enlarged lymph glands. It is particularly common in the elderly and requires urgent antibiotic treatment.

❺ Do the rashes occur on pressure areas?

The diagnosis of bedsores is usually obvious because the sufferer is bed- or chairbound and the sores appear on those areas subject to unrelieved pressure. The skin will be numb, red and shiny to begin with, but later on large, ugly ulcers and holes may develop, particularly over the buttocks, heels, elbows and shoulder blades.

❻ Is the rash confined to the nose and cheeks?

The red rash of rosacea affects the middle part of the face, often producing a bulbous red nose with pimples as well as a tendency for the skin to flake. The cause is not known, although the chronic use of steroid creams on the facial area will certainly bring on the condition. It is commonest in middle-aged women and affects approximately 1 in 500. It is made worse by alcohol and hot, spicy foods. Although it is a nuisance cosmetically, it is not serious in any other way. Long-term treatment with tetracycline antibiotics will often improve the condition.

SUMMARY
RASHES

POSSIBLE CAUSE	ACTION
Rashes with blisters	
Impetigo	Antibiotic ointment or tablets.
Shingles	Acyclovir antiviral treatment.
Chickenpox	Antihistamines or oily calamine lotion for itching, antibiotics if there is secondary infection with bacteria.
Rashes with blotches	
Measles	Antibiotics only if there is secondary infection, for example, in pneumonia.
German measles	Symptomatic treatment only.
Meningitis	Urgent hospital admission.
Blood poisoning	Urgent hospital admission.
Other rashes	
Psoriasis	Coal-tar preparations, steroid preparations.
Medication	With your doctor, identify and discontinue drug responsible.
Scarlet fever	Antibiotics.
Erysipelas	Antibiotics.
Bedsores	Appropriate nursing measures, water beds, bed frames.
Rosacea	Antibiotics.

ITCHING

Itching can be experienced with or without an accompanying rash. When it occurs without a rash it is known as pruritis and can be localized to particular areas or it can be generalized, covering the entire body.

❷ Is there any yellowing of the eyes and skin?

The yellowing of the skin and eyes seen with jaundice is due to the deposition of browny-yellow bile pigments in the skin itself. The bile pigments can also set up an irritation that results in itching. Usually yellowing of the whites of the eyes, darker urine and pale motions suggest the underlying problem, which may be a blood disorder, liver damage or obstruction of the bile ducts that carry bile away from the gall bladder towards the intestine.

❷ Have you lost weight and do you feel constantly thirsty?

The high blood-sugar levels characteristic of diabetes predispose the sufferer to irritation and infection of the skin which commonly causes itching. Recurrent itching in the genital area in both men and women is not an uncommon early feature of undiagnosed diabetes, which often runs in families. *Consult your doctor immediately if you have this combination of symptoms.*

❷ Do you feel weak and tired?

With both anaemia and leukaemia itching may be an early symptom. Itching lasting more than a few days in the absence of any rash or redness requires investigations, including blood tests, to unmask the underlying problem. Additional symptoms may include aching muscles, pallor, bruising for no apparent reason, unexplained high temperature and frequent infections.

❷ Is the itching confined to moist, sweaty areas?

Occasionally, fungus infections can be present on the skin without there being an obvious rash. Nevertheless, there will still be itching as the fungal elements spread into the deeper layers of skin and produce irritation.

❷ Are you taking any medication?

Itching can sometimes be an allergic response to certain medications, when it often occurs without any obvious rash being present. Almost any drug can produce this effect, including diuretics, antidepressants, antibiotics and antihypertensives. Even creams and gels to be rubbed into the skin, some of which are prescribed to relieve itching, may contain chemicals and other synthetic substances that actually make the irritation worse.

❷ Are you or could you be pregnant?

Many women, even in early pregnancy, notice itching, particularly over the backs of the fingers and hands and on the trunk. It is hormonal in origin and settles after the baby is born.

❷ Are you particularly anxious at present?

The nervous system has a powerful influence over the skin and ongoing anxiety can cause itching in its own right, so that itching can sometimes represent one of the physical symptoms of anxiety. However, because the itching leads to scratching, the end result is the release of chemicals in the skin that set up further irritation, completing the vicious circle.

WITH A RASH
❷ Has the rash appeared after eating a particular food or coming into contact with a particular substance?

Undoubtedly, the commonest cause of a red,

itchy rash is an allergy of some kind. The list of possible causes is endless, but the problem is usually due either to something you have eaten or to something your skin has come into contact with. Whatever the cause, the result is a raised, blotchy rash that is intensely itchy. Scratching can lead to irritation of the apparently unaffected skin around the rash, causing a similar outbreak in that area.

❷ Is the itching in a moist part of the body?

Fungal infection is a common problem that tends to affect the groin, armpits and between the toes. There will usually be a red rash covered by a degree of scaling, with or without peeling, and the outer ring of the rash tends to advance gradually as times goes on. Such infections are not terribly contagious, as is often thought, and may be treated easily with antifungal preparations.

❷ Is the itching much worse in bed or after a hot bath?

Scabies produces an intensely itchy rash with little scabs. It tends to be a lot worse in bed at night when you are warm. Scabies rashes usually affect the creases of the skin, for example between the fingers, the wrists, the groin area, the armpits and around the buttocks. This 'infestation', as it is called, is almost always picked up through sleeping in dirty bedlinen used by someone else with scabies, or through close physical contact. Treatment involves application of an insecticide, which should be used after immersion in a warm bath.

❷ Is the itching restricted to hairy areas of the body?

Lice live on the hairs of the body and so can affect the scalp, pubic hair and/or body hair. The lice themselves feed on blood, which they obtain through the outer layers of the skin, and it is this activity that produces the itching. The problem is treated with an insecticide lotion.

❷ Are there any blisters containing watery-looking fluid?

The chickenpox rash consists of small, itchy blisters that rupture and ooze on to the surface of the skin. It is intensely itchy, especially in adults and particularly when it affects the eyelids, the lining of the mouth or the inside of the vagina. It is caused by the chickenpox virus and unless there is secondary infection with a bacteria, antibiotics are not required.

❷ Is the rash violet-coloured?

In the condition known as lichen planus, the cause of which is unknown, there are flat-topped, shiny patches that can be incredibly itchy. They are violet in colour with occasional white streaks and the centre of the patches tends to be a little sunken. The patches can affect any part of the skin, although the commonest site is the wrists.

❷ Is the rash confined to the trunk?

Pityriasis rosea starts with a single 'herald' patch swiftly followed by the appearance of numerous other reddish-brown, scaly patches running along the lines of the ribs on the front and back. It may be slightly itchy. The cause is unknown, but it tends to settle down within two to three months if left alone.

❷ Is the itching down the sides of the fingers and toes worse during cold weather?

The red, swollen and itchy spots known as chilblains are commonly suffered by people with cold fingers and toes and tend to occur along the sides of the digits. They can in fact be intensely itchy, and may go on to form blisters with secondary infection.

SUMMARY
ITCHING

POSSIBLE CAUSE	ACTION
Without a rash	
Jaundice	Treat underlying condition. Antihistamines.
Diabetes	Control blood sugar and treat skin infection. Antihistamines.
Anaemia	Treat underlying cause. Correct anaemia with dietary adjustment, tablets, injections or, if severe, transfusion.
Leukaemia	Chemotherapy. Bone-marrow transplant.
Fungus infection	Antifungal preparations.
Medication	With your doctor, identify and discontinue drug responsible. Antihistamines.
Pregnancy	Will settle after childbirth, but mild hydrocortisone cream may be used in the meantime.
Anxiety	Avoid scratching, antihistamine preparations if necessary. Anxiety-management counselling.
Cancer	Treat underlying cause. Antihistamines.
With a rash	
Allergy	Avoid trigger factor, antihistamines.
Ringworm	Antifungal preparations.
Scabies	Insecticide lotion.
Lice	Insecticide lotion.
Chickenpox	Antihistamines, antibiotics if secondary infection present.
Lichen planus	Steroid creams.
Pityriasis rosea	Mild hydrocortisone cream, antihistamines.
Chilblains	Keep warm, avoid temperature changes, antihistamines, mild cortisone preparations.

LUMPS AND SWELLINGS

There are a huge number of conditions that can cause lumps and swellings to develop on the surface of the skin. Most of these are usually quite obvious to the individual concerned, and if the swellings are in exposed areas such as the face, the cosmetic result is usually the predominant worry.

❷ *Do you have any raised moles that have changed in any way?*

Moles are quite normal. Most people would find, if they actually bothered to count them up, that they had somewhere between 100 and 200 over the entire surface of their body. Usually moles are quite flat on the surface of the skin, like freckles, but some are raised and may sport long hairs from their surface. The important thing is to recognize if a mole changes at all. If moles enlarge in size, or if they irritate, bleed, become surrounded by little satellite areas of pigmentation or if the surface pigmentation alters, it suggests changing biological behaviour that just might represent the early stages of cancer. Cancer arising in a mole is called a malignant melanoma and the incidence of this condition is increasing at an alarming rate in this country, especially in relatively young people. So, if you have a mole that has changed in any way, especially if it is larger than the blunt end of a pencil, or a mole you are concerned about for any reason *it is very important to ask for your doctor's opinion as early treatment is essential.*

❷ *Is there a lumpy birthmark?*

Birthmarks come in all shapes, sizes and forms, some lumpy, some not. A common lumpy birthmark is the strawberry naevus, which tends to develop in the first few weeks of life in a newborn baby, reaching its maximum size by the age of six months. After that it decreases in size until it resolves quite spontaneously by the age of three or four. They can sometimes look quite alarming, but the good news is that they do disappear without any treatment being required, and without leaving any residual marks on the skin.

❷ *Are there painful lumps on the feet?*

Hard corns are located on the toes and tend to be pea-sized with a hard centre. Soft corns are found between the toes and are kept soft by the moisture in this area. Sometimes there will be inflammation and infection underneath the corn that may require treatment with antibiotics. A callus is an area of thickened skin, for example on the palms of the hands of a manual worker, and is usually painless. Corns tend to ache on pressure.

❷ *Do you have one painful, red lump?*

A boil is a hard, red, hot, tender and painful lump that can, if traumatized, exude an infected, waxy material. They tend to appear in clothed or dirty areas of the body such as the neck and buttocks.

❷ *Is there one or more lump containing a watery-looking fluid?*

Blisters can arise from bacterial, viral, or fungal infections or from infestation with insects, as in scabies. Chickenpox and athlete's foot can also produce blisters on the skin. Blisters may also arise after scalds or burns or even from exposure to strong sunlight when no protection has been used.

❷ *Is the lump dome-shaped and in a hairy area of the body?*

Sebaceous cysts tend to occur in hairy areas of the body such as the armpits, the chest in men, and the pubic area. They tend to be fairly firm and when examined closely have a tiny indentation in the top where the duct of the sebaceous gland is blocked. They may gradually become larger as time goes by and are usually painless. Occasionally they can become infected, in which case exudation of the creamy, cheesy material contained within the cyst occurs. Larger ones may be removed surgically under local anaesthetic.

❷ Is the lump hard and fleshy?

Warts are greyish, firm growths, usually painless and insensitive, and can range in size from a pinhead to an inch across. They can occur on any part of the body, but are usually found on areas such as the soles of the feet, when they are called verrucae, or on the fingers.

❷ Is the lump red and itchy?

Weals are temporary itchy lumps on the skin and are round and red with a whitish centre. They are allergic in origin and are particularly seen in people who suffer from eczema, asthma and hay fever.

❷ Are the lumps flattish and yellow?

Xanthelasmata are flat or slightly raised painless nodules that tend to arise around the eyes and are associated with high circulating levels of blood cholesterol. They contain deposits of yellow fatty material and may also appear on the knees, elbows, palms and heels. Anybody who develops such yellowish deposits would be well advised to see a doctor to check blood-cholesterol levels in order to ascertain whether any treatment is required.

❷ Have you been suffering from acutely painful joints, particularly the big-toe joint?

Gout usually causes extreme pain in the big toe and other joints, but it may also produce lumps in the skin that represent collections of uric-acid crystals. These lumps, which tend to appear on the ear and over various joints such as the elbow, are called 'tophi'.

❷ Has the lump grown quickly in size, irritated or bled?

There are a number of malignant conditions of the skin that can produce swellings, often with accompanying irritation and bleeding. They tend to occur in older people with fair skin who have been employed in outdoor work in hot climates for prolonged periods. Hopefully, the recent growth in awareness about the dangers of exposure to ultraviolet light will reduce the incidence of skin cancer, especially as malignant melanoma (the cancer involving pigmented moles) is still very much on the increase. *Any skin lump that ulcerates, bleeds, irritates or enlarges should therefore be looked at as soon as possible* by a doctor to rule out the possibility of skin cancer. Early diagnosis is vital since invasion of surrounding tissues and spread to distant sites in the body occurs relatively swiftly. When caught early enough, wide surgical excision of the malignant skin lump is often curative, although in some cases radiotherapy is offered as additional insurance against recurrence.

❷ Are the lumps apparent along scar tissue resulting from an operation for breast cancer?

Recurrent breast cancer may spread to various sites of the body, including the skin, and patients who have had a mastectomy as part of their previous treatment often experience nodules of secondary breast cancer along the line of the mastectomy scar. Usually there will also be enlarged lymph glands in the armpit area and possibly in the neck. If you do experience these symptoms, you should consult your doctor as soon as possible.

SUMMARY
LUMPS AND SWELLINGS

POSSIBLE CAUSE	ACTION
Moles	Keep under observation; report any changes to the doctor.
Birthmarks	Strawberry birthmarks resolve spontaneously without treatment, other birthmarks may require surgery or laser treatment.
Corns and calluses	See a chiropodist.
Boils	Local or oral antibiotics, surgery for larger ones.
Blisters	Identify cause and treat.
Sebaceous cysts	Surgical excision of larger ones. Smaller ones removed for cosmetic reasons only.
Warts	May resolve spontaneously, otherwise chemical, diathermy (burning) or cryotherapy (freezing) treatment.
Weals	Antihistamine treatment.
Xanthelasmata	Check blood cholesterol.
Gout	Skin tophi may be removed surgically.
Skin cancer	Surgery and/or radiotherapy.
Breast cancer	Medical and surgical treatment.

SORES AND ULCERS

Sores and ulcers occur whenever there is a breach in the continuity of the top layers of the skin or mucous membrane. On the legs they are usually the result of poor circulation to or from the ankles, heel or toes. In the mucous membranes they commonly occur in the mouth, stomach or in any part of the small or large intestine. The skin of the genitalia may be ulcerated as a consequence of certain sexually transmitted diseases, including syphilis, whilst the cornea, the clear window at the front of the eye, can develop ulcers as the result of viral or bacterial infection. Ulcers come in many shapes and forms, shallow or deep, and can be acutely painful or completely insensitive. A painful ulcer is sometimes referred to as a sore.

❷ Do you suffer from adolescent-type spots?

Acne spots generally appear on the face, neck, back and chest. In severe cases some of the spots can produce large cystic masses that ulcerate, producing infections and subsequent scarring. This can be prevented by adequate provision of long-term, low-dose antibiotics, or, in very severe cases, by the prescription of isotretinoin, a derivative of vitamin A. This very potent medication is only given under supervision in hospitals and should never be taken by pregnant women.

❷ Do the sores occur on pressure areas?

Bedsores are red, shiny patches of skin that occur on pressure areas such as the buttocks, heels, elbows and shoulder blades in people who are bed- or chairbound. If neglected, continued pressure will further upset the circulation and lead to large sores and ulcers.

❷ Do you have bad varicose veins around your ankles?

Varicose veins allow blood to 'stagnate', thereby effectively depriving the overlying skin of oxygen. The resulting varicose ulcers are particularly common in the elderly. Preventing varicose veins in the first place is obviously helpful, and surgical support stockings and putting your feet up whenever possible are both good measures. Good nursing care may enable the varicose ulcers to heal up, albeit gradually, although it is essential that bacterial infection must be eliminated first. Severe cases require surgical stripping of the veins or at least the injection of sclerosing agents to get rid of them.

❷ Are your feet always cold? Do you suffer cramp in your calf muscles on walking only a few yards?

People with these symptoms who have deep, raw-looking ulcers with steep edges are usually suffering from ischaemic ulcers. These occur in legs where there is partial or complete blockage of the arteries that supply the skin with nourishment (ischaemia means an inadequate blood supply to part of the body). They tend to be deeper and more difficult to heal than varicose ulcers, and often require some sort of surgery to correct the problem.

❷ Is the ulcer on an exposed area of the body?

Neglected skin cancers, which are always more likely to crop up in an area of the body exposed to the sun's ultraviolet rays, can ulcerate and enlarge. The problem might start with a tiny spot that irritates or bleeds before appearing to heal over with a dry crust. This soon falls off and the underlying spot oozes fluid again, gradually enlarging as the cycle is repeated. The appearance of such an area should be treated with a high degree of suspicion.

Always consult your doctor as soon as possible if you experience this symptom.

❷ *Have you developed a soft, painless ulcer in the genital region following unprotected sex?*

These days syphilis is relatively rare, with only something in the region of 1,500 cases per year being reported. It begins with a soft, painless ulcer on the skin of the genitals, on the tongue, or over the testicles. These ulcers are extremely slow to heal and antibiotic treatment is required to prevent the infection spreading elsewhere in the body with much more serious consequences.

SUMMARY
SORES AND ULCERS

POSSIBLE CAUSE	ACTION
Acne	Antibiotic creams and tablets, ultraviolet-light exposure, vitamin A derivative (isotretinoin).
Bedsores	Adequate nursing care, bed frames, water bed.
Varicose ulcers	Treat varicose veins, elevate legs, elastic stockings, nursing care, surgery.
Ischaemic ulcers	Surgery.
Skin cancer	Surgery and/or radiotherapy.
Syphilis	Appropriate antibiotics.

12

CHILDREN'S SYMPTOMS

Although children can suffer from the majority of disorders that adult patients are prone to, they are not always able to tell us what is wrong. Nor do they have the experience of previous pain to make any sense of what is happening to them. Thus the pain of an ear infection will be expressed by crying and screaming. A child with a bladder infection probably won't complain of burning when urinating, but will become obviously uncomfortable with a high temperature. A baby with a viral infection will not be able to complain, but may develop a telltale bright red rash. For this reason, I have chosen to cover below some of the commonest symptoms seen between the ages of three months and six years.

CRYING

All babies cry at various times, some more than others. However, crying that becomes very loud and persistent, with an element of desperation in it, is quite a different matter and is obviously a cause of great concern.

❷ *Could your baby be hungry?*
Think about when you last fed your baby and whether the usual amount of feed was taken. Was your baby sick after the last feed? If your baby has become constantly hungry and is not satisfied with milk, it could be time for weaning.

❷ *Is your baby thirsty?*
Your baby may be drinking normal amounts of fluids, and I don't mean just milk, but juices and water as well, but if the weather is very hot or the room is very warm, or if the baby is wearing a lot of clothing, a lot of fluid may have been lost through perspiration. Similarly,

if your baby has a high temperature, there is a risk of dehydration, and in the early stages, your baby will certainly let you know that he or she is thirsty by crying.

❷ *Could your baby be uncomfortable?*
Babies don't like to lie for too long in dirty or wet nappies. It can cause irritation and soreness of the skin, leading to nappy rash. Alternatively, your baby could be tired, having missed a nap, or feeling anxious, isolated or bored. Usually changing the baby's nappy, a little bit of comfort and a nap will work wonders.

❷ *Could your baby be in any pain?*
If it isn't so much crying as screaming, and in crescendos at that, your baby may be in pain. Common sources of pain are ear infections, teething, severe nappy rash and colic.

❷ *Is there a high temperature?*
Children have a relatively immature

315

temperature-regulating mechanism and can often show temperatures up to 104°F (40°C). High temperatures can be due to trivial illnesses like cold viruses, or to something more serious such as meningitis. With a straightforward cold, children often perk up quite quickly when the temperature comes down. With meningitis, however, the child will be disinterested in his or her surroundings, may vomit, may be distressed by bright lights, may have the characteristic purple rash, may be completely off feeds, and is likely to become increasingly drowsy or even unconscious. *If you are in any doubt whatsoever, a doctor's opinion must be sought as soon as possible* as early treatment can often mean the difference between mental and physical handicap and full recovery or even between life and death.

You should also ask yourself if your baby's crying sounds unusual; if he or she cries when being fed, highlighting the possibility of a throat infection; if there is any diarrhoea, suggesting a bowel upset (gastroenteritis) or food intolerance; if the baby's nose is running, indicating a cold, measles or a foreign body up his or her nose; if there is any coughing or wheezing, which could be due to a chest infection or asthma; if the urine is very strong smelling as the result of a bladder infection; if the motions are loose, hard or bloodstained, suggesting gastroenteritis, food intolerance, constipation or other bowel disorders; if a baby under a year old is drowsy or floppy, which suggests a more serious underlying problem such as dehydration or meningitis; and whether his or her lips or fingers have turned blue, which could indicate a heart condition. If there is vomiting and/or diarrhoea together with the high temperature, there is the possibility of dehydration, so it is vital to make sure that your baby's fluid intake is adequate. Finally, in children under five the biggest risk of a high temperature is the possibility of febrile convulsions.

SUMMARY
CRYING

Possible Cause	Action
Hunger	Feed your baby.
Thirst	Cool the baby and the room if necessary. Give fluids and check temperature.
Discomfort	Change the nappy, comfort the child, encourage sleep.
Pain	Medical examination and treatment.
Illness	Don't hesitate to call your doctor.

CONVULSIONS

Children can experience convulsions or seizures in the same way that adults can, so it is worth consulting the section on seizures. However, children under the age of five are particularly prone to seizures as a result of high temperature. These are known as febrile convulsions. They do not mean that the child has epilepsy, but they should *always* be brought to the attention of a doctor as soon as possible.

Febrile convulsions are common, with about one child in twenty suffering one or more attacks. They tend to run in families, are not usually serious, and generally occur between the ages of six months and five years. The seizures themselves, which understandably are very frightening to witness, are identical to those occurring for other reasons, but occur only as the result of a sudden rise in the child's temperature. Common infections likely to cause such fevers include tonsillitis, ear infections, measles and flu. It is thought that an immaturity of the temperature-lowering mechanism in the child's brain cannot cope adequately with the sudden rise in the temperature. As a result, susceptible brain cells become excitable and discharge inappropriate electrical signals to the muscles of the young child's body, producing the so-called convulsion.

During the seizure, the child becomes unconscious. Then the arms and legs go stiff for a few seconds before starting to jerk and twitch uncontrollably. The face may grimace and twitch as well. Occasionally urine is passed and the tongue bitten. The seizure is usually over well within five minutes, after which time the child gradually comes round, again over a period of five minutes or so.

However, the child will not be quite back to full alertness for a while longer and may be irritable, drowsy and complain of a headache.

The symptoms of the infection producing the fever in the first place will still be apparent too, so it is unrealistic to expect the child to recover completely too soon.

It is important to note that most febrile convulsions last for less than five minutes, so a more prolonged attack should be investigated further to rule out an underlying cause other than a fever. Similarly, an attack affecting only one side or part of the body, suggesting to a doctor a single area of scarring or abnormality within the brain, would indicate a condition other than febrile convulsions, which are characterized by an overall overexcitability of the brain.

Although extremely disturbing for the parents who witness the febrile convulsion, it is important to realize that children who suffer such seizures are otherwise completely normal and that they will have suffered no harmful effects as a result of the seizure. A second attack will occur in about 30 to 40 per cent of cases, usually within six months, and again, purely as the result of a high temperature. By the age of five, the child will almost certainly have grown out of the tendency to suffer these convulsions and only a very few children go on to develop recurrent seizures (epilepsy) in adulthood.

Factors that can make the possibility of recurrent seizures more likely, however, include any condition that may have rendered the brain or nervous system more susceptible to irritation, thereby lowering the threshold for convulsions, for example birth trauma, cerebral palsy and meningitis. A family history of epilepsy will also increase the chances of epilepsy in a child, but this is by no means invariable. In fact, even children with all these factors only have a 10 per cent chance of recurrent seizures in the future.

SUMMARY
CONVULSIONS

POSSIBLE CAUSE	ACTION
Any convulsion	Remove any nearby objects that could be hazardous. Do not restrain the child or force anything between the teeth. After the convulsion lie the child on his or her side with the head lower than the body in case of vomiting. Cool the child down urgently by cooling the room, cool sponging the skin, cool drinks and cool bedding. Call the doctor if this is the first seizure. Call the ambulance if it lasts more than five minutes. In hospital, tests may be done to exclude a more serious underlying cause such as meningitis. Anticonvulsant drugs can be used to bring prolonged seizures under control.
Febrile convulsions	Prevent temperature from rising early on in an infection by cooling down the child (see above). Paracetamol syrup. Antibiotics, anti-convulsants from the doctor.

RASHES

Rashes are extremely common and notoriously difficult to diagnose without experience. Many parents expect doctors to make the diagnosis over the telephone from a description of the rash but there are so many different possible causes and so many similar-looking rashes that the only real way to tell is for a professional to take a good look.

Even then it is not always easy to make the diagnosis, but the following check list of questions should help you establish whether the problem is due to one of the common rash-producing conditions:

❷ Does the child have a cold and is he or she miserable and with a blotchy rash?

Measles is a highly infectious virus infection that can on rare occasions be dangerous. It appears one to two weeks after initial contact with the virus. The child will be very miserable with a runny nose, red eyes and a cough. A blotchy red rash will appear on the face and then spread over the rest of the body. Temperatures in measles can go as high as 104°F (40°C) and older children complain of headaches. Symptoms last about three to five days before the rash appears, but the child will have been infectious since early on in the incubation period, which begins 8–14 days before the onset of the rash. The rash itself lasts 4–5 days, during which time the child remains infectious. Approximately one in 15 children with measles will develop certain complications such as bronchitis, pneumonia, seizures, deafness or even encephalitis (inflammation of the brain). Many doctors prescribe antibiotics to deal with such secondary bacterial infections despite the fact that these are not at all effective against the measles virus. However, with the new MMR vaccine, which is offered to all children, we should see far fewer cases of measles infection in the future.

❷ Is the rash pale pink and did it start behind the ears?

Unlike true measles, there may be no cold symptoms with German measles, which usually develops 14–21 days after contact with the illness. However, occasionally there may be a slight runny nose with mild swelling of the glands at the back of the neck and behind the ears. Within a day or two a pale pink rash will develop, often starting behind the ears, then spreading to the face and trunk. It usually lasts for 2–3 days before clearing up, although the child will be infectious for four days following the onset of the rash. Many children develop rubella with no symptoms whatsoever, in which case only blood tests can confirm that they have had the infection. Again, the new MMR vaccine should prevent outbreaks of rubella in the future.

❷ Does the rash consist of tiny, itchy blisters?

Chickenpox appears 14–21 days after contact with the virus. It may cause a slight temperature with a mild headache but often there are no symptoms whatsoever until the spots appear. These last 7–10 days and look like tiny blisters on a red base. They can appear anywhere on the body including the mouth, inside the eyelids, inside the ears, the vagina and the anus and up the nose. The blisters are intensely itchy as they pop and crust over and the person is infectious until all the crusts have dried up.

❷ Does your child have a sore throat and deep red, flushed cheeks?

Scarlet fever, or 'scarlatina', produces a sore throat with a widespread red rash 1–5 days after initial contact with the infection. The tongue looks furry, the child has a high temperature and may experience tummy pain and sickness. The rash is deep red, usually first appearing on the chest and back, but later spreading to the rest of the body. It is caused by a toxin made by the bacteria responsible for the infection and lasts 4–5 days. Antibiotics are required. The child will be infectious for four days after the onset of the rash.

❷ Is the rash reddish-purple and is your child floppy, drowsy and vomiting?
In one particular form of meningitis caused by the meningococcus bacterium a purply-red rash sometimes accompanies the more usual symptoms of a high temperature, neck stiffness, vomiting, high-pitched crying, discomfort when looking at lights, and a headache. *This is a very serious combination of symptoms and requires the most urgent admission to hospital for further investigations and treatment.*

❷ Is there a localized circular patch of scaly skin anywhere on the body?
Fungal infections of various kinds can produce circular scaly rashes confined to one small area of the skin. The circles gradually enlarge over a period of weeks and the condition is spread by close physical contact. Washing hands can prevent the condition, but, once developed, simple treatment with antifungal cream is usually enough to eradicate the problem.

❷ Is the skin dry, scaly, thickened and itchy in places?
Eczema is an extremely common condition with approximately five million sufferers in the UK alone. It often runs in certain families and can be accompanied by hay fever and/or asthma. One common type of eczema seen in children that tends to arise during the first two years is atopic eczema. In this, the symptoms initially appear on the face, scalp and nappy area, later involving the skin creases at the wrists, the elbows, the back of the knees and around the ankles. The fingers and hands are

often affected. The usual symptoms include redness of the skin, dryness and scaling, intense itching and weeping of the skin with small blisters. Often, there is also secondary bacterial infection with crusting and discharge.

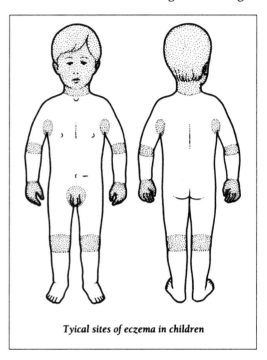

Tyical sites of eczema in children

❷ Is the rash red, scaly and itchy and worse on the scalp, face, chest and back?
This is seborrhoeic eczema and is so called because it appears mainly in areas of the body where sebaceous glands are plentiful. On the scalp it is the predominant cause of dandruff, producing thick, yellowy, crusty layers. It may also appear around the neck, on the hairline, behind the ears, on the face and under the armpits. It tends not to be quite so itchy and troublesome as atopic eczema, but is nevertheless unattractive and worrisome to parents. The good news is that both types often settle down completely as the child grows up, with 90 per cent of children being clear by the age of eight.

❷ Is the rash intensely itchy and does it come and go?

A blotchy red rash is just one of the reactions that can be caused by an allergy in a child, the others being asthma, hay fever, food intolerance, vomiting and diarrhoea. Eczema which is also intensely itchy but produces dry, scaly patches, can be 'endogenous', coming from within due to an hereditary condition, or 'exogenous', triggered by some external factor such as detergents, wool or rubber. In this respect it can be closely associated with an allergy. The things to avoid include coloured and perfumed soaps, bubble baths, lanolin-containing creams, biological washing powders, woollen clothes, passive smoking, excessive house dust, medicated bandages, strong shampoos, and certain foodstuffs, including dairy products, wheat-containing foods, orange juice and tomatoes. Other products can produce allergic reactions too but these are amongst the commonest. In addition, colouring agents and additives are increasingly thought to be responsible for allergic symptoms.

SUMMARY
RASHES

POSSIBLE CAUSE	ACTION
Measles	Symptomatic treatment unless complications arise, in which case antibiotics necessary.
Rubella (German measles)	No treatment required.
Chickenpox	Antihistamines for itching.
Scarlet fever	Antibiotics.
Meningitis	Emergency hospital admission and treatment.
Fungal infection	Antifungal creams.
Eczema	Avoid precipitating factors if applicable, moisturizers and emollients, mild cortisone creams, evening primrose oil. Consider Chinese herbal medicine.
Allergy	Identify trigger factor and avoid. Antihistamines.

PAINFUL EARS

A child suffering from ear pain will often pull or rub the ear in question, and may also be generally unwell. Occasionally the ear canal will produce discharge, which may be yellowy-green or bloodstained. In addition, you may have noticed that your child isn't hearing as well as normal and that he or she doesn't respond to spoken commands. There are a number of common conditions that could be responsible for the pain.

❷ *Does your child have a runny nose and a high temperature?*

The typical virus throat infection characteristically causes sneezing, a runny nose, watery eyes and a high temperature.

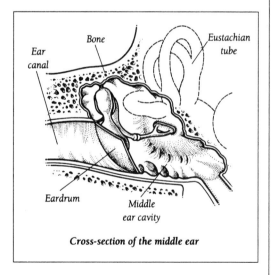

Cross-section of the middle ear

These symptoms are often accompanied by blockage of the Eustachian tube running between the back of the nose and the middle-ear cavity, and a build-up of fluid behind the eardrum, producing pressure changes in the middle-ear cavity and leading to temporary hearing problems and pain. This condition is known as otitis media and is the commonest cause of painful ears in children.

❷ *Are there any teeth coming through?*

There is no doubt that as growing teeth cut through the gums, referred pain may be felt in the ears. Children with this problem may pull frantically at their ears, but when examined by a doctor will show no evidence of any abnormality there whatsoever. However, in the mouth there will be telltale signs of emerging teeth cutting through the sensitive gum, and as more saliva tends to be produced at this time, children often dribble more.

❷ *Is the ear canal red, flaky or blocked?*

Inflammation of the outer ear canal (otitis externa) is usually the result of infected eczema of the skin in that area or of a build-up of wax and skin flakes. It is usually itchy rather than painful, although both symptoms can be experienced simultaneously.

❷ *Is there any swelling in front of the ear(s)?*

Hopefully, the advent of the MMR vaccination means that mumps, which is a virus infection, will become less common. In the meantime, however, the commonest symptom is a tender swelling just in front of and underneath the ear on one or both sides of the face. The swelling and inflammation of the salivary gland is a result of the virus infection itself.

❷ *Could your child have pushed something small into his or her ear?*

Small children are quite keen on pushing small objects like beads, sweets or toys into their ears. A foreign body lodged inside the ear canal will cause inflammation and infection, followed by a painful discharge. If you are suspicious that this may have happened, *do not under any circumstances attempt to clear the ear out yourself.* This could push the foreign body further inside and cause damage to the sensitive eardrum. Instead, ask your doctor to examine the ear with an auriscope. This allows clear visualization of the entire ear canal and makes careful removal of any offending object a safe procedure.

SUMMARY
PAINFUL EARS

POSSIBLE CAUSE	ACTION
Cold viruses	Decongestant nose drops for no longer than 10 days without consulting your doctor, antibiotics if secondary infection with bacteria occurs.
Teething	Pain relief.
Otitis externa	Anti-inflammatory and antibiotic eardrops following cleaning-out of the ear.
Mumps	Pain relief.
Foreign body	Removal of foreign body by doctor. Treat any underlying infection.

SORE THROAT AND BLOCKED NOSE

There are two main areas of glandular tissue at the back of the nose and throat, namely the tonsils and the adenoids. Both of these are the first line of defence against infection from outside. When they are faced with invading organisms, they swell and inflame, initiating the first stage of the fight against disease. Many of the infections that produce tonsillitis and adenoiditis are viruses and bacteria, and antibiotics are effective against the latter. It is difficult for the doctor to tell which of the two is responsible but generally when there are constitutional symptoms of severe illness such as a high temperature and prostration, antibiotics are given to prevent any possible complications. Operations to remove these glands (tonsillectomy and adenoidectomy) are not carried out as much as they used to be, but when the glands are extremely large and there is blockage of the airways causing difficulty swallowing and speaking, there is a good case for carrying out the surgery. If the infections are particularly recurrent, resulting in six or more episodes in a year, the ear, nose and throat surgeon may also feel that the operation is justified. Furthermore, if the child is subject to febrile convulsions and these are precipitated by frequent tonsil or adenoid infections, surgery again is worth considering.

❷ Does your child have a high temperature and is he or she reluctant to eat or drink?

Tonsillitis causes sore throats with pain and difficulty swallowing, a decreased appetite and a high temperature. When you look at the back of the throat, the tonsils are obviously swollen and red and may be covered in white spots. These are areas of pus. The glands in the neck are often swollen, the child's breath may be bad and there may be abdominal pain too as the abdominal glands also swell (mesenteric adenitis). Tonsillitis is rare in children under a year old but common between the ages of two and 12 as children come into contact with scores of other children of the same age.

❷ Does your child snore and is he or she not hearing very well?

When the adenoid glands swell there may be partial or complete obstruction to the nasal passages, leading to mouth breathing and snoring. Furthermore, the glands obstruct the Eustachian tube connecting the back of the throat to the middle-ear cavity, causing catarrh, ear infections and 'glue ear'. In this condition, sticky fluid builds up behind the eardrum, resulting in temporary deafness.

SUMMARY
SORE THROAT AND BLOCKED NOSE

POSSIBLE CAUSE	ACTION
Tonsillitis	Antibiotics. Consider tonsillectomy.
Adenoiditis	Consider surgery (adenoidectomy) in severe cases or where hearing is affected.

WHEEZING

A wheeze is a high-pitched whistling sound made when breathing, usually when breathing out. It is caused by a narrowing of the respiratory tubes within the lungs and may be loud enough for others to hear or only audible for a doctor through a stethoscope placed on the patient's chest. Asthma is the commonest disorder producing wheezing, but there are two other conditions that should be excluded.

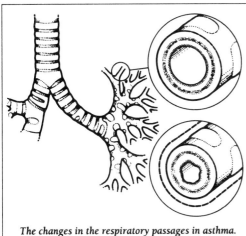

The changes in the respiratory passages in asthma. The normal airtube (top) contracts, and the inner lining swells and is congested with mucus (below)

❷ Does your child have a cold and a high temperature?

Infections of the respiratory passages due to viruses and bacteria can cause inflammation of the passages' sensitive lining, resulting in the production of fluid and phlegm. As this narrows the airway, wheezing may result. Common examples of such infections include bronchitis in older children and bronchiolitis in younger children and babies.

❸ Could your child have inhaled a small object such as a bead or a peanut?

Small children have a habit of putting things other than food in their mouths. Between 18 and 36 months this experimentation is common and may lead to a child swallowing or inhaling a small object. When inhaled, these foreign bodies can partially or totally obstruct the passage of air in and out of the lungs. Partial obstruction produces a wheeze, but total obstruction will be silent.

❸ Does your child often become wheezy?

Approximately one in five children will wheeze at some time, but wheezing does not necessarily mean asthma until there have been recurrent bouts of wheezing in response to upper respiratory infections or other triggers over a period of time. Sometimes, however, wheezing can be minimal during the early stages, in which case a dry and particularly persistent night-time cough, one of the commonest symptoms of asthma in childhood, may be more obvious. Shortness of breath is another common symptom. Asthma is about twice as common in boys than girls and other siblings may well be affected, perhaps also by hay fever and/or eczema.

To help keep asthma under control, it is therefore important to be aware of the various factors that commonly trigger an asthmatic attack. The commonest of these is a viral or bacterial infection causing inflammation of the sensitive lining of the respiratory passages, as is seen in bronchitis for example. Many asthmatics also find that exercise of a vigorous nature will bring on their wheezing. Having said that, however, exercise is generally good for asthmatics as it develops the heart and lungs and the muscles of the ribcage. If necessary, treatment can be given before any exertion to prevent wheezing from occurring. Another trigger is cold air, which acts as an irritant to the muscles encircling the respiratory passages, making them go into a spasm and narrowing the passageways so that there is a high-pitched sound when air goes through

325

them. Environmental pollution, including sprays, gases and car-exhaust fumes, can trigger attacks too. Asthma is also associated with allergies, so that children who are susceptible to allergies and develop hay fever and eczema also tend to suffer from asthma. Common allergens include house dust and house-dust mite, pollen, feathers, animal fluff and certain foods such as strawberries, shellfish and peanuts.

Because of known precipitating factors like dairy products, it is advisable, particularly if there is a family history of asthma, that the child is breast-fed as a baby if at all possible, and for as long as possible. Cows' milk should

be avoided for at least a year. Food additives and preservatives also tend to cause problems. Some medications can also bring on wheezing as an allergic reaction in someone already suffering from asthma. Finally, it is important to remember that not only can excitement and emotional upset bring on an asthmatic attack, but the fear caused by the attack itself can worsen the situation.

However, medication for asthmatics is very effective and includes anti-allergic preparations to prevent the trigger factors from producing an attack in the first place, bronchodilators to open up the respiratory passageways, and steroids to inhibit inflammation.

SUMMARY
WHEEZING

POSSIBLE CAUSE	ACTION
Infection	Antibiotics if appropriate.
Foreign body	Urgent removal by means of a flexible telescope.
Asthma	Identify and avoid trigger factors. Avoid passive smoking. Exercise (preceded by preventative medicine). Medication, including anti-allergic preparations, bronchodilators and steroids.

STOMACH PAIN

Stomach pain in children is extremely common. Children often learn to complain of tummy pain as an excuse to avoid some unpleasant activity or task such as going to school or being asked to do something they don't want to do. Pointing to their tummy button, they say to their parents that it hurts there, but usually their appetite is unaffected and when they are distracted from the problem they are often as right as rain. Nevertheless, there are a number of relatively common physical conditions that need to be excluded before it can be assumed that the tummy pain is no more than a figment of the child's imagination.

❷ Does the pain happen every evening after milk feeds in a baby under four months?

Colic is the name given to the apparent abdominal pain experienced by babies up to the age of about four months. Characteristically, the baby is absolutely fine and happy during the day but during the early hours of the evening begins to cry incessantly, screaming at times, drawing his or her legs up and looking extremely distressed with a flushed, red face. This may go on for 2-3 hours at a time and is obviously alarming for the parents. It tends to be more common in babies who are bottle-fed, who have been given cow's milk before the age of 12 months, or who have been started on solids at an early age. It is also seen more often in children of mother's who smoke. Nobody knows the real cause, but it is thought to be due to immature function of the intestine and a failure of the muscular wall of the intestine to push food waste along. The result is trapped air that distends the intestinal wall, causing a painful spasm. Although the condition tends to disappear by itself by the age of four months, there are a number of things parents can do.

First of all, adequate winding of the baby after bottle-feeding is useful for bringing up any trapped air. Massage of the baby's tummy using your fingers can also be soothing and can actually disperse trapped air and encourage normal bowel function. Checking the teat size on bottles is also important as teats that are either too large or too small can precipitate the problem. Breast-feeding is best for the first three months if possible and semisolids should not be encouraged until after the age of three months. Theoretically cow's milk should be avoided until after the age of one and if certain foods seem to cause the problem in children over the age of 3–4 months then these should obviously be avoided. Some people also believe that certain foods eaten by mother may cause colic if she is breast-feeding as the substances may be transmitted to the baby in the breast milk. Infacol is one of the few medicines that can be prescribed to a baby under the age of six months and can be very effective in certain cases. If in doubt, the doctor or health visitor should be an excellent source of further help and advice.

❷ Is your child suffering from sickness and diarrhoea?

Gastroenteritis is a very common cause of tummy pain and is accompanied by diarrhoea and vomiting. It is caused by a virus and is spread in much the same way as the virus causing the common cold. For this reason, it tends to go round a community, leading to small epidemics.

❷ Has your child got a sore throat or a cold?

Abdominal gland enlargement (mesenteric adenitis) is the result of infection elsewhere in the body producing swelling of the glands in the abdomen, just as tonsillitis causes swelling in the glands of the neck. The glands swell quickly, causing pain, there may be a slight fever present and the child may also have signs of infection elsewhere, for example, earache, a sore throat or a cough. The pain is usually felt in the navel area and tends to stay there. The pain is not severe, touching the abdomen does not produce much of a problem, and the child will rarely be flushed. However, the condition is sometimes extremely difficult to distinguish from appendicitis, so a doctor's opinion should be sought. In fact, because mesenteric adenitis mimics that condition so completely, occasionally a child is admitted to hospital for observation only to have a perfectly normal appendix removed.

❷ Is your child completely off his or her food with pain in the lower part of the belly?

Appendicitis is a common condition, especially in children and young adults, with approximately one in 500 people being affected every year. It is the commonest surgical emergency of all but often puzzles doctors initially because symptoms are not always obvious in the early stages. Classically, the condition starts with a coming-and-going type of stomach pain that begins at the belly button and then shifts to the right lower corner of the abdomen. It then becomes a constant ache that gradually grows more severe, making sitting up or turning impossible. Alternatively, initial symptoms can be very trivial, so that the child runs about, eats and drinks until quite late on. Generally speaking, a child with acute appendicitis goes completely off his or her food and stops drinking, has a coated tongue, usually with a strange smell to the breath, looks flushed and may have a fever. Some children will also feel and actually be sick and others may have diarrhoea or constipation. Because the result of an untreated inflamed appendix is perforation of the wall of the appendix, leading to the very serious condition of peritonitis, which requires *urgent* surgical intervention, *any child who is off his or her food with unexplained abdominal pain lasting more than a couple of hours, especially if there is a high temperature, should be seen by a doctor straight away.* Parents should also discourage the child from having anything to eat or drink prior to the doctor's arrival because if a general anaesthetic does become necessary to remove the appendix, vomiting will then be less of a problem.

SUMMARY
STOMACH PAIN

POSSIBLE CAUSE	ACTION
Colic	Winding, massage, breast-feeding, Infacol.
Gastroenteritis	Fluid and mineral replacement.
Mesenteric adenitis	Observation and rest.
Appendicitis	Surgery.

DIARRHOEA AND VOMITING

Diarrhoea and vomiting are both common symptoms in children. Most babies bring up a bit of milk, and some bring up a lot, without any distress whatsoever. In fact, generally speaking, vomiting is far more common and much less of a problem in children than it is in adults. However, if your baby is vomiting very frequently or violently and there are other signs of illness, alarm bells should ring and your doctor should be contacted for further advice. Young children can lose a great deal of fluid and minerals quite quickly if they are frequently sick, especially if they have diarrhoea at the same time.

The motions of young babies are naturally runny and yellowy-orange, but again, if there is anything unusual about the stools and if there are any other signs of illness, further advice must be sought. A baby suffering from sickness and diarrhoea, especially if the weather is hot and he or she has a fever, is likely to lose significant amounts of fluid in a very short space of time. Dehydration is potentially life-threatening and immediate fluid replacement is required. Rehydrating fluid can be purchased over the counter and given by parents for even short-lived and trivial conditions, but in any situation it is worth avoiding formula milk and concentrating on clear fluids. Frequent nappy changes are also recommended as the acid content of loose, watery stools can irritate the skin around the baby's bottom and produce severe nappy rash. Barrier creams are therefore also worth using.

❷ Does your child have a high temperature?

Infections of the ears and throat are often associated with diarrhoea and vomiting as well as with a fever. The vomiting and diarrhoea are secondary to the respiratory infection but both

require treatment. Alternatively, viruses and other organisms can strike solely at the intestine, producing gastroenteritis, for example, which tends to go round a community, leading to small epidemics.

Parasites such as giardia can produce a form of food poisoning that causes chronic diarrhoea, sometimes lasting several weeks. Like other organisms that affect the bowel, giardiasis is transmitted through contaminated food and is particularly common in the Third World. 'Waterworks' infections can also begin with vomiting and it may be that investigation of the cause of the vomiting uncovers the underlying kidney or bladder infection.

❷ Is the sickness brought on by travelling?

Fortunately, children tend to grow out of travel-sickness, but in the meantime they may be helped by preventative treatment taken before a journey.

❷ Does a particular food or drink always trigger the symptoms?

Various food allergies can produce sickness and diarrhoea together with abdominal pain. Common culprits include dairy products, shellfish, strawberries, peanuts and various food additives. A careful evaluation of everything in a child's diet is necessary to eliminate the cause. Your doctor or health visitor will certainly be able to advise you about the likelihood of food intolerance in a particular case, although only full investigation, possibly with referral to a paediatrician, allergist or expert in clinical ecology, can confirm the precise diagnosis.

❷ Is there forceful and dramatic vomiting in a baby of about six weeks?

In the condition known as pyloric stenosis, the ring of muscle that closes off the bottom end of the stomach thickens, causing a build-up of pressure in the stomach following a feed. Because of this, the milk that cannot pass into the intestine is brought up. It occurs mainly in boys between three and eight weeks of age and the vomiting can be so forceful that it travels several yards across the room (projectile vomiting). As the condition progresses the vomiting becomes more frequent and more dramatic, eventually leading to dehydration. Surgery is usually required.

❷ Is your child listless, floppy, and disinterested in his or her surroundings? Do you instinctively feel something more serious is wrong?
Very often, parental instinct is spot-on, and the cause of long-standing diarrhoea and vomiting will come down to a serious underlying condition. With appendicitis, for example, vomiting may precede the development of abdominal pain or a high temperature. Diarrhoea may or may not be a feature. With meningitis there will often be vomiting, with or without diarrhoea, and usually in conjunction with a high temperature, headache, neck stiffness, drowsiness, photophobia (discomfort when looking at bright lights) and, at times, a purply-red rash. *If meningitis is even suspected, immediate examination by a doctor and treatment are required.* It may save your child's life.

SUMMARY
DIARRHOEA AND VOMITING

POSSIBLE CAUSE	ACTION
Infection	Mineral and fluid replacement. Identify underlying infection and treat appropriately. Antibiotics should be avoided in most cases.
Travel sickness	Prevent with antihistamines, hyoscine.
Food allergy	Identify cause(s) and avoid.
Pyloric stenosis	Surgery.
Serious condition	Admit to hospital for further medical and/or surgical treatment.

NAPPY CONTENTS

Babies' stools can vary greatly in colour, especially if the baby is bottle-fed, starting off greenish, changing to a yellowy-orange and then becoming greyish-green. Bottle-fed babies' motions tend to be quite firm and smelly, whereas babies who are breast-fed have much looser, runnier stools. Seen from day to day motions can change in colour and consistency quite a lot. If there is any significant change such as a particularly bad smell or very liquid diarrhoea, further help is recommended from either your health visitor or doctor. As far as frequency is concerned, some babies will fill a nappy during or after each feed, whereas other babies will go several days producing nothing. Babies who produce extremely hard, rock-like motions and cry when they are passing the stool are constipated and you should seek a little further advice regarding diet and fluid intake. In obstinate cases glycerine (soapy) suppositories are very effective.

NAPPY RASH

Most babies will develop a degree of nappy rash at some point. It may be more of a general soreness than a rash but in either case it is caused by irritation of the skin, the result of ammonia-like substances that are produced when urine and stools are left on the baby's skin for any length of time. Cleaning your child's skin is important, but use ordinary water or nonmedicated wipes rather than soap. The child's skin should be exposed to the air to dry as much as possible and nappies should be changed on a very regular basis. Barrier creams are useful but if the rash gets very bad and will not clear up of its own accord various creams and ointments are available to abolish infections such as thrush and to reduce the inflammation in the skin. Sometimes nappy rash is worse if there are other areas of eczema on the body but generally speaking the treatment is along similar lines to the above, with the possible addition of 0.5 per cent hydrocortisone cream.

BEDWETTING

Most children learn to control their bladders during the daytime somewhere between the ages of two and four. Night-time control is established a little later, between the ages of two and five. About 85 per cent of children are dry at night by the age of five. When a child older than five continually wets the bed at night and there is no physical cause for it such as a bladder infection or a problem with the nervous system, then he or she has a medical condition known as nocturnal enuresis, or bedwetting. Some children have never been dry at night by the age of five, whereas others have been dry for some time but start wetting the bed again later on (secondary enuresis). Approximately half a million children between the ages of six and 16 wet the bed at some time and there are actually up to 70,000 adults aged 20–25 who report occasional problems. The truth is that in some families, bladder control is established much later than in others, and if the parents used to wet the bed until they were quite a bit older than it's likely that the children will too.

TREATMENT

Easy though it may be to become angry and frustrated at yet another soaking mattress and sodden bedding, showing anger or punishing a child are big mistakes. The child is asleep when the bedwetting occurs and has no conscious control over the problem. He or she is already anxious enough about it and would certainly be dry if it was simply a matter of choice. Reassurance and understanding are needed, and a gentle 'Don't worry, it's all right' goes a long way. It's always better to praise a child after a dry night and to say that lots of children have the same problem. It really isn't worth reducing the amount of fluid you give your child as not only doesn't it work, but it wrongly punishes a thirsty child. Having said that, fluids such as tea, coffee, colas and other fizzy drinks should be avoided because they contain caffeine, which is a stimulant and increases urinary flow. Many parents still believe that getting their child up when they themselves go to bed so that the child can empty his or her bladder late at night is a good idea, but this is disruptive for the child and may be counter-productive. Any older child frightened of the dark may be better with a night light or at least a light in the corridor outside the bedroom, but some may prefer a potty in the room rather than have to face the trek down a long dark corridor. Another way of dealing with bedwetting is to use a reward system. Each night the child is dry, he or she places a star on a chart and when there have been three dry nights in a row, a gold star is awarded.

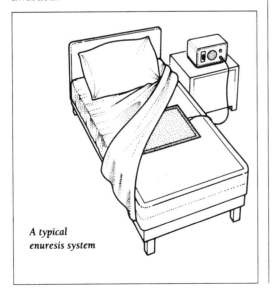

A typical enuresis system

Enuresis alarms can also be used, but they are really only useful in children over the age of seven who can get up when the alarm rings, put the light on and take themselves to the toilet. They are electrical devices that are triggered when the little pads attached to them, which are placed between two layers of underpants, become in the least bit moist. At this point, the alarm sounds, waking the child, who then realizes it is time to get up and empty his or her bladder. They can be bought from a chemist or borrowed from many NHS health visitors or enuresis clinics in hospitals.

Finally, there are at least two medical preparations that are very useful in treating bedwetting, namely imipramine taken in syrup form, and vasopressin, which is a nasal spray. Both may be initially very successful in stopping the bedwetting, but unfortunately the problem tends to recur when the medication is discontinued. Having said that, a few children will get a psychological boost from the good effect that it has during the course of treatment and may continue to remain dry after therapy.

❷ *Has your child never been dry at night?*
Control of the bladder depends on how fast the nervous system matures. This varies from child to child and is largely determined by heredity. If your child is over the age of five and has still not developed night-time bladder control and there is no underlying physical reason for this, he or she will be said to have primary enuresis. Following the treatment measures above should prove very helpful.

❸ *Does your child want to pee more often than usual?*
One of the commonest reasons for continued bedwetting, especially when the child has previously been dry, is a bladder infection. This is much more common in girls than in boys because they have a shorter urethra (the tube

from the bladder to the outside), and this allows infections from outside to creep in. The child may experience burning or stinging when passing water, but often the first sign is continual bedwetting, possibly with a high temperature and backache. In every case of bedwetting over the age of five, bladder infections should be excluded by way of a laboratory examination of a urine sample. Although rare in boys, these infections are still seen and the same tests should be performed.

Some children are born with congenital abnormalities in the kidney and bladder system so that there are not enough tubes, too many tubes or abnormal valves in the tubes, interfering with the normal drainage of urine. Frequent infections together with recurrent and persistent bedwetting problems should therefore be further investigated.

❸ Is your child constipated?

Constipation can produce bedwetting as a full rectum can push forwards against the base of the bladder, irritating it and interfering with the valve that allows the passage of urine. Treating the constipation with dietary measures or laxative suppositories can solve the problem.

❹ Is your child unduly worried?

A child under any degree of stress and anxiety is liable to wet the bed. Stress leads to muscular tension and can therefore cause bladder contraction even at night. Nightmares are also more common in anxious children and these too can lead to bedwetting.

❺ Is your child excessively thirsty and losing weight?

Diabetes can often manifest itself initially as bedwetting. The rise in the blood sugar caused by the lack of insulin makes the kidneys produce far more fluid than normal with the result that the child will pass much greater quantities of urine than is usual. The bladder capacity is overwhelmed by this volume and bedwetting at night may well be the result. The urine can be checked for sugar, which will be immediately apparent. A blood test can then reveal the exact level of glucose in the blood and usually treatment with insulin will be required. Children with uncontrolled diabetes are always thirsty.

SUMMARY
BEDWETTING

POSSIBLE CAUSE	ACTION
Primary enuresis (no underlying physical cause)	General measures, reward systems, enuresis alarms, Vasopressin or Imipramine.
Bladder infection	Antibiotics.
Constipation	Dietary adjustment, laxative suppositories.
Diabetes	Insulin.
Stress	Reassurance and counselling.

LIMPING

Limping describes an uneven type of walking where the weight is carried more on one leg than on the other. Usually it is caused by pain in one or other leg, although painless limps are also possible. If there is pain, it may help to show where the problem lies but caution is required because pain can be experienced away from the site of the underlying cause. Furthermore, there may be muscle strain as a result of the limp and this can produce pain in other areas. Any limp that persists for more than 24–48 hours and does not have an obvious, simple explanation should be investigated further.

❷ Has the child tripped over or fallen?

Simple injuries, particularly of the foot or knee, are the problems most likely to cause a short-lived limp. Usually the cause is obvious, but sometimes the pain may not occur when the child initially trips as it may not be noticed in the heat of the moment. It is not unusual for it to come on the following morning after a good night's sleep.

❷ Are the shoes the right size?

Tight or narrow shoes can compress the bones of the feet, causing a child to limp.

❷ Are there any hard lumps on the soles of the feet?

Verrucae are warts on the soles of the feet. They can be pushed inwards into the soft tissues, causing pain when walking.

❷ Are any of the joints swollen, red or hot to touch?

Children can develop different types of arthritis, just as adults do, and inflammation of any of the joints of the lower limb, the hip, the knee, the ankle or the small bones of the feet may produce limping.

❷ Is there any pain in the groin or thigh?

Perthe's disease of the hip is a problem of the upper end of the thigh bone where it forms the hip joint with the pelvic bone. In this condition, the cartilage that covers the end of the bone is inflamed. It is more common in boys, who usually complain of a pain in the groin or the thigh. The symptoms may start quite suddenly or else appear gradually over a few days or months.

❷ Is there tenderness just below the kneecap?

The tendons of children who grow very quickly may not be able to keep up with fast bone growth, with resulting inflammation (tendinitis). This is particularly common just below the kneecap over the bony prominence to which the thigh tendon is attached, and is known as Osgood-Schlatter's disease.

❷ Is there muscle wasting?

Thankfully most people are now vaccinated against polio. Those who are not or whose immunity wanes as a result of not having booster vaccinations may develop polio, particularly if they travel to parts of the world where it is endemic such as the Mediterranean. Paralysis may follow the acute infection, which is characterized by headache, fever, diarrhoea and loss of appetite. If the muscles of the legs are involved, a permanent limp may result.

❷ Has your child never walked properly?

Damage to one side of the brain during either pregnancy or childbirth may result in cerebral palsy. This produces some degree of weakness in one side of the body and is associated with a degree of spasticity (rigidity) in the affected muscles. It is usually diagnosed at birth, but sometimes may only become apparent in early childhood.

❸ Has your child been slow in starting to walk properly?

In congenital dislocation of the hip, the socket of the hip joint is not properly formed, enabling the top of the thigh bone, the femur, to slip out or dislocate. Girls are more often affected than boys and if one girl in the family suffers there is a higher risk that her sisters will too. All babies are checked at birth for this condition and if there is a slight click when the hip is moved, further investigations with X-rays are carried out so that orthopaedic treatment may be given. However, dislocation that is not discovered at birth may only show up when the child begins to walk, usually later than normal, and limping becomes obvious.

❸ Is there swelling and tenderness over any area of bone, especially where there has been a previous injury?

Infection that enters a bone from the outside, often as the result of a fracture, can set up a chronic infection in the bone itself (osteomyelitis) causing a limp.

❸ Is there any unexplained swelling or pain in a bone?

Very rarely, a tumour of the bone in the lower leg may produce a painful limp. To put things in perspective, I have been in general practice for more than 14 years, seeing 200 patients every week, and I have never seen a case.

SUMMARY
LIMPING

POSSIBLE CAUSE	ACTION
Injury	Rest, pain relief.
Ill-fitting shoes	Attention to footwear.
Verrucae	Salicylic acid plasters, cryosurgery, chiropody.
Arthritis	Medical and/or surgical treatment.
Perthe's disease	Bedrest initially, splinting, possible surgery. The condition often resolves spontaneously.
Tendonitis	Rest and heat.
Polio	Physiotherapy, caliper splints.
Cerebral palsy	Physiotherapy, caliper splints.
Congenital dislocation of the hip	Splinting, traction, surgery.
Osteomyelitis	Long-term antibiotics. Surgery.
Bone tumour	Surgery. Radio- and/or chemotherapy.

BEHAVIOURAL PROBLEMS

All children behave differently. Some children are as good as gold, others, sometimes in the same family with the same upbringing, can be particularly awkward. Also, what some parents consider to be bad behaviour will be perfectly acceptable to others. Nevertheless, there will always be times when the behaviour of any child begins to get you down, irritates or worries you. When this happens, rather than getting upset or becoming angry, it is worth staying calm and working out exactly what the problem might be. There are a number of factors to consider. First of all, ask yourself how much of a problem it really is. Are you just very tired and frustrated and have come to your wits' end with what is actually normal behaviour in a child? If so, the answer probably is that you need a good night's sleep and a bit of a break. If the child really is being troublesome and fretful, he or she could be having nightmares. Is there another baby on the scene making the first child jealous? Has there been a change of house, a change of play group or a different child minder? Has your child become used to sleeping in your bed and is now being asked to sleep in his or her own room? Have you been paying too much attention to tantrums, thereby rewarding your child for having them? Finally, when does the difficult behaviour occur? Is it when your child is bored, particularly excited, hungry or just plain tired?

WHAT TO DO

At the end of the day parents have to tackle the problem their way. A lot of advice is available, but most people will handle the same situation in a slightly different way. Whatever you do, you need to persevere with the policy you have decided upon and be consistent. There is no point whatsoever in Mum embarking upon certain rules, only to have Dad change them. Try not to overreact to hassles, but communicate with your child and explain what is right, what is wrong, what is good and what is bad. Praise good behaviour wherever possible rather than simply punish bad, and think about offering a system of rewards when things are going particularly well. Generally speaking, no child cannot be 'trained' to behave politely and obediently, provided loving, firm and consistent handling is exercised.

❷ Is your child particularly bad at mealtimes?

Parents often complain that their child won't eat. Often it is partly because the child is snacking frequently and is simply not hungry at mealtimes. Snacks should therefore be seriously limited unless each meal is eaten up with relish and enjoyed. It certainly isn't worth force-feeding a child. This distresses the parents much more than the child and in many ways the child is actually achieving something with this in the form of attention. Personally I think picking at and pushing food around on the plate for ever and a day should not be allowed. Instead mealtimes and eating should be fun and enjoyable, so perhaps it's worth putting less on the plate in the first place. It is also worth thinking about inviting children round who are good eaters so that your child can pick up these good habits. There is no doubt that a child may be totally unimpressed with what an adult does, but will copy another child. However, children who are little tykes otherwise have a habit of eating extremely well in the presence of an adult who is not a parent. For this reason, grandparents often have more luck in persuading a child to eat than the parents do. If a child is particularly choosy about food, rather than struggle too much with forcing everything down, there is no harm in giving foods that he or she will definitely take, provided that new foods are introduced slowly and gradually. Again, inviting children who don't have eating problems round can be helpful because your child may be eager to copy what they do.

❷ Is your child awake all night?

A child who refuses to go to sleep is one of the biggest problems parents can face. Firstly and most importantly, establishing a sleep routine for the child is a good idea. If a child can come to recognize that a certain time of night is bedtime, and that a certain sequence of events leads up to it, then in a short period of time, generally around two weeks, he or she will come to realize that this is not a punishment but something nice. For example, a good routine could be a bath at 6 or 7 o'clock with games played in the water, then being dried and dressed in nightclothes, then the feed, then a little story followed by lights out in the bedroom. If this happens each day in exactly the same way, a reflex will be established that allows the expectation of sleep and compliance. If the child won't be left when you turn out the light and leave the room, you may need to leave for a few minutes and then go back in to reassure him or her that you are still around. The problem is that each time you go back in when the child has been crying, he or she will realize that bellowing and hollering actually pay. Be firm and persistent and soon you will get them out of the bad habit of not sleeping. It may seem difficult at first, but sometimes you have to be cruel to be kind. Finally, if you think your child is afraid of the dark or just bored, then think about having glow plugs in the bedroom or at least a dimmer switch on low, give them little comforters like cuddly toys or soft material to hold, and think about playing some soft music. Make sure there are pictures on the wall to look at or mobiles hanging from the cot to provide distraction.

❷ Does your child have tantrums?

Temper tantrums are a common behavioural problem, with something like 20 per cent of children aged between one and a half and two having one or two tantrums every day. They tend to happen when the child becomes frustrated at not being able to do what he or she wants to do. For example, if you child can't express his or her feelings with a limited vocabulary, or can't reach some tempting toy or object, he or she will often feel infuriated. But difficult though a tantrum may be to manage, especially if it happens somewhere in public, as they often do, a firm but understanding approach is important from the outset. First of all, it is worth making sure that the child isn't just tired or hungry. If that is the case, then a bit more sleep or a good feed usually work wonders. Occasionally there may be jealousy at the arrival of another baby, which can make the older child feel frustrated or that his or her own position in the family is threatened. In this situation a little bit of extra affection and re-assurance is important. It is also necessary to appreciate that children of any age can have an off day and feel discontented, just like an adult. Sometimes a child having a temper tantrum can be distracted from it if you can draw his or her attention to some other exciting and enjoyable pastime. It is vital to stay as calm as possible and to be consistent. A child that gets his or her way through a temper tantrum will only be encouraged to behave similarly again, so do make it clear that this behaviour won't be tolerated and don't try to bribe the child out of his or her behaviour with the promise of sweeties or toys as this just leads to bad-tempered children with rotten teeth. This is particularly important when a tantrum happens in public, where maximum embarrassment to the parents can occur.

❷ *Is your child endlessly on the go?*

Many children are overactive but very few are truly 'hyperactive'. Hyperactivity is a word much overused by modern parents and only a very small percentage of children are genuinely affected by this condition.

However, most children are at times incredibly energetic and active, sometimes bordering on the restless, chaotic and unmanageable. These children are often bright and intelligent and intensely curious about the world around them. They require a rigorous daily routine to give them a framework in which to work, and obviously this has to be imposed upon them by the parents. They also need quality time from whoever is looking after them and one-to-one communication and game-playing can reap very large dividends.

Because they become quickly bored by the mundane tasks parents have no choice about, such as shopping, queuing in the bank or visiting the doctor's surgery, try wherever possible to keep these trips short and organize your own life in a way that will cause the least boredom and frustration for your child. It is important to reiterate the laws of right and wrong, and discipline is probably even more important in an overactive child. Just so that he or she doesn't rebel against this discipline, however, it is worthwhile letting your child have at least one opportunity every day to run free and wild. Take your child out to the park or to a bumper castle; rule off a separate area of the playroom where noise and damage don't matter; give the child time to burn him- or herself out. This also teaches your child that there are other places in the house that must be respected. If this kind of activity is done at set times of the day, it further establishes a routine that can help your child start to make sense of his or her life.

SUMMARY
BEHAVIOURAL PROBLEMS

POSSIBLE CAUSE	ACTION
Refusal to eat	No snacks. Don't force-feed. Limit mealtimes. Invite children who are good eaters to meals. Invite others to administer meals. Introduce new foods gradually.
Refusal to sleep	Establish routines. Supply low lights, favourite cuddly toys, soft music, mobiles above cot.
Tantrums	A firm, consistent and loving approach. Constant reinforcement of 'right' and 'wrong'. Distraction techniques in early stages.
Hyperactivity	Establish routines. Reinforce ideas of right and wrong. Exclude additives, colourings and stimulants from the diet.

338

INDEX